PIONEERS OF CARDIOLOGY IN CANADA 1820–1970

To George Wyse
With warmest Regards
Harold Segall

PIONEERS OF CARDIOLOGY IN CANADA 1820–1970

The Genesis of Canadian Cardiology

Harold N. Segall

M.D., C.M. (McGill 1920), F.A.C.P., F.R.S.A.,
F.A.H.A., F.A.C.C., D.Sc. (Hon. McGill)

Hounslow
Press

Hounslow Press
A Division of Anthony R. Hawke Limited
124 Parkview Avenue
Willowdale, Ontario, Canada
M2N 3Y5

ISBN 0-88882-105-0

Design / David Shaw & Harrison Shannon
Composition / Accurate Typesetting Limited
Manufacture / T.H. Best Printing Co. Ltd.

Contents

To the Pioneer Patients,
those who volunteer to undergo new, more or less risky
diagnostic or
therapeutic procedures;
and to
those men and women of medicine and surgery
in whose ethics, judgements and skills,
the Pioneer Patients entrust
their fates.

There is no cause from whose nature some effect does not follow.

Baruch Spinoza

History is the essence of innumerable biographies.

Thomas Carlyle

The true student is a citizen of the world, the allegiance of whose soul, at any rate, is too precious to be restricted to one country.

William Osler

Within the infant rind of this weak flower
Poison hath residence and medicine power.

William Shakespeare:
Romeo and Juliet

Acknowledgements

The minutes of the annual business meeting of the Canadian Cardiovascular Society in Quebec City on December 1962 contain the following item:

> Archives: There was considerable discussion about the desirability of preserving records of the Society. It was moved by Dr. D. S. Munroe and seconded by Dr. P. Marion that Dr. H. Segall be appointed Chairman (with power to add) of the Standing Committee on Archives. Carried.

To the members present at that meeting and especially to Munroe of British Columbia and Marion of Quebec, I have incurred a debt of gratitude. An amateur historian, they entrusted me with an important task which I have greatly enjoyed.

I exercised the powers to add in 1972. By then I had accumulated minibiographies of 71% of the members. I invited one member in each province to join the committee and assigned him the task of examining the minibiographies of his province in search of errors of omission or commission that I may have made. The following men accepted the invitation and performed their tasks admirably.

D. S. Munroe, B.C.
Robert Fraser, Alberta
David Baltzan, Saskatchewan
R. E. Beamish, Manitoba
W. Bigelow, Ontario
Lea Steeves, Maritimes
John Keith, Ontario
Paul David, Quebec
Yves Morin, Quebec
Jean Gratton, Quebec

Because of the membership's slow response rate to my calls for the questionnaires, secretarial work was done periodically with longish quiescent intervals. The following ladies performed the tasks of typing and retyping the several drafts: Mrs. Marie Clark,

Miss Lois Garth, Miss Gloria Berlin, Miss Rita Tchalekian and Mrs. Joyce Granich. Each shared my special interest in the work, leaving me in their debt for efforts beyond the routine of the work.

Editing was initiated by Harvey Blackman, who completed the first quarter of the manuscript; the remaining three-quarters was edited by Mrs. Norma Alt. Final editing and proofreading was done by Mrs. Olive Koyama, who also composed the Glossary, and both the index of names and the index of subjects were composed by Mr. Dana Cook. I'm deeply appreciative of the zeal with which these tasks were carried out.

The Councils and executive officers of the society were ever helpful and patient in awaiting the completion of the book. Dr. Robert E. Beamish, a former president, keenly interested in the project from its inception, continually gave whole-hearted encouragement. Dr. Henry Mizgala provided wise guidance in matters financial, Mrs. Dolores Lourenço, the Executive Secretary, assisted in tasks related to the Archives. My very sincere thanks are extended for these supportive influences.

I am especially appreciative of and grateful to the Hannah Institute for the History of Medicine for very friendly encouragement and for a "feasibility grant" which paid for most of the initial editing of the final draft.

Dr. Charles G. Roland, Hannah Professor of Medical History at McMaster University, on whom I depended for frank uninhibited criticism, was more effective than he might imagine in shaping my decisions when faced with dilemmas. I seek to express very special thanks to Dr. Roland.

To Miss Marie Atkinson for her assistance in translating French responses to the questionnaire, I offer warmest thanks.

For the meticulous care with which he exercised his exceptional skills, I am grateful to Mr. David Travers who photographed the collection of stethoscopes for the picture in the jacket design.

The acid-free paper on which the book is printed is a gift from two paper companies in honoured memory of their former presidents, the late Mr. Douglas W. (Doug) Ambridge of Abitibi-Price Inc. and the late Mr. J. Bruce Brown of Intercity Paper Company. They gave vigorous leadership in the founding and early development of their respective provincial Heart Foundations (Ontario and Quebec) and the national, the Canadian Heart Foundation. To the two companies I seek to convey my deep appreciation and warmest thanks.

Since its arrival at McGill in 1929 the Osler Library has been a great joy to visit. The friendships with the librarians, the late Dr. W. W. Francis, and with Miss Cecile Desbarats and more recently with Dr. E. H. Bensley, Dr. Philip Teigen and Dr. Faith Wallis, I count as precious experiences. The rich resources of the Library and its excellent personnel served this project very effectively.

Mr. David Shaw of David Shaw and Associates designed the book and orchestrated its production. I feel most grateful to him and to Harrison Shannon for the great devotion they gave to the project.

To Mr. Tony Hawke of Hounslow Press who will market and distribute the book, I offer warmest thanks for his enthusiastic cooperation.

Introduction

At the Annual Meeting of the Canadian Cardiovascular Society in Quebec City in December 1962, I rose to suggest that the Society should have an Archives Committee in order to avoid neglect and loss of precious documents related to the Society's origins and development. Predictably, I was appointed Chairman with power to add. I found the school exercise book with the names of all those who attended the organization meeting in Winnipeg on 24 June 1947 and other irreplaceable items, and initiated the collection of archives.

Presently, thinking about the task of someone who would undertake to make use of the archives to write an account of the beginnings and the evolution of cardiology in Canada, I found what was available woefully inadequate. Information about the careers of all those who practised cardiology in Canada would be needed to provide the necessary pool of facts. Accordingly, in 1965 a questionnaire was composed and sent to each member (Figs. 1 and 2). A disappointingly small number of responses trickled in. A second mailing was made in 1968, and a third in 1971. Eventually 371 of the 481 members did respond. I felt frustrated but people familiar with the practice of questionnaire techniques consider 71% very good.

The questionnaire has three parts: (1) curriculum vitae, (2) four special questions which when answered would reflect the socio-economic conditions and the professional milieu in which the person was educated and in which the career of cardiology developed, and (3) the bibliography. All respondents provided more or less complete curricula vitae. Relatively few paid serious attention to the special questions, and about two thirds provided their bibliographies. The four special questions were:

> In addition to the data inserted in the questionnaire it would be most helpful if you would add supplementary remarks dealing with at least the following four items:
>
> A. How you arrived at the decision to specialize in cardiology. It would be of interest to mention at what stage of

your education you began to consider the study of cardiology seriously.

B. What experience you had in planning and in carrying out your plan for special training; the obstacles you met with and how you overcame them; the influences which led you to choose the place where you practice cardiology; the year in which you bought your first electrocardiograph.

C. What role, if any, did membership in the Canadian Cardiovascular Society play in the development of your career.

D. Please do mention extracurricular activities, community services, hobbies, etc.

Voulez-vous avoir l'obligeance de répondre aux 4 questions suivantes afin de nous donner des renseignements complémentaires à ceux que vous avez fourni dans le questionnaire:

A. Comment en êtes-vous arrivé à la décision de spécialiser en cardiologie. Pouvez-vous indiquer à quelle étape de votre formation vous avez commencé à considérer sérieusement de vous spécialiser en cardiologie.

B. Quels obstacles avez-vous dû surmonter lors de l'élaboration de projects en vue d'études spécialisées et comment y êtes-vous arrivé. Quelles ont été les influences qui vous ont amené à choisir le lieu ou vous pratiquez maintenant la cardiologie. En quelle année avez-vous acheté votre premier électrocardiographe.

C. Quel rôle a joué La Société Cardiovasculaire du Canada dans le développement de votre carrière.

D. Voulez-vous décrire brièvement vos activités en dehors de vos occupations professionnelles, par exemple, travail de service communautaire, si vous avez des passe-temps, etc.

Initially it was thought that it would be a good plan for a book on the genesis of cardiology in Canada, to write a succinct account of the evolution of knowledge about the cardiovascular system, and to follow this with minibiographies of all the members of the Canadian Cardiovascular Society. The first draft (completed in 1972) did not please anybody. The absence of 29% of the members, the obvious contrast between the few serious responses to the four special questions and those that were inadequate made this plan seem impractical.

Eventually the decision was made to base the story of the genesis of cardiology in Canada on the available responses. To a large extent these are quoted in full, providing not only the facts but also some telling clues about the nature of each individual as a person. This element greatly outweighs in importance whatever advantage might be gained from editing and paraphrasing to render the book more evenly composed as literature. This view finds strong support in a thought by Carl Sandburg, expressed in the last two sentences of the foreword to his four-volume biography, *Lincoln – The War Years:*

> Sometimes I regret that I have generally used the . . . "three dots of elision" for unimportant matter omitted in quotations. However, I have never been able to stifle suspicions that any "tearing of text from context" in a letter or document . . . any act of selection of what is deemed 'essential' or 'significant' in distinction from what is not . . . has always a touch of the hazardous and very often of the arrogant. . .

Please type or write in block letters.

Surgeons and non-clinicians please alter questions to suit your case and answer accordingly.

CANADIAN CARDIOVASCULAR SOCIETY ARCHIVES

FULL NAME______________________________
Surname Given Names

ADDRESS________________ ________________
Office Home

DATE OF BIRTH__________ PLACE OF BIRTH__________

FATHER'S NAME__________ MOTHER'S NAME__________

WIFE'S MAIDEN NAME__________ NAMES OF CHILDREN__________

EDUCATION

ELEMENTARY SCHOOL__________ YEAR_____

UNIVERSITY__________ DEGREE_____ YEAR_____

MEDICAL SCHOOL__________ DEGREE_____ YEAR_____

OTHER DEGREES__________

CERTIFICATIONS__________

POSTGRADUATE EDUCATION (Arrange chronologically)

APPOINTMENTS (Arrange chronologically)

UNIVERSITY__________

HOSPITALS__________

OTHERS__________

MEMBERSHIP IN SOCIETIES:

BIBLIOGRAPHY:

Fig. 1 Questionnaire in English

Vous nous obligeriez en dactylographiant ou en écrivant en lettres moulées.

Les chirugiens et les non-cliniciens sont priés d'adapter les questions à leur situation particulière et de répondre selon le cas.

ARCHIVES DE LA SOCIÉTÉ CARDIOVASCULAIRE DU CANADA

NOM____________________
Prénoms

ADRESSE__________ __________
Bureau Résidence

DATE DE NAISSANCE__________ LIEU DE NAISSANCE__________

NOM DU PÈRE__________ NOM DE LA MÈRE__________

NOM DE L'ÉPOUSE__________ NOM DES ENFANTS__________

ÉDUCATION

ÉCOLE SECONDAIRE__________ ANNÉE_____

UNIVERSITÉ__________ DIPLÔME_____ ANNÉE_____

FACULTÉ DE MÉDECINE__________ DIPLÔME_____ ANNÉE_____

AUTRES DIPLÔMES__________

CLASSIFICATION__________

ÉTUDES DE SPÉCIALISATION (Énumération chronologique)

NOMINATIONS (Énumération chronologique)

UNIVERSITÉ__________

HÔPITAUX__________

AUTRES__________

SOCIÉTÉS SCIENTIFIQUES DONT VOUS ÊTES MEMBRES

BIBLIOGRAPHIE:

Fig. 2 Questionnaire in French

CHAPTER ONE

Our European Heritage

Cardiology received its greatest stimulus from the achievements of William Harvey (1578-1657). In 1628, in his modest little book entitled *De Motu Cordis et Sanguinis in Animalibus* (The Movement of the Heart and Blood in Animals) he describes for the first time in medical history how the heart functions as a pump which maintains the circulation of the blood in the arteries and veins. How did it come about that he made this discovery?

He had the good fortune of birth into an affluent family (Power, 1897). His father Thomas Harvey, a well-to-do merchant, played an important role in his city, Folkestone, as a jurat (alderman) and also (in 1600) mayor. He married first at the age of 26 in 1575; his wife, Julia Jenkin, died a year later soon after giving birth to a daughter. A little more than a year after this he married Joan Halke (or Hawke). When their first child, William, was born Thomas was 29 and his wife 23 years old. In biographies of William Harvey we find that about all that is known of his mother is to be read in an inscription on a brass tablet in the parish church at Folkestone. Said to have been composed by her husband or by her eldest son, it reads:

> A.D. 1605 Nov. 8th died in the fiftieth year of her age Joan wife of Tho. Harvey. Mother of seven sons & 2 daughters. A Godly harmless woman; A chaste loving Wife: A charitable quiet Neighbour: A comfortable frendly Matron: A provident diligent Hvswife: A careful tender-hearted Mother. Deere to her Hvsband: Reverenced of her Children: Beloved of her Neighbours: Elected of God. Whose Soule rest in Heaven, her Body in this Grave: To her a happy Advantage: to hers an unhappy Loss. (Power, 1897)

William Harvey's good fortune also included considerable longevity; he lived to the age of 79 years and two months (1 April 1578 to 3 June 1657), five years longer than his father and seven longer than his brother Eliab. His seven other siblings had shorter lives. Not the least of advantages he enjoyed during his student years was adequate financial support from his father. Later in life, he had good advice and practical assistance in the management of his business affairs from his brother Eliab, a successful merchant who had acquired considerable wealth. Nor did William lack some influence at court; his brother John (1582-1645) rose to the position of servant-in-ordinary to King James I. Furthermore, on 4 November 1604 William married the daughter of Dr. Launcelot Browne who was physician to Queen Elizabeth and her successor, James I.

During Harvey's almost four score years England experienced much political turmoil. He was nine years old when he witnessed his father's preoccupation with preparing Her Majesty's navy for its historic encounter with the Spanish Armada in 1588. He became physician-in-ordinary to King Charles I in 1631 and remained his friend all his life. What anguish he must have felt during the civil war which culminated in the execution of Charles I in 1649!

Because Harvey chose to inscribe himself in Gonville and Caius College at Cambridge it may be inferred that at the age of 16 he had already chosen to study medicine, this with his father's consent. In 1557 Dr. Caius had pioneered in England the teaching of the anatomy of the human body. Caius obtained a charter which permitted the masters and fellows of the college, once a year, to obtain the bodies of two criminals who had been condemned to death and executed in Cambridge to be used for dissection "with a view to the increase of knowledge of medicine and the benefit of Her Majesty's lieges, without interference on the part of her officials" (Power, 1897). However, it is not known whether such dissections, named "Anatomies," were practised at Cambridge during Harvey's sojourn there; he graduated Bachelor of Arts in 1597. In a novel based on the life and times of William Harvey, the author (Weiss, 1975) composes a graphic and dramatic description of such an "Anatomy" attended by Harvey and his fellow students.

Soon after graduation, Harvey travelled through France and Germany en route to Padua, then the leading centre for the study of medicine; Galileo was a member of Padua's university faculty at that time, and about half a century earlier (1538-1543) Vesalius (1514-1564) taught human anatomy there and wrote his epoch-making *De Fabrica Corporis Humanis*, published in 1543. When Harvey arrived in Padua (1597) he met a worthy disciple of Vesalius, namely Fabricius of Acquapendente (1537-1629). A close friendship developed between this very good and popular teacher and his devoted pupil Harvey, in spite of, or perhaps because of, the wide age difference of 41 years. At that time Fabricius was engaged in an intensive study of the venous valves (Saunders, 1978). These valves first appeared in medical literature in Charles Estienne's book *De Dissectone Partum Corporis Humani* (About dissection of parts of the human body) in Paris, 1545. Their presence was subsequently confirmed by Gambattista Canano (1515-1579) who spoke of them to Vesalius in 1546. Amatus Lusitanus (Jean Roderigo) (1511-1568) wrote of his observations in the dissections of twelve human bodies and of animals during which he demonstrated venous valves in the presence of "a large assembly of learned men" (1547). Fabricius Acquapendente appears to have rediscovered the valves in 1574 and eventually wrote a small treatise on them in 1603. Amatus and Canano mentioned that the valves functioned to impede reflux of blood, but Vesalius did not agree. He believed they simply strengthened the venous wall. Other authorities even denied their existence.

Harvey knew of their existence because of his close association with Fabricius and, in the spirited, unfettered thinking characteristic of Padua during the Renaissance, he confirmed the opinions of Amatus and Canano. He emancipated himself from the Galenical Concepts (Siegel, 1968) of the functions of the heart and blood vessels. He used the existence of venous valves as the point of departure for the logical development of his concept of the physiology of the cardiovascular system. This historical fact is well documented in a statement by Robert Boyle (1627-1691), in *A Disquisition about the Final Causes of Natural Things* published in London in 1688 (Keynes, 1953):

> And I remember that when I asked our famous Harvey, in the only Discourse I had with him, (which was but a while before he dyed) what were the things that induc'd him to think of a circulation of the Blood? He answer'd me, that when he took notice that the Valves in the Veins of so many Parts of the Body, were so Plac'd that they gave free passage to the Blood Towards the Heart, but oppos'd the passage of the Venal Blood the Contrary Way: He was invited to imagine that so Provident a cause as Nature had not so Plac'd so many Valves without Design: and no Design seemed more probable, than That since the Blood could not well, because of the interposing Valves, be sent by the Veins to the Limbs; it should be sent through the arteries, and Return through the Veins, whose Valves did not oppose its course that way.

The established teaching of Galen considered the blood in the arteries and veins as performing a to-and-fro motion, almost static.

Harvey, with due respect for Aristotle, Hippocrates and Galen, all of whom he greatly admired, replaced this concept by that of blood circulation. The second important element after the function of the venous valves, which he adduced to prove this idea, was the calculation of the total volume blood present in the body, the output per heart beat, and the amount which circulated per unit of time. He measured the amount of blood in the heart of a human adult cadaver and found over two ounces. The following quotation from *De Motu Cordis* (Harvey, 1628) deals with his calculations:

> If in one beat, the heart emits two drachms, then in a thousand beats during half an hour, the total is twenty pounds ten ounces, and if it is an ounce at each beat, eighty three pounds four ounces have been transfused in one half hour from the Veins to the arteries.

Translated into metric parlance this represents 227 ml per minute for one drachm and 990 ml for one ounce per beat at a rate of 33 per minute, which is about a third of the known circulation rate, calculated by modern methods, for a heart rate of about 70 per minute for a man at rest. The large volume of blood which passed through the heart in the course of one day rendered the concept of circulation self-evident. Yet few of his peers accepted his ideas; some actively disagreed, and most paid little or no attention to his work. However, over the next 29 years of his life the majority of authorities came to agree with him, recognizing the great importance of his achievements.

Harvey did not demonstrate the capillary circulation in the lungs. He depended on his logical hypothesis, that blood passed through such channels from the pulmonary arteries into the pulmonary veins. He probably did not know that during his lifetime the methods by which capillaries were discovered were being developed. A primitive microscope, the by-product of Galileo's telescopes, did magnify small objects but produced hazy images. Thus, although Galileo demonstrated the microscope in 1610, not until improved lenses became available after 1650 did the instrument lead to important discoveries during the second half of the seventeenth century. In 1660 Malpighi of Bologna (1628-1694) (Singer, 1956) the founder of histology, in his treatise *De Pulmonibus* (1661) described the movement of blood in capillaries of the frog's lung (which is almost transparent and thus a favourable tissue for this purpose) confirmed Harvey's hypothesis.

The next important event in the study of cardiovascular physiology occurred in 1733 with the publication of Stephen Hales' treatise on haemostatics (Hales, 1733). For the first time in medical history, Hales measured an animal's arterial pressure.

> In December I caused a Mare to be tied down alive on her back. She was fourteen Hands high [56 inches] and about fourteen years of Age, had a Fistula on her Withers [shoulders], was neither lean nor yet lusty; Having laid open the crural [femoral] artery about three inches from her Belly, I inserted into it a brass Pipe whose bore was one sixth of an inch in Diameter; and to that, by means of another brass Pipe, which was fitly adapted to it, I fixed a glass Tube, of nearly the same Diameter, which was nine Feet in Length: Then untying the Ligature on the Artery, the Blood rose in the Tube eight Feet three inches perpendicular above the Level of the left Ventricle of the Heart: but it did not attain to its full Height at once: it rushed up about half way in an Instant and gradually at each Pulse twelve, eight, six, four, two, and sometimes one inch: When it was at its full Height, it would rise and fall at and after each Pulse, two, three or four Inches; and sometimes it would fall twelve or fourteen Inches, and hover there for a time and the same Vibrations up and down at an after pulse, as it had at its full Height; to which it would rise again after forty or fifty pulses.

In this connection, I give way to the temptation to relate a personal reminiscence.

In the autumn of 1923, Dr. Paul Dudley White, my chief, set up a booth for measuring the arterial pressure of visitors to a Boston community fair which took place in Mechanics Hall. The general public was not yet aware of this medical method. I worked at the booth for several hours that day. The manometer was a long glass tube, 1 cm in diameter and 3 metres high; the fluid was water tinted red with litmus. The heights attained were 13 times the level reached in the usual mercury manometer. Thus for a pressure of 120 systolic the red water rose to 1.56 metres. I explained this to each person who volunteered for the arterial pressure measurement.

Stephen Hales knew of the mercury manometer but did not mention it in connection with arterial blood pressure measurement. Almost a century later, J. L. M. Poiseuille (1799-1869) made arterial pressure the subject of his doctoral thesis. He used a mercury manometer to measure the arterial pressure of a dog (Poiseuille, 1828), precisely two centuries after the publication of *De Motu Cordis.* Subsequent progress towards measuring arterial pressure in humans moved less slowly. First, however, knowledge about arterial pressure in animals was to be extended by the epoch-making work of Carl Ludwig (1816-1895). In 1847 he invented the kymograph (Ludwig, 1847) which is here most conveniently described in his own words as translated into English (Geddes, 1970):

> In order to secure a good value from Poiseuille's mercury manometer, and in order to get the time-relations of the changes in pressure, put a staff-like float on the mercury at the upper end of which is a pointer. Let the fluctuations be written on a surface which passes by the pointer with a uniform speed. In this way one secures curves, the height of which is an expression of the blood pressure and the duration of which is an expression of time.

This epoch-making apparatus became standard equipment in all physiological and pharmacological laboratories. Carl Ludwig did more than invent this very important technique; he attracted pupils from all over the world. Garrison comments (Garrison, 1929):

> Ludwig was perhaps the greatest teacher of physiology who ever lived. He had over 200 pupils, of all nationalities, and most of the younger generation of investigators in his science were trained by him.... Most of his important discoveries were published under the names of his pupils, some of whom, as von Kries relates, "sat on the window sill, while Ludwig and his faithful assistant Salvenmoser did all the work."... His object was to form capable investigators while carrying out his own ideas.

One could make a good case for the idea that the impetus which Harvey gave to the study of physiology found the first worthy response only with the advent of Ludwig 250 years later. Sir William Bayliss (Bayliss, 1924), in his great book *Principles of General Physiology,* states categorically that "Exact investigation of the phenomena of the circulation was impossible until Ludwig (1847) invented the graphic method of recording blood pressure." Ludwig's pupils became the researchers and teachers of the next century, one of the most, if not the most, fruitful period in the history of medicine related to cardiology. Modifications of the kymograph to improve its accuracy as an instrument of precision were made by Ludwig and others.

Although Karl Vierordt (1818-1884) was the first to adapt Ludwig's kymograph for clinical study of the human pulse (1853), his apparatus had gross defects which Marey did much to correct

(Marey, 1881). A number of others contributed special modifications, all of which used strips of smoked paper as the recording surface, until Ozanam (1824-1890) introduced an ink-writing lever on plain paper mounted on the usual cylinder (Ozanam, 1886). One of the most efficient models of a sphygmograph was constructed by James Mackenzie (1853-1925) and his friend Mr. Shaw, the watchmaker. The process involved a roll of paper, several yards in length, on which a continuous record could be made with ink-writing levers for time marking and for three simultaneous pulses: arterial, venous and hepatic. This apparatus, which was easily portable, provided important technical advantages over all the others. Mackenzie named it "a clinical polygraph" (Wilson, 1926), but it was known throughout the world as the "Mackenzie Ink Polygraph." Mackenzie, a general practitioner in Burnley, a suburb of Manchester, began his study of the pulse using the Dudgeon model of sphygmograph, and accomplished most of what appears in his book on the pulse (Mackenzie, 1902) using short strips of smoked paper for recording. He demonstrated how very much could be achieved when this physiological apparatus was applied to the investigation of clinical problems in the patient's home, the doctor's office, or the hospital.

About fifty years before Harvey began his medical career, Vesalius (1514-1564) had been teaching anatomy at Padua. In 1543, he published his classic work *De Fabrica Humani Corporis*, the first highly accurate description of the human body. This provided Harvey with knowledge of fundamental importance for his thinking about the physiology of the cardiovascular system. He probably knew of the 1555 revised edition of the *Fabrica* in which Vesalius describes the venous valves but erroneously attributes to them the function of giving added strength to the wall of the vein. Vesalius corrected many serious errors found in the Hippocratic and Galenical teachings. His pupils and other men of the Renaissance, emancipated from the Galenical dogmas, examined the phenomena of nature in search of understanding the functions of the human body.

The ancients looked at signs of disease in animals and extrapolated from these bits of knowledge to account for the dynamics of symptoms of illness in humans. The newly emancipated Renaissance men ignored the ancient taboos and performed autopsies on deceased patients whom they had observed and treated. These early pioneers had to brave the opposition of the entrenched establishment. The taboos concerning the performance of post-mortem examinations were significant obstacles. Jean Fernel (1506-1588)

(Garrison, 1929), the leading physician in France in the latter part of the sixteenth century, published in 1554 what appears to be the earliest treatise on the correlation between clinical appearance of disease and what was found at post-mortem examination as a clue to explain symptoms. The section of his book *Medicina* which dealt with this theme was entitled "Pathologica." Fernel also corrected many errors of the ancients.

In 1749 Jean-Baptiste Senac (1693-1770) published a two-volume work entitled *Traité de la Structure du Coeur, de Son Action et de ses Maladies* (A treatise on the structure, the functions and diseases of the heart) (Herrick, 1942). This book embodied his many years of careful work in correlating the clinical with the pathological features he had observed in patients. He reached out for methods of sharpening his diagnostic skills. In an era when physicians did not examine the body in the purposeful search for physical signs, he practised the art of careful palpation of cardiac pulsation to estimate the position and the size of the heart. He noted unusual prominence of neck veins associated with enlargement of the right heart.

What is rightfully considered a great event in the history of medicine occurred fifty-five years before Laennec invented the stethoscope. In 1761 there appeared Giovanni Battista Morgagni's monumental work, *De Sedibus et Causis Morborum per Anatomen Indagatis* (About the seats and causes of disease investigated anatomically) (Morgagni, 1761). When these five volumes on clinico-pathological correlations were published Morgagni (1681-1771) was 79 years old and had been a professor of medicine at Padua for 54 years. The lucidity of his style of writing in the form of letters made for precision in his descriptions of both clinical and anatomical abnormalities. Morgagni's teachers (Herrick, 1942), Bonetus (1679), Albertini (1672-1733), Valsalva (1715-1771) and others also had made significant contributions in this field and he cited their observations. Thus his five volumes allude to nearly all current knowledge of this nature which had accumulated by 1761. His work inspired subsequent generations of physicians; indeed his method continues to be a basic element in both undergraduate and post-graduate continuing medical education at present.

Albertini (1672-1733) wrote in 1729: "I know from long attentive observation in dissection of bodies after death, that diagnosis is the branch of healing art in which the greatest number of mistakes are made." Before Senac, he sought methods of improving the skill of clinical diagnosis. He palpated the cardiac apical pulsation of the chest, he noted thrills, and he tried to estimate heart size and thickness of ventricular walls (Herrick, 1942).

In 1729 Albertini was 57 years old, a professor of medicine at Padua. In that year Leopold Auenbrugger (1722-1809) (Neuburger, 1922) was seven years old, the son of a wealthy landlord in Graz, Austria. After preliminary education in his home city Auenbrugger went to Vienna to study medicine. Graduating in 1752, he remained in Vienna, and associated with the Spanish Hospital and the University. In 1754 he invented and began to use percussion as a clinical method, and seven years later published his classic treatise on clinical percussion, *Inventum Novum*. This work did more than demonstrate the value of a clinical method of examination. It finally revived an attitude adopted by Hippocrates but essentially neglected for over 2000 years (400 BC to 1808 AD). The Hippocratic method of succussing (shaking) the chest to elicit a splashing sound in cases which suggest the presence of fluid and air in the pleural cavity, bears witness to the fact that Hippocrates had invoked a special procedure plus the sense of hearing as a diagnostic method. He searched for clinical signs. Briefly mentioned through the centuries are references to analogous methods, e.g., percussing the abdomen to distinguish between ascites and air distention of the bowels, or tapping the skull with a stick in search of evidence of fracture.

Auerbrugger's merit resides in the fact that he did a systematic study of percussion in search of clinical signs of various diseases of the lungs and the heart. He worked with his method for seven years before publishing his observations. The preface to his small yet epoch-making book merits being quoted in its entirety as it reflects the spirit of the times (Neuburger, 1922):

> I here present the Reader with a new sign which I have discovered for detecting disease of the chest. This consists of the Percussion of the human thorax, whereby, according to the character of the particular sounds thence elicited, an opinion is formed of the internal state of that cavity. In making public my discoveries respecting this matter, I have been actuated neither by an itch for writing, nor a fondness for speculation, but by the desire of submitting to my brethren the fruits of seven years' observations and reflexion. In doing so, I have not been unconscious of the dangers I must encounter; since it has always been the fate of those who have illustrated or improved the arts and sciences by their discoveries, to be beset by envy, malice, hatred, detraction and calumny.
>
> This, the common lot, I have chosen to undergo; but with the determination of refusing to every one who is actuated by such motives as these, all explanation of my doctrines. What I have

written I have proved again and again, by the testimony of my own senses, and amid laborious and tedious exertions; — still guarding, on all occasions against the seductive influence of self-love.

And here, lest any one should imagine that this new sign has been thoroughly investigated, even as far as regard the diseases noticed in my Treatise, I think it necessary candidly to confess, that there still remain many defects to be remedied — and which I expect will be remedied — by careful observation and experience. Perhaps, also, the same observation and experience may lead to the discovery of other truths, in these or other diseases, of like value in the diagnosis, prognosis and cure of thoracic affections. Owing to this acknowledged imperfection, it will be seen, that in my difficulties, I have had recourse to the Commentaries of the most illustrious Baron Van Swieten as containing everything which can be desired by the faithful observer of the nature; by which means I have not only avoided the vice of tedious and prolix writing, but have, at the same time, possessed myself of the firmest basis whereon to raise most securely and creditably, the rudiments of my discovery. In submitting this to the public, I doubt not that I shall be considered, by all those who can justly appreciate medical science, as having thereby rendered a grateful service to our art, — inasmuch as it must be allowed to throw no small degree of light upon the obscurer diseases of the chest, of which a more perfect knowledge has hitherto been much wanted.

In drawing up my little work I have omitted many things that were doubtful, and not sufficiently digested; to the due perfection of which it will be my endeavour henceforth to apply myself. To conclude, I have not been ambitious of ornament in my mode or style of writing, being contented if I shall be understood. December 31, 1760.

This 1824 translation from the original Latin is by John Forbes, translator of the Laennec book on mediate auscultation in 1821.

It appears that Auenbrugger celebrated New Year's eve of 1760 by writing this preface after having prepared the treatise for publication. A few of his contemporaries praised his thesis and others spoke and wrote disparagingly, but the great majority, at home and abroad, simply ignored the work.

This neglect was interrupted by Nicholas Corvisart (1755-1821), Napoleon's favourite physician and Laennec's teacher. A French translation by Rosière de la Chassagne of the *Inventum Novum* had been published in 1770, but it too had been ignored. Corvisart discovered the Latin book, translated it into French, and published it in 1808, a year before Auenbrugger's death at the age of 86. When Corvisart revised the first edition (1806) of his popular book on *Diseases of the Heart* he included observations made with percussion (Corvisart, 1818).

Auenbrugger described the technique of percussion as follows: (Neuburger, 1922): "The thorax ought to be struck slowly and gently, with the points of the fingers brought close together and at the same time extended." So far no accessory instrument belonged to the clinical technique of invoking the sense of hearing in search of physical signs. It remained for Réné Théophile Hyacinthe Laennec to invent the first diagnostic instrument, a simple paper tube — an improvisation for estimating the heart rate because the radial pulse was too weak to be felt satisfactorily. The distinguished medical historian Max Neuburger has suggested that the impulse to use percussion derived from Auenbrugger's boyhood observation of how adults estimated by percussion the level of wine in the barrels (Neuburger, 1922). Auenbrugger does mention this practice in his treatise but does not directly attribute his discovery to his boyhood experiences. He does not mention the precise circumstances under which he began to use percussion as a clinical method. Fortunately, Laennec had a good sense of history and devoted a paragraph to those mental processes which led to his invention (Laennec, 1819). The following is this author's (Segall, 1954) translation:

> In 1816 I was consulted by a young person who presented general symptoms of heart disease and in whom palpation and percussion resulted in little information for the elucidation of the case. As the age and sex of the patient did not warrant the kind of examination I referred to above [immediate auscultation] I happened to recall a well-known acoustic phenomenon; namely, if one applies the ear to one end of a beam of wood, the scratch of a pin made at the other end is readily heard. I imagined it might be possible to take advantage of this property of bodies in this particular case. I therefore took a quire of paper, made a tight roll of it and applied one end to the precordium and placing my ear at the other end, I was as much surprised as I was delighted to hear the beatings of the heart in a much clearer manner than I had ever heard them by direct application of the ear to the chest.

Laennec related that he first saw a physician apply his ear to the chest in order to listen to the beating of the heart, when his colleague

Gaspard-Laurent Bayle (1774-1816) performed this type of clinical auscultation one day on ward rounds with Corvisart and his pupils. Laennec adds that their Chief never used this method, but did remark that he had on many occasions "heard the beating of the heart by listening near the chest." Laennec further states that Bayle practised immediate auscultation relatively rarely. He reminds us that the method was described by Hippocrates, and adds that after witnessing Bayle's auscultation he also practised it when palpation of the radial or cardiac pulsation was not satisfactory. Thus only after the incident which led to his invention of the instrument did he fully explore the effectiveness of auscultation as a diagnostic method. He at first named the instrument "le cylindre," and shortly after making a wooden model — a tube — he coined the name *stethoscope* (Webb, 1928). He chose this name in consultation with his uncle Guillaume François Laennec, Professor of Medicine and Dean of the Faculty at Nantes. It is derived from the Greek word for chest, *stethos*, and the word *skopein*, to observe, to look out at, to examine. The name "cylindre" described the anatomy of the instrument; the term stethoscope reflects its function, and is by far the preferable name.

Carl Ludwig's 1847 invention of the kymograph initiated a chain of progress which led to the creation of an instrument for recording pulses (radial, jugular, hepatic, etc.) at the bedside in the patient's home, in the doctor's office, or in the hospital. The polygraph represents the first clinical instrument to develop from experimental physiology. But the stethoscope had a strikingly different ancestry. Its invention was inspired by a clinical diagnostic problem, the difficulty Laennec experienced in estimating pulse rate because the radial artery and the cardiac pulsation were difficult to feel. In this case, by serendipity, a physician with a well-prepared mind created the method of systematic clinical auscultation in search of diagnostic signs. The practice of medicine thus changed radically (Thayer, 1931). Physicians sharpened their thinking with the additional clinical evidence gathered by purposeful searching for objective signs. They applied all five senses, aided by these new instruments. The invention of medical instruments, which derive from progress in other fields of science, physics, chemistry, and engineering, continues to the present time. The story of cardiology in Canada begins with those men who went to study in Europe during the nineteenth century and transplanted the "new medicine" into this country.

CHAPTER TWO

Canadian Pioneering

The earliest recorded evidence of some special interest in heart disease in Canada appears in a historic case report by Andrew Fernando Holmes of Montreal. He had performed an autopsy on a cyanotic young man of 22 and reported a congenital abnormality of the heart — Cor Triloculare Biatriatum. Dr. Maude Abbott (1869-1940), Assistant Curator of the McGill Medical Museum, brought this case report into the limelight from the *Transactions of the Edinburgh Medical Chirurgical Society for 1824,* and she published it with her interesting comments in the *Montreal Medical Journal* of 1901. The illustration she used to depict the course of the circulation within the heart is of historic interest, as it was drawn by Dr. W. Tait Mackenzie, the pioneer of sports medicine famous for his sculptures of athletes during their performances. Abbott had found this heart among some unlabelled specimens in the McGill Medical Museum; William Osler guided her in identifying it and drew her attention to Holmes' report. It formed the cornerstone, so to speak, of her famous collection of congenital heart-disease cases in the McGill Medical Museum. It is also *the* cornerstone of cardiology in Canada.

Holmes was one of the four members of the staff of the Montreal General Hospital who in 1823 founded the first Canadian medical school: the Montreal Medical Institution. Construction of the Montreal General Hospital's new building on Dorchester Street had begun on 6 June 1821. Eleven months later, on 3 May 1822, eight patients were transferred from the Hospital's first site on Craig Street, where it had begun to function in 1819, to the new building. This structure continued to form part of the Hospital's complex until 1955, when the institution moved to its present location on Cedar Avenue. In January 1823, the Board of Governors granted permission for an advertisement to be published announcing the formation of a medical school, the Montreal Medical Institution, which was incorporated into McGill University as its first faculty in 1829. The lectures started in the second week of November, 1823. Dr. Holmes was assigned to teach chemistry, pharmacy, and botany (MacDermot, 1950).

Dr. Andrew Fernando Holmes was born in Cadiz (1797), where his parents had been taken by a French frigate as captives from a British vessel on which they had been travelling from Britain to Canada. They and their son, then four years old, eventually came to Canada (1801). Holmes was educated in Montreal and began his study of medicine as an apprentice of Dr. Daniel Arnoldi. He also studied in Edinburgh, where he obtained the degree of M.D. in 1821, and then returned to Montreal. Perhaps clinical auscultation had not yet become an important subject during his sojourn in Edinburgh; the case of Cor Triloculare Biatriatum that he reported in 1823 was well described but his report made no reference whatever to clinical auscultation, even though the case was published eight years after Laennec's invention of the stethoscope and five years after the appearance of Laennec's book, *Traité de l'Auscultation Médiate et des Maladies des Poumons et du Coeur.* In a valedictory address delivered to McGill medical students on 8 May 1850, Holmes said:

> It is now about thirty years since Laennec first announced his great discovery to the French Academy, and it is much less since the practice of auscultation has become general. Like most other improvements, it met with opposition at its first introduction, but this has now quite disappeared and its only obstacle is that which it shares with all other objects of pursuit, the labour necessary for acquiring expertness in its application. It has not only given precision to our diagnosis of diseases of the chest, it has led to the discovery of others not previously suspected. (Holmes, 1850)

Holmes was a slender man of medium height, with the slight stoop of a scholar. He had an enquiring mind, and worked diligently late into the night, as a rule going to bed after 2:00 a.m. It would be very useful to know in what year he began to use a stethoscope. He died in 1860 (suddenly while at his desk in the evening), and there were at least ten years during which he taught medical students the art and science of clinical auscultation.

The story of the introduction of the stethoscope in Canada begins with the logical assumption that Pierre Beaubien was the first to bring a Laennec model of the instrument with him when he returned to Canada from Paris in 1826. Pierre Beaubien was born near Trois Rivières on 13 October 1796. His education in Canada ended with his graduation from the Collège de Montréal in 1816. In that year, shortly before his twentieth birthday, he sailed for Paris to study medicine. He became associated mainly with l'Hôpital de la Charité where he enjoyed the special friendship and patronage of the surgeon, Joseph Recamier (not the husband of the famous Madame Recamier). This was the year of Laennec's invention of the stethoscope. Laennec was then working at l'Hôpital Necker (Segall, 1967); four years later (1820) Laennec returned to his alma mater, l'Hôpital de la Charité. The Hospital annals record that when Laennec made his ward rounds in 1822 he was followed by sometimes as many as fifty students. Particular reference is made to "a student from Newfoundland" who was one of his followers (Kevran, 1960). Newfoundland was not then a province of Canada, but that student, not Pierre Beaubien, may have been the first to bring a stethoscope to what is now Canada.

Pierre Beaubien returned to Montreal in 1827 and began to work at the Hôtel-Dieu. No evidence has been uncovered to show that he used a stethoscope or taught auscultation to others. His thesis for the doctorate (1822) provides some clues to his interests at that time. The title "Rheumatisme Articulaire" suggests it might contain descriptions of heart murmurs related to rheumatic heart disease. In the preface he states that he chose this subject for his thesis, first, because he had spent time with M. Fouquier, a physician of l'Hôpital de la Charité in Paris, where there were many cases of rheumatic fever, and secondly, because he expected to practise medicine in Canada where the disease was very common. "Mostly affected," he claims in his thesis,

> are those who work in the open, under rigorous climatic conditions, such as farmers who stand and walk a great deal in water in the course of their day's work; labourers who often must gather in the harvest in wet weather; the workers who collect the maple sap in the spring. While doing so, they are obliged, by the nature of the operation to stand in melting snow and ice for a whole day and sometimes for several successive days without a change of shoes.

In his thesis, there are no references to clinical auscultation by Beaubien himself. He mentioned the use of the stethoscope only once, and he did not do the listening himself. The patient had been examined by his colleague, M. Senn, who kindly supplied Beaubien with the clinical story. Included is the fact that M. Senn had percussed the chest and had found some dullness below the left breast region. He therefore used the cylinder of M. Laennec and could not hear any breath sounds over the dull area. The patient recovered from the acute phase of the illness (Beaubien, 1822).

It would appear that Beaubien did not share the enthusiasm of some other foreign students for the stethoscope. Were it possible to examine some of the clinical notes he made during his medical career in Montreal, perhaps evidence of his interest in clinical auscultation might be uncovered.

In the first half of the nineteenth century, the stethoscope worked a revolution in medical education and practice. Despite the importance of this invention, however, its universal acceptance was not immediate. A very perceptive comment on the slow pace at which clinical auscultation entered into the life of the medical profession was written by Oliver Wendell Holmes (1809-1894) in 1836. In that year, the Boylston Medical Committee of Harvard University set the following question for a prize essay: "How far are the external means of exploring the condition of the internal organs to be considered useful and important in medical practice?" The 27-year-old Holmes won the prize with his essay (Holmes, 1836) in which he wrote:

> The treatise of Laennec on mediate auscultation was translated by Dr. Forbes, in 1821; and thus the new methods of direct exploration can only be said to have been before the English and American public for the space of fifteen years. It is to be remembered that in the very city where they originated, the discoveries of Laennec were not at once received without opposition. Thus in the first edition of the *Dictionary of Medicine,* in twenty-one volumes, the author of the article *Auscultation* estimated so very modestly the importance of the new method of exploration, that after reading it, one might have been tempted to throw the stethoscope into the receptacle which holds the scale of Hippocrates and the balance of Sanctorius. It was from this article that Dr. Good derived one of his two authorities for undervaluing auscultation. Unfortunately, the author and editors had committed so serious an error, that in the second edition of the *Dictionary of Medicine,* now publishing, it had been thought necessary to suppress it entirely, although its author is still one of the collaborators, and a popular professor in the School of Medicine; and the treatise which has taken its place is from the hands of one of the most ardent admirers of Laennec.
>
> If the arts of direct exploration struggled with difficulties in Paris, it might well be supposed that they would fight their way

with tenfold labour into general acceptation in medical communities where novelty excites and concentrates attention with less activity. This has been the case in our own country; and at the present day it is well known that some practitioners of a certain merit, and particularly some who pride themselves on strong sense and intuitive sagacity, habitually neglect and depreciate the value of the physical signs, even of thoracic disease.

Several causes have been combined to produce this indifference and disbelief. We need not mention the reasonable scepticism with which those who have often been deluded by novelties, regard almost every innovation. But, if with the most startling novelty, and with extravagant promises, an invention comes forward which demands the laborious training of a sense hitherto uncultivated in its more delicate capacities, bearing in one hand an instrument which is to be the practitioner's inseparable companion, and in the other a treatise full of new terms and peculiar doctrines, is it to be supposed that the schools of Sydenham and Cullen would consent, without a struggle, to recommence their education and remodel their nosology?

It was perfectly natural that they should look with suspicion upon this introduction of medical machinery among the old hard-working operatives; that they should for a while smile at its pretensions, and when its use began to creep among them, that they should observe and signalize all the errors and defects which happened in its practitional application. And erroneous conclusions are formed by those who employ direct exploration, as well as others.

They are not always sufficiently careful in their examinations, any more than other people in their investigations; they draw positive conclusions from insufficient premises, as often as other observers. There is sometimes a tendency in those who have long employed the physical signs, to carry their observation to that infinitesimal minuteness which the tare and tret, inseparable from the mass of evidence, may render nugatory.

The first Canadian medical journal, *Le Journal de Médecine de Québec,* had a brief existence (1826-1827). In its first volume, which consisted almost entirely of excerpts from European literature, there is one article which mentions percussion and another which refers to Laennec's clinico-pathological studies of tuberculosis, but none mention the stethoscope or auscultation. Percussion appears in an article entitled "Reflexions sur la Mort Subite" (Reflections on

Sudden Death) presumably by Dr. X. Tessier who founded the journal. He states (our translation):

> Another method which the moderns have revived with great benefit, in all diseases of the chest, is percussion of this cavity which when it contains an organic abnormality within its space, sounds badly, giving only a dull sound, *tamquam percussi femoris* (as though the thigh were being percussed) over the region which it occupies.

Did Tessier know of Laennec's communication to the Academy of Medicine on mediate auscultation in 1818, and of the first edition of the book on this subject in 1819? He selected for publication in the same volume of the *Journal de Médecine de Québec* several paragraphs from a book of 260 pages by Sir Alexander Crighton on the treatment of "several varieties of pulmonary consumption." Crighton states:

> The author was led to think, that various forms of consumption, were curable, from the observations of Mr. Laennec of Paris, who discovered that tubercles in the lungs sometimes are softened, evacuated and cicatrized. The profession is certainly much indebted to the pathological observations of this eminent Frenchman, and we except that we shall have an opportunity at some future period, of showing that this is not the most essential service which he has rendered to humanity in his researches on diseases of the lungs.

Laennec's book on mediate auscultation with the stethoscope appeared in 1819 and was translated into English in 1821. It is a matter of historical record that English physicians showed the earliest and greatest enthusiasm for auscultation. If Crighton did make any reference to auscultation in his book, Tessier did not consider it of sufficient importance to quote in 1826, the year in which Laennec's second edition of *Mediate Auscultation* was published.

Little evidence has been found of a Canadian who enthusiastically practised and taught auscultation during the first half of the nineteenth century. There are some indications that Francis Badgley (MacDermott, 1950:64) did much, perhaps more than any other individual, to introduce clinical auscultation in Canada. Badgley was born in Montreal in 1807. His father, a wealthy fur trader, made possible his son's education in London, Edinburgh, Belfast, Dublin, and Paris. Francis Badgley obtained his degree from the Royal

College of Physicians and Surgeons of Edinburgh at the age of 20. Auscultation, by 1827, was being practised and taught in Edinburgh by several prominent men — Cullen, Stokes, Clarke, Commins, and others. Badgley must have been influenced by them. After leaving Edinburgh, he practised medicine in Kensington, London, until 1842, when he returned to Montreal. The following year, together with several colleagues, Pierre Beaubien among them, he founded l'Ecole de Médecine et Chirurgie de Montréal, the first French medical school in Canada. He resigned from the school in 1850, and was appointed a professor to the faculty of McGill. Thus, he taught both in French and in English at the first two medical schools of the country.

In the 1849-1850 volume of the British American Medical and Physical Journal there is an unsigned review of the second edition of Henry Bowditch's *The Young Stethoscopist, or the Student's Aid to Auscultation* (Bowditch, 1846). The reviewer seems well informed and writes authoritatively, saying:

> We do not think very highly of the above treatise as we do not consider it capable of communicating any but the most superficial knowledge on the subject. It cannot bear comparison with the treatises of Walshe, Cowen, Raciborski, Barth and Roger, André and Hughes, but as the work has reached a second edition it would appear to have become a favorite with the class of readers for whom it was intended.

This review could very well have been written by Badgley who was, most likely, the main force in introducing auscultation to Canada and in promoting it, since he probably taught it at both medical schools in Montreal. Moreover, he went to live and practise in Toronto in 1850, and he must have had some influence in advancing the use of auscultation there.

CHAPTER THREE

Beginnings of Specialization

Some degree of specialization existed in the division of responsibilities for teaching among the four founders of McGill Medical School. Dr. William Caldwell lectured on the Principles of Medicine, Dr. John Stephenson on Surgery, Dr. William Robertson on Midwifery and Diseases of Children and Dr. Andrew F. Holmes on Chemistry, Pharmacy and Botany. However, in his private practice, each man functioned as a general practitioner in the broadest sense. The laity expected the doctor to perform operations, to be an obstetrician, to diagnose and treat non-surgical conditions. When occasion required or demanded it the doctor performed an autopsy to search for an explanation of clinical symptoms and signs or as in a medico-legal case. In the course of time each man developed a reputation for excellence as a surgeon, or obstetrician, or medical diagnostician and therapist. The appellation "specialist" was not in common use; it began to appear in the English language, according to the *Oxford Dictionary*, in 1856.

The career of Robert Palmer Howard exemplifies how surgery gradually diminished and eventually (in 1880) ceased to play any significant role in the practice of a pioneer medical internist. Howard greatly enjoyed the study and the teaching of medicine, both at the bedside and as a good and popular lecturer. He was an effective leader in the development of the Montreal General Hospital, the McGill Medical School, the medical societies, and the introduction of necessary public health measures by government legislation. He taught and inspired William Osler, who revered him as a great teacher.

Howard was born in Montreal on 12 January 1823, the son of Robert Howard and Margaret Kent who had emigrated from Ireland a few years before. Following completion of his secondary school education (in Montreal), he worked in his father's mercantile establishment for several years until he entered McGill Medical School. In 1848 graduated with the degree M.D. During the next year he studied in Dublin, London, Edinburgh and Paris. In Dublin at the

Meath Hospital he witnessed the brilliant work and teaching of Robert Graves (1796-1853) who supplanted the "walking on the wards" by what he had witnessed during his post-graduate studies on the Continent, namely, assigning patients to senior students who were responsible to the physician. "Walking on the wards" consisted of a crowd of students following the professor and his assistants around from bed to bed. Graves had recently published his classic book *Clinical Lectures on the Practice of Medicine* (1843). He promoted radical therapeutic reforms, the elimination of bleeding, purgation and starving from the treatment of fevers. He went so far as to suggest as his epitaph: "He fed fevers."

In 1848 William Stokes, the friend and colleague of Graves at Meath Hospital, was 44 years old. In 1825, shortly before graduation at Edinburgh, he had written a treatise entitled *Introduction to the Use of the Stethoscope* inspired by the recent appearance of Laennec's book on *Mediate Auscultation*. In the controversy over the significance of clinical auscultation Stokes fervently affirmed its great value. In 1828 he published *Two Lectures on the Application of the Stethoscope* and in 1837 a book on *Diseases of the Chest*. Only a few years after Howard returned to Montreal, Stokes' book on *Diseases of the Heart* appeared (1854). Howard, always an earnest reader of the latest in books and journals, surely bought a copy. Later in life he spoke of his indebtedness to these two teachers, Stokes and Graves, in a period of the 19th century that was Dublin's "golden era" of medicine.

In London, visiting University College Hospital and its new, most modern medical school, Howard found a great pioneer, a student of Laennec, in the person of C. J. B. Williams. In 1825 Williams, together with other English physicians, had been in Paris to learn about the stethoscope and clinical auscultation. He worked enthusiastically with the new method on his return to London, first at St. George's Hospital and later (in 1839) as Professor of Medicine and chief of the department at University College Hospital. He studied the physiology of the heart sounds experimentally, did much writing of books and articles, and taught at the university and at meetings of scientific societies (Williams, 1884). Howard must have enjoyed learning from and with him. Other great teachers in London at that time, to mention only a few, were Thomas Hodgkin, Samuel Wilks, Richard Bright, and Thomas Addison (a great admirer of Laennec).

In Edinburgh Howard fulfilled the requirements for becoming a fellow of the Royal College of Physicians. The initials F.R.C.P. (Edin.)

would look good on his curriculum vitae when he was to become a candidate for an appointment on the staff of the Montreal General Hospital and on that of McGill. Paris also had great clinical teachers, notably Gabriel Andral who carried on the Laennec tradition, including the editing of new editions of *Mediate Auscultation*. One of the most popular teachers, attracting many students from North America, was Pierre-Charles-Alexandre Louis. His statistical methods of identifying disease syndromes were widely adopted. All told, Howard spent a profitable year in Europe.

In 1823, the year of Howard's birth, the Montreal Medical Institution had begun to function as the first medical school in Canada at the newly built Montreal General Hospital. A very good description of how this hospital came into being was written in 1839, in *Hochelaga Depicta, The Early History and Present State of the City and Island of Montreal* (Newton Bosworth, ed.; 1839). The following quotation reflects the flavour of conditions in Montreal during the second and third decades of the 19th century:

> The various charitable institutions connected with the Roman Catholic establishments of this city, were several years since found inadequate to the increasing wants of the population, either from their own limits, the restriction of admission to particular cases, or the reluctance of the Protestant part of the inhabitants to enter them. On all these accounts a new establishment, of a more general and extensive character, became desirable. The increase of emigration, too, which, since the termination of the war in 1815, brought to our shores vast numbers of persons who were incapable of reaching their destination, being overtaken by sickness on their passage, or detained by poverty on their arrival, and unable to procure either support or medical attendance from any funds of their own, made an urgent appeal to the benevolent inhabitants of our cities, and prompted them to devise means for the relief of these miserable exiles. An association of females in Montreal, designated as the Ladies' Benevolent Society, was formed expressly for the relief of the indigent emigrants, who were sought out and relieved with an assiduity which cannot be too highly commended. The concern for these objects soon became so general among the inhabitants, that, in 1818, a fund of 1200 pounds was raised to relieve the wants of these sufferers and the poor of the city; and a soup kitchen was opened, where these philanthropic ladies personally superintended the distribution. But more than this was needed and the

> ladies pressed upon the attention of the Committee entrusted with the disbursement of the money collected, the cases of sick, who needed, but were not able to procure, medical aid. Dr. Blackwood, a young gentleman who had retired from the army in which he had been a surgeon, and some other medical gentlemen of the city, agreed to give their professional assistance, provided a house could be obtained where the most necessitous cases of sick poor could be relieved. The late Isaac Winslow Clark, Esq., then Deputy Commissary General, and an active member of the Committee, obtained from the Governor, the Duke of Richmond, a quantity of condemned barrack bedding. A small building, of four apartments, in the St. Joseph Suburbs, was then hired, and called House of Recovery. Small as it was, and inadequate to meet the numerous cases that needed relief, it became the germ of the noble institution which redounds so greatly to the benefit and honour of the city of Montreal.

Thus the seed for the Montreal General Hospital was planted. The initial small operation soon declared itself as very inadequate. This led quite quickly to the collection of money for building a hospital. The cornerstone was laid on 6 June 1821 and the hospital began to receive patients on 1 May 1822. The first annual report stated that: "In the year ending 1 May 1824 there had been received 254 Protestants and 216 Roman Catholics; outpatients 254 Protestants and 110 Catholics." In 1823 the medical staff consisted of five men. H. P. Loedel, the youngest, played little part and unfortunately died of typhus in 1825. The remaining four established the Montreal Medical Institution in 1823, the first medical school in Canada. All four were Edinburgh graduates — John Stephenson (1797-1842), Andrew Fernando Holmes (1797-1860), William Caldwell (1782-1833), and William Robertson (1784-1844). In 1829 the medical school was incorporated into McGill University as its first functioning faculty (MacDermot, 1950).

Some clues to what Howard contributed to cardiology are found in his bibliography (Howard, 1983). At the very beginning of his career, before he was appointed to the hospital or university he prepared an erudite dissertation entitled *Observations Upon Diagnosis of Cardiac Disease* which was published in 1850 (Howard, 1850). This ranks as one of the earliest and probably the first Canadian contribution to the study of heart disease with the aid of percussion and auscultation. Five years later, A. F. Holmes, who had mentioned the delay in recognizing the value of auscultation in his valedictory address of 1850, published clinico-pathological observations on several cases in which he had observed heart murmurs with the stethoscope. At present, more than 125 years later, one notes with pleasure that Holmes emphasized caution in making excessively pessimistic prognoses of heart disease. He cited his own observations and refers to analogous cases and opinions by Corvisart and Stokes, in patients who presented gross clinical signs of heart disease and lived into the seventies and at autopsy presented an enlargement of the heart and severe deformities of heart valves (Holmes, 1855).

Howard's enthusiasm for clinical auscultation appears also in a clinical lecture to McGill students in which he used symbols to describe heart sounds and murmurs. In 1819 Laennec had used musical notes to describe a venous hum he heard over the jugular vein. In 1861 William Gairdner of Glasgow published *A Short Account of Cardiac Murmurs* in which he used vertical lines to illustrate sounds and murmurs crossing a horizontal line representing time. Howard probably read this article, for the illustrations in his lecture are similar to those in Gairdner's article. About a hundred years later, I wrote about the evolution of such graphic symbols (Segall, 1962). My special interest in this aspect of clinical auscultation arose out of the work in initiating a cardiac clinic at the Montreal General Hospital in August 1926.

William Osler, 1849-1919

Howard was at or near the peak of his career in 1870 when William Osler came from Toronto to complete his undergraduate education in medicine at McGill. At this time Howard was 47 and Osler 21 years old. They soon discovered that they were kindred spirits, enthusiastic students of medicine and the humanities. A close friendship developed which, given their ages, had the quality of a father-and-son relationship. Osler later spoke of this in his farewell address to American and Canadian students, later published as one of the essays in *Aequanimitas* (Osler, 1914) under the title "The Student Life." A few quotations will serve to suggest the mood in which Osler spoke: "Except it be a lover, no one is more interesting as an object of study than a student."

On the fourth page we find the following:

> The hardest conviction to get into the mind of a beginner is that the education upon which he is engaged is not a college course, is not a medical course, but a life course for which the work of a few years under teachers is but a preparation.

A little further on, discussing excessive narrowness of attitude, he declares:

> The best preventive to this is to get denationalized early. The true student is a citizen of the world the allegiance of whose soul, at any rate [price] is too precious to be restricted to a single country.

And there are these few lines from Cowper which Osler declared he never tired of repeating to a medical audience:

> Knowledge and wisdom, far from being one
> Have oft-times no connexion. Knowledge dwells
> In heads replete with thoughts of other men;
> Wisdom in minds attentive to their own.
> Knowledge is proud that he had learned so much;
> Wisdom is humble that he knows no more.

In the final portion of the essay a long paragraph begins with the following two sentences: "Of the *student teacher* every faculty affords examples in varying degrees. It goes without saying that no man can teach successfully who is not at the same time a student." Osler then describes the character of the student-teacher and ends with the following reminiscence.

> In my early days I came under the influence of an ideal student-teacher, the late Palmer Howard, of Montreal. If you ask what manner of man he was, read Matthew Arnold's noble tribute to his father in his well-known poem, "Rugby Chapel." When young, Dr. Howard had chosen a 'path to a clear-purposed goal,' and he pursued it with unswerving devotion. With him the study and teaching of medicine were an absorbing passion, the ardour of which neither the incessant and ever-increasing demands upon his time nor the growing years could quench. When I first, as a senior student, came into intimate contact with him in the summer of 1871, the problem of tuberculosis was under discussion, stirred up by the epoch-making work of Villemin and the radical views of Niemeyer. Every lung lesion at the Montreal General Hospital had to be shown to him, and I got my first-hand introduction to Laennec, to Graves, and to Stokes, and became familiar with their works. No matter what the hour, and it usually was after 10 p.m., I was welcomed with my bag, and if Wilks and Moxon, Virchow, or Rokitanski gave us no help, there were the *Transactions* of the Pathological Society and the big Dictionnaire of Deschambre. An ideal teacher because a student, ever alert to

> the new problems, an indomitable energy enabled him in the midst of an exacting practice to maintain an ardent enthusiasm, still to keep bright the fires which he had lighted in his youth. Since those days I have seen many teachers, and I have had many colleagues, but I have never known one in whom were more happily combined a stern sense of duty with the mental freshness of youth.

The students of Osler's graduating class could compete for three prizes. Osler did not win any of them. He presented his thesis together with a study of pathological specimens which included 33 microscopic and other preparations which he presented to the McGill Medical Museum. He was awarded a special prize at convocation. Some months later, when he was in London at University College he received a letter from Howard, a long letter concerning his choice of a specialty in which there is also the news that the dean, Dr. Wright, had arranged for Osler to go to the bookseller, Nock, and select the books of his prize. He was advised to have printed on them "Graduation Prize Awarded to William Osler, etc." This letter reveals yet another critical point of Osler's career at which he had to make a far-reaching decision. The course of his career as a student was no streamlined affair.

Until he was eighteen years old his education was intended to prepare him to become an Anglican minister. At this age, as a student at Trinity College in Toronto he bought the 1862 edition of Sir Thomas Browne's *Religio Medici*. He had heard readings from this classic during evenings with his teacher at Weston School, the Reverend William Arthur Johnson, the enthusiastic naturalist who introduced Osler to biology. The influence of this book may well have led him to change course from doctor of divinity to doctor of medicine (Segall, 1985). Osler entered medical school at the University of Toronto in 1868, while continuing to attend the lectures and enjoy the friendship of Dr. James Bovell, who delivered lectures on theology and also on physiology and medicine. In 1870, probably on the advice of Dr. Bovell, he transferred to McGill which had better facilities for students to work in the hospital than Toronto could offer at that time. Another important crisis developed after graduation in 1872. Before his departure for London he had chosen to become an ophthalmologist. A few months later Howard, in the letter mentioned above, wrote to him about the likelihood that Dr. Morgan, a distinguished London ophthalmologist, was planning to settle in Montreal. This and the fact that another McGill graduate, Dr. Frank

Buller, was already studying ophthalmology in London and would also settle in Montreal led Osler to accept Howard's advice that he should prepare to enter general practice to earn his living and also to have an academic career at McGill.

In choosing ophthalmology, Osler had sought to find a lifestyle that would not deprive him of free time in which to enjoy his academic avocations. He did accept his teacher's advice, perhaps with some reluctance, as he recalled that Dr. James Bovell had tried to practise general medicine and also work as a physiologist and failed.

On 6 July 1874, soon after Osler's return to Dundas, Howard wrote to him that he had been appointed "Lecturer upon the Institutes of Medicine" (physiology, histology and pathology). In a fragmentary draft of Osler's reply there is:

> I do not accept without some diffidence, still I hope to be able to work up a decent set of Lectures. I am glad it is only a Lectureship. It not only sounds better (as I am so young) but to my English friends Saunderson, Sharpey, Klein, etc. it will seem more in keeping with what they know of my attainments. It now remains to be seen whether with teaching and private practice I can follow up any original work. Of course, I shall try hard.

For two years he was active in the Montreal General Hospital both as a pathologist and clinician, before he was officially appointed the first pathologist of the hospital in 1876.

Among the large mass of Osleriana that has accumulated no item is now more useful and helpful than Maude Abbott's classified bibliography of Osler's writings (Abbott, 1939). In it we find that the earliest clinical item related to cardiology appears to be a paper he read before the McGill Medical Society of Montreal on 24 November 1877 on "The Influence of Position for Hearing Heart Murmurs." This was not published but was mentioned by title (Osler, 1877). The first article which has considerable relevance at present was published in 1880, "On a Remarkable Heart Murmur, Heard at a Distance from the Chest Wall" (Osler, 1880). It is now recognized as most likely the first report of the clinical syndrome associated with mitral valve prolapse (Segall, 1976).

In 1884 Osler left McGill to become professor of medicine at the University of Pennsylvania. He had been invited to deliver the Goulstonian Lectures in 1885 and assembled material for his classic study of malignant endocarditis. The selection of the lecturer as specified by Dr. Goulston who donated £200 to found the Lectureship in 1632 called for picking "one of the four youngest fellows" of the Royal College of Physicians of London. Osler had been made a Fellow in 1883 and remained the youngest and also the most recently elected in 1885. Reading his lectures today reveals the point of departure for the evolution of current knowledge about malignant endocarditis. An exhaustive study of the literature and thorough study of his own experience with 103 cases provided the facts for his interpretation with his keen insight (Osler, 1885). In 1884 most medical textbooks contained little or nothing on the subject. The clinical diagnosis was made in only about half the cases. Almost forty years later Dr. Emmanuel Libman, a world-renowned authority on endocarditis, wrote of these lectures: "There is nowhere in the literature such a masterly exposition of the pathology, the clinical picture, and the diagnosis of endocarditis" (Libman, 1926).

In discussing the little that was known of endocarditis bacteriology, Osler announces the appearance on the horizon of the beginnings of the modern era. He states that although he found "micrococci a constant constituent of the vegetations," the proven relationship of the bacteria to the disease remains uncertain. Of the recent work on clinical blood cultures, he stated:

> No conclusive culture experiments have yet been made. Grancher (*Journal de Médecine de Paris*, December 20th, 1884) has cultivated a microbe from the blood, taken during life with all necessary precautions, but apparently not in series, and no inoculations of animals were made. Cornil (*l'Abeille Medicale*, December 22, 1884) has made cultures on gelatine, but apparently no special results have been reached.

In the final few sentences he asks the precisely relevant questions which, for the most part, were answered during his lifetime:

> In the first place, we do not yet know with sufficient accuracy the frequency of occurrence of microbes in simple endocarditis. Are they constantly present, or only in forms associated with special disease? Secondly, we want full information of the various forms of micro-organisms occurring in secondary endocarditis and of their relation to the microbes assumed to be the cause of primary disease. And thirdly, we are only at the threshold of inquiries relating to the culture of these organisms, to the microscopic characters of their growth and the possible experimental production of endocarditis.

In 1889, the year in which he became Professor of Medicine at Johns Hopkins University, Osler wrote the section on Congenital Heart Disease for Keating's *Cyclopedia of Children's Diseases* (Osler, 1889). He composed a miniature monograph on congenital heart disease in twenty pages. He drew on European literature to delineate clinico-pathological patterns and wherever possible introduced comments or case reports out of his own experience, chiefly during the Montreal period (1874-1884). In telling how she came to write the monograph on congenital heart disease for *Osler's Modern Medicine*, Dr. Maude Abbott alludes to having asked Osler how to deal with the subject; his reply was "statistically." It seems likely that his idea arose, at least in part, from what he learned in writing those twenty pages. Dr. Abbott's classic monograph consisted of 103 pages.

Osler's textbook, *The Principles and Practice of Medicine*, first appeared in 1892. Indeed the brief "note" in lieu of preface is dated January 1, 1892. It proved to be an excellent way of starting that new year. He exercised his taste for epigraphs by placing these two opposite the first page of the list of contents:

> Experience is fallacious and judgement difficult.
>
> *Hippocrates*
>
> And I said of medicine, that this is an art which considers constitution of the patient, and has principles of action and reasons in each case.
>
> *Plato:* Gorgias

Osler's text contained 1079 pages, of which 29 were for the index. To the cardiovascular system he devoted 100 pages. Reading them now underlines the fact that Osler addressed his teaching to physicians who had only percussion and auscultation with the stethoscope as aids to their five senses in their search for clinical signs. The apparatus for measuring arterial pressure, X-rays, and the string galvanometer were on the verge of being invented or discovered. Osler mentions the sphygmograph once but no illustration of any kind appears on these 100 pages. He had access to books on diseases of the heart such as Bramwell's (1884) which contains much information on arrhythmias depicted in numerous sphygmographic illustrations. He chose not to dwell on this subject matter. The arrhythmias are discussed in terms of what could be found by examining the pulse with the fingers and in listening to the heart sounds. The clinico-pathological experience he accumulated during the Montreal period appears in numerous anecdotal references to interesting cases. The last revised edition of his textbook, written with the assistance of Thomas McCrae, appeared in 1916. In this edition, the section on the cardiovascular system covers 102 pages and there are six sphygmographic illustrations, one illustration depicting the special conduction system, and two schematic drawings to illustrate concepts of physiology. Electrocardiography is not mentioned, but X-ray examination is recommended not as a routine method but in special cases. As will be seen in the chapter on the introduction of electrocardiography in Canada, the first paper on this subject by a physician in Canada appeared in 1914. However, Osler did play a significant role in the training of the first Canadian (1913) in this discipline and in the purchase of an apparatus for the Montreal General Hospital (1914) (Segall, 1987).

In 1896 Osler delivered a series of seven lectures on angina pectoris to the graduate class at Johns Hopkins. The lectures first appeared in the *New York Medical Journal* of that year (Osler, 1896). He then made some modifications of the manuscript and they were published in a book which he dedicated to Professor William T. Gairdner, "in token of the appreciation which your Cis-atlantic brethren feel of the value of your life and work in our profession" (Osler, 1897). This book continues to be quoted, as it has been in the past 86 years, by most authors on this subject. In the course of these lectures, Osler often refers to observations he made during his Montreal period. He discusses the remarkably great rarity of angina pectoris at that time: "During the ten years I lived in Montreal, I did not see a case of the disease either in private practice or at the Montreal General Hospital." Nor was this true only of Montreal. He saw only four cases of angina pectoris during seven years at Johns Hopkins Hospital although there was "an unusually large 'material' in diseases of the heart and arteries, and with many cases of heart pain of various sorts." He adds statistics which indicate that in private practice the condition is less rare than in hospitals. In his own private practice he collected sixty cases, "forty of which may be regarded as true angina." This clinical experience, well recorded in his notes, forms the basis of these lectures. He describes the gross features and innumerable nuances of symptomatology of cardiac pain in the texture of his lively discussion. He explores with Oslerian insight the complex relationships between what was known in 1896 of anatomy and physiology (including biochemistry) and the symptoms and signs of angina pectoris. He has eloquent comments on the physician's task of meeting the needs of the patient, the family and friends and the need for advances in knowledge of etiology, therapy and prognosis. These lectures contain the seeds of the progress that has occurred over the past 86 years. The first lecture contains the main features of the history of knowledge about angina pectoris, and in the remaining lectures there are allusions that make the book one of the best, if not the best, documentary of the subject up to 1896. Little wonder that it continues to be quoted in current medical literature.

Osler preached in favour of general internal medicine in medical education; the wide interests revealed in his bibliography reflect this point of view. However, he seems to have devoted very special attention to the cardiovascular system (Segall, 1986). His own contributions to *Osler's Modern Medicine* (1908) included 160 of the 505 pages in the section on the cardiovascular system. He wrote the following chapters: *Acute Endocarditis, Diseases of the Arteries, Aneurysm, Diseases of the Valves of the Heart* (with Alexander G. Gibson, the pathologist at Oxford). He also wrote the chapter on *Raynaud's Disease, Angioneurotic Oedema, and Scleroderma*. The only other chapter he wrote, *The Evolution of Internal Medicine*, serves as an introduction to the seven volumes of monographs by leading authorities at the turn of the century.

John George Adami, 1862-1926

After Osler's departure Howard, who had been appointed Dean in 1882, further advanced his tendency to encourage specialization. The Institutes of Medicine were separated into Pathology, for which Dr. Wyatt Johnston was appointed, and Physiology for which Dr. Wesley Mills became the Professor. Howard also repeatedly drew attention to the need for enlarging the city's hospital facilities to meet the demands of a rapidly growing population, even after the addition of a new wing to the Montreal General Hospital. Some time in 1885 he suggested that a hospital be built in honour of Queen Victoria's Golden Jubilee (1887) (Howell, 1934). This challenge was met by his friends, the cousins Sir Donald Smith (later Lord Strathcona) and Sir George Stephen (later Lord Mount Stephen), who offered to donate the $500,000 for the purpose. These two were leaders among the entrepreneurs who built the Canadian Pacific Railway, and the first president of the Royal Victoria Hospital, Sir John Abbott, Maude Abbott's cousin, was the solicitor of the group. The city gladly donated the land on Mount Royal and the Royal Victoria Hospital project was set on foot. While the architects planned a building with a façade which resembles that of the Edinburgh Infirmary and the builders did their jobs, the board of directors guided by leading medical men composed the professional staff. Quite naturally they "raided" the General Hospital; however, for the pathologist they looked to the Mother Country and found John George Adami. They chose exceedingly well.

The memoir written in 1930 by Mrs. Marie Adami, his widow, begins "John George Adami was born at Ashton-on-Mersey, Lancashire, on January 12, 1862. The name is of Italian origin and was well known in Italy in the sixteenth century." His family roots include practitioners of medicine and surgery on both paternal and maternal sides. The genealogy of his mother, Sarah Ann Ellis Leech, started with John of Bosden, who was born in about 1400 and was given the name "John the Leche by reason of his profession;" an early connection with the cardiovascular system, for John used leeches for blood-letting. One of George's uncles, Dr. Daniel Leech, was on the medical staff of the Royal Manchester Infirmary and Professor of Materia Medica and Therapeutics at Owens College of Victoria University. George's father did well in the business world. George was the second of nine children, five sons and four daughters. His education at school was supplemented by travel on the continent when he accompanied his father.

At eighteen Adami entered Cambridge University at a time when Michael Foster, a pupil of Thomas Huxley, was creating a renaissance in the study of biology at Cambridge (Foster became its first Professor of Physiology in 1883). Adami, inspired by Foster, became an enthusiastic student of biology and began his professional career as assistant to C. S. Roy who had been appointed Professor to fill the newly founded chair of Pathology in 1883; Roy's forte was experimental medicine. Adami's official title in 1888 was University Demonstrator in Pathology. During the next four years Roy and he explored the physiology of the cardiovascular system. They published a series of papers on "Heart Beat and Pulse Wave" using the sphygmograph in clinical studies as well as in experimental animals. Their article on "Remarks on Failure of the Heart from Over-strain" was published in 1888, and in 1892 (the year in which he came to Montreal) they published "Contribution to the Physiology and Pathology of the Mammalian Heart" — the fifteenth item in Adami's bibliography.

Adami arrived in Montreal in November 1892 to fill the post of the first Professor of Pathology at McGill. He remained until the autumn of 1915 when during World War I he went on active service in the medical corps of the Canadian army. In the previous 23 years, building on what Osler had initiated, he founded the Department of

Pathology of McGill University and also created the Department of Pathology of the Royal Victoria Hospital. Fresh from the buoyant scientific atmosphere of Cambridge with his own rich endowment of personal charm, skill as a public speaker and, at age 30, experience in worldly matters from extensive travel, he was equal to the great tasks he undertook. He played an important role in planning the construction and equipment of the new hospital. After Sir Donald Smith donated $50,000 to endow the chair of Pathology at McGill, Adami became the first Strathcona Professor of Pathology. He saw to the endowment of two scholarships which helped him attract young workers for his department. He lost no time in introducing himself to the Montreal medical profession for in 1893, his first Canadian article, published in the *Montreal Medical Journal*, bears the title "Modern Pathology." His bibliography contains 119 items between 1893 and 1915. They deal with a wide variety of subjects which reflect the enquiring mind of a pathologist who considered this discipline an integral part of general biology, an educator who sought to improve the system and the art of university instruction, a medical scientist keenly interested in public health measures for the prevention of disease and the promotion of good health, and a scholar interested in history, especially medical history.

The first article related to the cardiovascular system appeared in the *Montreal Medical Journal* for 1894-95 entitled "Notes upon Cardiac Hypertrophy." In 1909, an article on "Nature of the Arteriosclerotic Process" marks Adami's special interest in this subject, and inspired Oscar Klotz (who joined his staff in 1903) to devote much of his life to the investigation of arteriosclerosis, first at McGill, then in Pittsburgh. Finally, in Toronto, Klotz influenced Lyman Duff (1904-1956), who later came to McGill to occupy the post of Strathcona Professor of Pathology. In 1950, Duff delivered the Louis Gross Memorial Lecture on "The Pathogenesis of Arteriosclerosis," an ideal point of departure for estimating what progress has been achieved in the three subsequent decades. A significant feature of the lecture, the precise identification of specific problems to be solved in search of understanding the biochemical and histologic dynamics of the processes involved in arteriosclerosis, makes it also a source of inspiration for the workers engaged in this research (Duff, 1951). Lyman Duff and his associates made important contributions to the investigation of arteriosclerosis. His untimely death at the age of 52 ended a great career.

Maude Elizabeth Seymour Abbott, 1869-1940

Both during her lifetime and since her death, Dr. Maude E. Abbott has remained the most famous Canadian cardiologist. How did this happen? The biographical memoir by Dr. H. E. MacDermot tells the story very well (MacDermot, 1941). Maude Elizabeth Seymour Abbott was born in St. Andrews East, Quebec on 18 March 1869. Her mother, Elizabeth Abbott, was the daughter of the Reverend William and Mrs. Abbott. When Maude was seven months old her mother died of tuberculosis. Maude's father, the Reverend Jeremiah Babin, abandoned his family, and Maude and her older sister Alice were officially adopted and brought up by their grandmother.

Excerpts of a diary which Maude kept at age 11 reflect a cheerful home with an abundance of friends and also reveal an early thirst for knowledge. An entry in the diary dated March 1884 gives insight into her character as it unfolded during her entire career:

> One of my day-dreams, which I feel to be selfish, is that of going to school. I know Alice would like it herself ever so much, but I do so *long* to go. And here I go again; once I begin dreaming of the possibilities and I become half daft over what I know will never come to pass. Oh, to think of studying with other girls! Think of learning German, Latin and other languages in general. Think of the loveliness of thinking that it entirely depended on myself whether I got on, and that I had the advantages I always longed for since Emma and I began to talk of it.
>
> Now I have worked myself up, and will be able to think of nothing else. I know I never can go and even if it were possible it would not be right. What geese some girls are. Why there are hundreds of them going to school and longing to get away from it, and lots who would envy us a governess . . .
>
> How dreadfully ashamed I should be of anyone knowing for an instant that I am not half thankful enough for what I have, but desire something more.

Maude Abbott surmounted the obstacles and, already fairly well prepared for school by the education she received at home, she entered a private school kept by Misses Symmers and Smith. In 1884 McGill finally decided to admit women to the Arts course, and having won a scholarship at the school Maude began her McGill studies in 1886 and graduated with high honours in 1890. Then she waged a valiant battle, aided by influential friends, to have McGill admit her to the Faculty of Medicine. Although her petition to the Faculty of Medicine did not succeed (McGill finally admitted women to Medicine in 1917), she was not deterred from her main purpose. She entered the Faculty of Medicine of Bishop's College. All the teaching took place in Montreal, some of the teachers were also on the McGill Faculty, and the clinical work was done at the Montreal General Hospital which was as closely affiliated with McGill as ever. She graduated in 1894, winning two prizes. Soon thereafter she went to Europe for post-graduate studies; she spent most time in Vienna (then the mecca for such work) after having spent a number of weeks in both London and Heidelberg and several months in Zurich. Her sister Alice, who accompanied her, studied music in each place. They remained in Vienna almost two years. Maude thought she might specialize in gynaecology and devoted considerable time to surgery and pathology related to this specialty. However, she also studied ophthalmology, general pathology, neurology, and general internal medicine.

On returning to Montreal in 1896 she was appointed to the medical staff of the Royal Victoria Hospital, the new institution which opened in 1894. She joined the department of pathology as Assistant Curator of the McGill Medical Museum and became Curator in 1901.

Some twenty-three years later, she reminisced about what appears to have been the most important event in her career:

> My first meeting with Dr. Osler was in December 1898, when I was sent by the faculty of McGill to Washington to see the Army Medical Museum and other institutions en route. Arrived at Baltimore and following the instinct that impelled nearly everyone where Dr. Osler was concerned, I sought him out, first, with my introduction. I found him at ten minutes to nine, just leaving his lecture room for the ward round which I was invited to join and [I] followed him with the usual crowd of students, interns and guests. The visit over, the procession had just left the wards when an unpleasant but certainly fortunate accident befell me, which threw me suddenly into a personal contact with him to an extent that even my connection with McGill was not likely to have gotten. Standing for a moment with my hands on the lintel of the half closed door, someone swung the other heavy half door to, crushing my finger and neatly extracting the nail. Dr. Osler's concern took the form, after the finger had been dressed by an intern, and a profitable morning given to me in the pathological department of his introduction, of an invitation to dinner that evening. "Come at quarter to seven," he said, in the hospital

> lunch room where I had been conducted at his request, "and be sure to take your rest this afternoon."
>
> The appointed time saw me at No. 1 W. Franklin St. as I was shown to Dr. Osler's study where I found him alone among his books. After a few minutes I ventured to ask him if he would give me a reprint of his "Internal Medicine as a Vocation." "Oh, you like reprints," he said, "come in here." And he led the way into a small room off his study which seemed to be completely lined with reprints arranged in piles on the shelves. "There you are," handing me one after another. *Thomas Dover, John Keats, William Pepper, Locke as a Physician,* until I had a great pile. "And this," he said, handling me a blue pamphlet, "is the one I like better than anything else I have written." It was an *Alabama Student.*

She goes on to describe the dinner in the company of his interns and students, and the demonstration by Osler of some books on the history of medicine, followed by a discussion of interesting cases and problems that had popped up during the week. Then she tells about her feelings:

> And then as I sat there with my heart beating at the wonderful new world that had opened so unexpectedly before me, he turned suddenly upon me, "I wonder now, if you realize what an opportunity you have. That McGill Museum is a great place. As soon as you go home look up the *British Medical Journal* for 1893 and read the article by Mr. Jonathan Hutchinson on "A Clinical Museum," that is what he calls his museum in London, and it is the greatest place I know for teaching students in. Pictures of life and death together, wonderful. You read it and see what you can do." And so he gently dropped the seed that dominated all my future work. This is but an illustration of how his influence worked in many lives.

Several years later, in 1905, Osler invited Maude Abbott to write the section on Congenital Heart Disease for *Osler's Modern Medicine.* He knew the nature of the task, for in 1889 he had written the chapter on "Congenital Affections of the Heart" for *Keating's Cyclopedia of Children's Diseases.* She asked him how she should treat the subject, and he replied, "Statistically." This she did.

In this monograph, a very significant contribution by Abbott to cardiology appears in the evolution of the system of classifying congenital cardiac anomalies. When she wrote the first edition she had collected 412 cases with autopsies mainly from European literature, some from American and Canadian sources, plus a few cases in the McGill Museum, most of which were collected by Osler (Abbott, 1907). She adopted an anatomical basis for their orderly arrangement in the statistical chart. In describing the clinical symptoms she invoked physiological concepts to some degree. An abrupt change from morphological emphasis to physiological-clinical dominance in the classification occurred in 1923. In that year she not only was thinking in terms physiological but also collaborated for the first time in her career with a physiologist. In 1923, she had consented to occupy the chair of Pathology at the Women's Medical College in Philadelphia for one year; she was prevailed upon to remain for a second year. In that year the monograph on "Cyanosis" by Lundsguard and Van Slyke appeared and she wrote a quite long, detailed review (Abbott, 1923). At the Women's Medical College physiology was being taught by Wilfred Dawson, B.A. (Oxon.), Acting Professor of Physiology. Together they published an article in the *International Clinics* (Abbott & Dawson, 1924) entitled "The Clinical Classification of Congenital Heart Disease, with Remarks upon its Pathological Anatomy, Diagnosis and Treatment." Henceforth congenital heart disease was thought of in terms of three types, Acyanotic, Delayed Cyanosis *(Cyanose tardive)* and Cyanotic. In this article they attempted to distinguish further between anatomical conditions which resulted in moderate or marked or extreme cyanosis. The adoption of the physiological basis for thinking of congenital heart disease made for improved clarity in understanding diagnosis, therapy and prognosis. She applied this method in the analysis of the thousand cases which she tabulated for the *Atlas* which was published by the American Heart Association (Abbott, 1936). In his foreword to the *Atlas* Paul Dudley White wrote:

> Senac, Peacock, Rokitansky, and Keith, one after another advanced our knowledge of congenital heart disease, but it was left to Maude Abbott, fired by a spark from Osler, to make the subject one of such general and widespread interest that we no longer regard it with either disdain or awe as a mystery for the autopsy table alone to discover and to solve. She has been the most important of the pioneers in establishing congenital heart disease as a living part of clinical medicine.

Although the work of the museum primarily concerned morphology, she had made a number of excursions into the field of physiology before 1923. The second item in Abbott's bibliography and the first concerned with matters cardiac is on *So-called Func-*

tional Systolic Heart Murmurs (Abbott, 1899). This project, suggested to her by Dr. Charles F. Martin in 1898, consisted of examining the clinical records at the Royal Victoria Hospital for the five years since the opening of the hospital in 1894. She assembled and analyzed over four hundred cases. Among her carefully stated conclusions there is this classic statement: "The examination of these cases yields results which are useful chiefly as a basis for further study, which may become valuable when conclusions drawn from them are confirmed by prolonged observation of individual cases by a single observer." In 1932, Dr. Paul Dudley White wrote to her of this article, "I have enjoyed reading [it] very much and [it] is just about as up to date today as it was when you wrote it."

Abbott's earliest introduction to the physiological methods of investigating cardio-respiratory regulation occurred in 1916, when she worked with W. M. Boothby on *The Difference Between the Carbon Dioxide Tension in Arterial and Venous Blood as a Diagnostic Sign in Cardiac Septal Defects* (Boothby & Abbott, 1916). In the light of what has since happened in the domain of intracardiac catherization this work represents truly precious pioneering. In the revised monograph on *Congenital Heart Disease* written for *Blumer's Bedside Diagnosis* (1928), she devotes sixteen pages to a detailed discussion of the state of the art and science of calculating the arteriovenous shunt in cases of cyanotic congenital heart disease. She begins by stating:

> The problem of congenital cyanosis still presents an almost unexplored field, but the plane of enquiry has shifted to an entirely new level; for the venous factors in its production have fallen, broadly speaking, into their correct etiological perspective. The credit for this does not, however, belong to any single observer. It is the indirect, but nonetheless definite, result of activities of that army of workers whose researches in the past thirty years into the changes in composition of the alveolar air, respiratory function of the blood, blood volume and of flow, vital capacity of the lungs and relative gaseous pressures, have revealed to us the extraordinary intimacy of co-ordination and delicacy of adjustments of the complex biological processes that take part in the cardio-respiratory mechanism.

She then mentions twenty references to critical work and in the last sentence of this paragraph adds, "Of fundamental importance to all these advances was the discovery made some twenty years earlier by Paul Bert of the physiological action of partial pressures of the gaseous contents of the blood" (Bert, 1878).

Another major component of her career, which grew out of that journey in December 1898, was the International Association of Medical Museums. Before Abbott's departure from Montreal, Dr. Wyatt Johnston who had been appointed pathologist at the Montreal General Hospital to fill the vacancy left by Osler had suggested that she should discuss with the curator of the Army Medical Museum the advisability of organizing a society of medical museum curators. In the course of the next few years she persistently pursued this objective and in 1906 an effective committee was assembled to found this association. Needless to say, Osler helped greatly in the project and was a member of the committee. Dr. Abbott was named the secretary-treasurer and also the editor of the Bulletin which was to be published. She continued to serve in both these capacities until the end of her life. Subsequently the name was changed in 1955 to International Academy of Pathology in order to be better identified with its primary objective of advancing teaching and research in pathology. The *Maude Abbott Memorial Lecture* is a regular feature of its annual meetings.

After Sir William Osler's death Maude Abbott began a series of memorial projects that engaged her intense and sustained interest during the remaining 21 years of her life. Only two items are mentioned here, namely the *Sir William Osler Memorial Volume. Appreciations and Reminiscences of Sir William Osler Bart. with a Classified Annotated Bibliography. Edited by Maude E. Abbott. Bulletin of the International Association of Medical Museums,* 1926, pp. 633, and the *Classified and Annotated Bibliography of Sir William Osler's Publications. Based on the Chronological Bibliography by Minnie Wright Blogg.* A second edition was published in 1939, a year before her death (Abbott, 1939).

Maude Abbott had William Osler as her inspiring hero from the time when she was twenty-nine years old, near the beginning of her career, to the end of her life in her 71st year. It can now be said that, like her hero, she too continues to be an important figure in the history of medicine. The renowned mural (Chavez, 1946) in the foyer of the National Heart Institute in Mexico City depicts the most important contributors to the evolution of cardiology throughout the world from 400 BC to 1944 AD. Only one Canadian and only one woman scientist appear in this company, both in the person of Maude Abbott. The only other woman is a nurse holding a cyanotic baby that Dr. Abbott is studying. Dr. Francisco Guerra, the distinguished medical historian, guided the artist, Diego Rivera.

CHAPTER FOUR

Physiology and Cardiology

Morphology appealed to Osler much more than physiology. During his post-graduate studies (1872-74) he had worked for some time with Burdon-Sanderson in the Department of Physiology at University College, London. On his return to Montreal, he was appointed Professor of the Institutes of Medicine which included physiology, histology and pathology. Although McGill provided a laboratory for biological experiments in the department of physiology, Osler's experience in Burdon-Sanderson's laboratory had not led him to acquire expertise in the use of kymographs, sphygmographs and related apparatus which stemmed from Carl Ludwig's school of physiology. He alluded to this in a letter he wrote to W. G. MacCallum in 1880 (Cushing, 1925):

> I followed the line of least resistance. There was always technique enough to do a good p.m. [post-mortem] but never enough to handle complicated apparatus. I never could get my drums and needles and tambours to work in harmony. After all, it [a good p.m.] makes a good basis for the hard work and for the teaching of bread-and-butter medicine to medical students.

One may now speculate about the difference that greater expertise in physiology would have made in the composition of his famous book, *The Principles and Practice of Medicine.* For more than four decades, it was the most influential medical book in the English-speaking world. In the physiological laboratory which McGill equipped in 1877, there were eleven microscopes. Osler had paid for some of them from his own pocket. (In those days the professor collected the fees and paid the expenses.) He used them for teaching histology: in the English schools of medicine this belonged to physiology.

At McGill several years later the "needles and the tambours" responded well to the skills of William Stairs Morrow (Segall, 1976). He was born in Halifax on Christmas Day, 1869. After graduating from Halifax Academy, he went to Edinburgh to continue his education at University College and Murchison College. He elected to study medicine at McGill and graduated in 1891. Following a year of postgraduate study with Professor Hurthle (a pupil of Carl Ludwig) in Breslau, Germany, he returned to Canada in 1892, and was appointed to the teaching staff in the Department of Physiology at McGill. It was Morrow who first introduced laboratory experiments performed by students as an important feature of the course in physiology at McGill. He was paid a small stipend and much to his chagrin he had to engage in some clinical practice in order to earn his living. He rose to the position of Assistant Professor of Physiology during the tenure of Professor Wesley Mills. In 1911, about a year after the death of Professor Mills, Morrow discontinued his connection with the McGill Department of Physiology and practised medicine as a heart specialist until his sudden death at the age of 51, in 1920. The obituary notice (Morrow, 1920) reveals that he died suddenly from "myocardial disease." He is described as a "cardiologist" and reference is made to his originality as a scientist, to the fact that he had been a prominent athlete in his youth, and that in later years he was especially interested in music and literature, and was well versed in the works of Browning.

Morrow's physiological researches were related to the study of venous pulsation. In 1900, he published an article on the rate of propagation of the venous pulse (Morrow, 1900). In 1906, at the meeting of the British Medical Association in Toronto, he read a paper entitled, "The Various Forms of the Negative or Physiological Venous Pulse." James Mackenzie, the outstanding British heart specialist, was also present at that meeting and delivered two papers: one on heart block and one on heart failure following long-continued high arterial pressure. Morrow's paper contained remarks to the effect that Mackenzie had misinterpreted some of the venous pulse tracings in his own book, *The Study of the Pulse,* particularly with respect to the meaning of the V wave in the jugular pulse. On his return to Burnley, 3 October 1906, Mackenzie wrote to his colleague, Dr. John Hay of Liverpool:

> When in Toronto, I found a physiologist, Morrow, on the warpath, but by sweet reasonableness I modified his sting. He read a paper at the physiological section, saying that we were all wrong, and in the enclosed letter and papers you will be able to get an idea of his objections to our view. I want you to read them carefully, say on your journey to Burnley, and we will discuss the different points here. His paper will be appearing by and

by in the *B.M.J.* and I want you to go for him for different reasons which I shall explain to you when you come to Burnley. (Amurlee, 1962)

Morrow's article was eventually published in two instalments under the title previously mentioned (Morrow, 1906).

Dr. Arthur Henderson of the McGill class of 1911, from whom I enquired about Morrow, remembered that he had a characteristic walk by which he was readily recognized. He also vividly recalled that Morrow shocked the "establishment." Although he was a Methodist, he was known to be an enthusiastic frequenter of horse races, and he smoked cigars. Henderson, as a McGill medical student, had consulted Dr. Morrow because he had been found to have a heart murmur. Morrow reassured him. Dr. Henderson related these reminiscences when he was in his eighties — good evidence of Dr. Morrow's valid diagnosis and therapy. Morrow wrote a number of clinical articles. Three in particular are noteworthy: "Respiratory Symptoms of Tobacco Poisoning and Its Experimental Investigation," (*B.M.J.*, 5 June 1897, p. 1406); "A Short Note on Irregularities of the Heart, in Association with Visceroptosis," (*C.M.A.J.*, 1918, 8, 1101-1104); "Heart Disease. A Functional Conception of Pathology as a Basis for the Diagnosis and Treatment of Heart Disease," (*C.M.A.J.*, 1919, 19, 497-518). The last article is of special interest to me because I found several reprints of it at the McGill Medical Museum in 1920 and, after reading it, I obtained Dr. Abbott's permission to keep one. In 1923, when I began work in Dr. Paul Dudley White's Department of Cardiology at the Massachusetts General Hospital, I read it again as an excellent review of cardiology. The present task of searching for the pioneers of cardiology in Canada led me to remember the name "Morrow." I knew nothing of Dr. Morrow's life or career until I engaged in this work on the history of cardiology in Canada. I read the lecture again in 1973 and found it an elegant description of the state of clinical cardiology in 1919. Dr. Morrow had delivered it at the sixty-fifth annual meeting of the Medical Society of Nova Scotia on 3 July 1918, a year and half before his death on 8 February 1920. He mentioned angina pectoris and narrowing of coronary arteries as one of the lesions related to it. He mentioned Sir James Mackenzie, but neither the name James B. Herrick nor the term coronary thrombosis appear in this essay. He stated: "In a few cases some further tests may suggest themselves such as [. . .] X-ray examination of the aorta for suspected aneurysm, or the elucidation of an arrhythmia by the graphic method or the electro-cardiogram." In 1919, the Mackenzie polygraph was more readily available than the electrocardiograph. Moreover, it was more efficient for recording arrhythmias. The electrocardiograph was limited by the technique of recording on a six-inch photographic plate for only six seconds at a time, whereas a continuous record for many minutes could be made with an ink-writing polygraph. Digitalis received much attention but no diuretics were discussed. Altogether, this paper serves well as a point of departure in examining the progress that cardiology has made in the half century between 1918 and 3 December 1967 when the first human heart transplant operation was performed. The functions of a cardiologist include the responsibility to teach both undergraduates and graduates. The paper which Dr. Morrow read before an audience of general practitioners and general surgeons marks him as a cardiologist who carried out these responsibilities very well.

Morrow occupies a significant position in the story of cardiology in Canada. At a time when it was the vogue to study pathology and bacteriology in preparation for a career as a physician or surgeon, he adopted physiology. This was a prophetic choice, when viewed from the vantage point of the 1970s or 1980s. His obituary states "It is due to his initiative and genius that the first laboratory of Practical Physiology was established in McGill University and was conducted by him for years with the greatest efficiency." Fortunately for anyone interested in the influence of physiology on the progress of cardiology in Canada, Dr. Morrow published a detailed account of one of his important achievements (Morrow, 1903). The first two paragraphs of this article reflect his pioneering spirit:

> The present is a time of transition in the teaching of practical physiology. There is no settled standard of what should be expected of a medical student in this subject. It seems well, therefore, for those who have reached even a very temporary halting place to state their position, so that others may derive benefit from their experience, or assist them by friendly criticism. Even those who are not devoting their time especially to physiology, but who are daily using it in the practice, or perchance the teaching of medicine, can help us in the solution of some of our problems if they will give expression to their views.
>
> The opportunity of taking a forward step was afforded us at McGill two years ago by the erection of a large addition to our medical building through the munificence of Lord Strathcona and Mount Royal. At about the same time the Faculty of Medi-

cine authorized the Professor of Physiology to spend between three and four thousand dollars on new apparatus. Advantage was taken of this combination of circumstances to reorganize the whole department. In the present account, however, it is intended to dwell especially on the provisions that have been made for students' practical work.

Additional comments on this article and other items of Dr. Morrow's bibliography appear in a biographical sketch published in 1976 (Segall, 1976). There is little doubt that he was the first Canadian physiologist-cardiologist, and as such his career began with his appointment as lecturer in the Department of Physiology at McGill in 1892.

CHAPTER FIVE

Clinical Measurement of Arterial Blood Pressure

The ancient medical practitioners took careful note of the arterial pulse. In China, the physician felt the pulse continually as he listened to the history of symptoms. What he felt with his fingers on the radial pulse he integrated with traditional concepts of illness and thus arrived at decisions for therapy and prognosis (Veith, 1972). Avicenna (AD 980-1037?) the great Persian "physician, philosopher, theologian, mystic, musician, poet and man of affairs," assembled knowledge of the pulse from Greek, Persian and Chinese sources, and in the translation by Gruner of Avicenna's *Canon of Medicine*, the subject of sphygmology occupies 50 pages (Gruner, 1929). In a paragraph entitled "Reason for feeling the pulse at the wrist," it is stated: "1. It is readily accessible; there is little flesh over it. 2. The patient is not distressed by exposing this part."

In China, the physician was restricted to the study of two radial pulses and to noting the state of the eyes and the tongue, because it was forbidden to expose the body of the female patient in any way. To aid in describing her symptoms, the doctor had an ivory, female nude model at hand so that the patient could point to the site of her symptoms.

Avicenna's specific instructions for the technique of feeling the pulse are followed by a paragraph on the "Emotional state of the Patient," and this by one on "The State of the Observer," namely: "The observer must be in a calm state of mind. He must be very attentive and free from the least distraction of thought. The body must be tranquil and the posture at ease ... his own state of health should be good." The varieties of pulse, the comparisons between normal and abnormal, and the significance of the numerous details and nuances are dealt with under titles such as "Duration of the Pulse," "Equality or Inequality," "Orderliness or Disorderliness," "Rhythm" described by analogy with music, "Dicrotic," "Fading or Failing," "Chord like pulse feels like a twisted chord," "Large pulse," "Hard pulse," and "Soft pulse." A number of paragraphs deal with the pulse as observed at different age periods: "late childhood," "early adult life," "elderly persons," and "old age." A number of pages are devoted to the effects of food, wine, sleep, athletic exercise, pregnancy, pain, anger, joy, delight, fear, etc.

William Harvey declared, "Go to the fountainhead, and read Aristotle, Cicero, and Avicenna" (Shah, 1966). In broad terms, knowledge about arterial pressure as estimated by the physician during examination remained much as Avicenna described it for the next 900 years, until the turn of the twentieth century. Poiseuille's mercury manometer (Poiseuille, 1828), Ludwig's kymograph (Ludwig, 1847), and Vierordt's valiant effort (Vierordt, 1853) laid the foundations. Finally, Hill and Barnard in London (Hill & Barnard, 1897) and, at about the same time, Riva-Rocci (1896) in Pavia, independently of one another, invented the pneumatic cuff. This capped by Korotkoff's discovery of the auscultatory method of measuring arterial pressure in 1905 (Segall, 1976, 1980) brought into existence the method now in general use. Even as late as 1905 the estimation of diastolic pressure by available methods, described and critically assessed by Theodore C. Janeway (1904), were at best cumbersome and unreliable. Once the basic instruments — the pneumatic cuff, the mercury or the anaeroid manometer (Breckenridge, 1977) (of H. H. Rogers) the binaural stethoscope and awareness of the Korotkoff sounds — were in place, clinical experience by many observers fine-tuned the technique and the method became reliable throughout the world.

When and how did this new method of arterial blood pressure measurement come to Canada? It appears that Harvey Cushing (1869-1939) was the first to introduce the Riva-Rocci method to North America. Dr. John Fulton's biography of Cushing includes the following extract from a letter Cushing wrote to Ralph Major in April 1930 (Fulton, 1946):

> I brought the first Riva-Rocci apparatus to this country from Pavia in 1901, when I came back from my year abroad and introduced it to the Johns Hopkins Clinic where Briggs and Cook subsequently modified it and got it put in a box. The original apparatus was of course simply home-made and was perhaps as good as any of the more recent ones. . . . But I am not sure that the general use of a blood pressure apparatus in clinical work has done more good than harm. Just as Floyer's pulse watch led to two previously unknown diseases, tachycardia and bradycardia, so the sphygmomanometer has led to the uncovering of the

diseases (God save the mark!) of hypertension and hypotension which have vastly added to the number of neurasthenics in the world.

The mental attitude of physicians, including clinical teachers, is well reflected in the following comment by a distinguished internist, Professor David Riesman of the University of Pennsylvania, in an address he delivered in 1931 on "High Blood Pressure and Longevity" (Riesman, 1937):

> When the late Dr. William Stanton of Philadelphia invented his mercury blood pressure instrument in 1903, I immediately began to use it with the same zeal and curiosity with which, presumably, the contemporaries of Laennec used the crude wooden stethoscope of his invention. Just as they heard things that must have seemed terribly ominous to them — so well brought out in the poem of Oliver Wendell Homes (Holmes, 1896) — so I often saw things in the manometer that sent a chill into my heart. When I observed a systolic blood pressure of 180 or 200 or higher, I became, not at all in keeping with my innate optimism, depressed as to the patient's future prospects. I was sure that individuals with such blood pressure were doomed. But as my years of practice lengthened I began to realize that there were worse things than high blood pressure. There were patients who, in spite of high blood pressure, survived for an unexpectedly long time and enjoyed good health and undiminished vigour for many years. That was a valuable lesson.

Dr. Stanton's introduction of the wider armlet made for greater accuracy (Stanton, 1903). However, in 1903, only the systolic level could be identified satisfactorily.

Serendipity played a dominant role in Korotkoff's discovery of the auscultatory method in November 1905, an important event in the history of methodology related to the measurement of arterial pressure.

Nicolai Serge Korotkoff (1874-1920) graduated in medicine with a Bachelor's Degree at the University of Moscow in 1898. He joined the surgical staff of the Military Medical Academy in St. Petersburg (Leningrad) in 1901. The Russian-Japanese War began in February 1904 and in May of that year Korotkoff headed a military surgical unit which functioned in Harbin, Manchuria. He had developed a special interest in vascular surgery and, as he was able to collect over 40 cases of arterial traumatic lesions, he decided to make this the subject of his doctoral thesis. Upon returning to civilian life in 1905, he began a study of the dynamics of collateral circulation in the physiological laboratory. One protocol in his experimental work required the absolute but temporary obliteration of arterial flow in a limb. He observed that palpation could fail to detect persistence of some flow after application of a constricting band. This led him to recall the teachings of Pirogoff for detection of an aneurysm which appeared to be a solid, nonpulsating mass. Pirogoff taught that listening with the aid of a stethoscope over such a mass would reveal a murmur of blood flow if it were an aneurysm. Korotkoff, therefore, listened over the artery just below the constriction and thus discovered what has since been known as the Korotkoff sounds (Segall, 1976, 1980). This method very significantly improved the precision and accuracy of clinical measurement of arterial pressure at diastolic as well as systolic levels.

Janeway's book on blood pressure (Janeway, 1904) contains what was known about systolic arterial blood pressure measurement before Korotkoff's critical discovery in 1905. Because the auscultatory method came into use gradually over a period of about 20 years, clinicians had acquired the habit of speaking of arterial pressure in terms of the systolic level alone. It required another 20 years to acquire the correct habit of measuring, recording and speaking of both systolic and diastolic levels.

When did arterial blood pressure measurements come to Canada? So far we have only some very slender clues. One of these resides in a Von Basch spring manometer which one of my teachers, the late Dr. Frederick Gault Finley (1861-1940), gave me. One evening in 1938, he attended a patient as my consultant. While driving to and from the house-call our conversation about medical history led him to invite me into his home, where he presented me with this instrument which had been invented by Von Basch in 1876. Dr. Finley told me of his studies in Germany and dwelt mainly on the teachings of Quincke, who had introduced spinal paracentesis and the study of spinal fluid. Dr. Finley was born in Australia and came to Canada with his parents in 1865. He obtained the degree M.B. in London and later at McGill in 1889 the degree of M.D.C.M. He became a staff member of the Montreal General Hospital and of the Medical Faculty of McGill, and served with great distinction until his retirement in 1924. An interesting contribution to cardiology which he made together with Dr. L. J. Rhea, the pathologist of the Montreal General Hospital, merits being mentioned here (Finley, 1921). He identified the clinical syndrome of kyphoscoliotic heart disease which was confirmed by pathological studies.

Thus it would appear that Dr. Finley measured systolic pressure in the 1890s with the Von Basch pioneering instrument. It consisted of a pelote filled with water connected by a tube to the spring manometer. The pelote was placed on the radial artery, and pressure was exerted to the point at which the pulse was obliterated; this identified the systolic pressure. Unfortunately, I do not remember any discussion of the precise year in which he began to use the more modern method.

An ever-so-slender but attractive and reasonable clue to the introduction of the Riva-Rocci cuff into Canada concerns William Stairs Morrow, Canada's first physiologist-cardiologist. In the course of writing this chapter I had to borrow Janeway's book on blood pressure (1904) from the McGill Library because, after an apparently *thorough* search for mine, I could not find it on any of my book shelves. Thus I discovered that Morrow's copy (his name was inscribed on the fly leaf) had found its way into the library as a gift from his estate. If we accept the reasonable conjecture that he acquired the book soon after its appearance he would have been the first, or among the first to use the Riva-Rocci apparatus in this country. As a second year medical student in 1916 I had first learnt how to measure blood pressure with the pneumatic cuff and a stethoscope, and first heard of the "Korotkoff sounds" in the physiology course at McGill — the very course of practical experiments for students which Morrow had instituted in 1903 and continued to develop until his retirement from teaching physiology in 1911.

However, some reservations about this conjecture arise from the fact that Morrow does not mention blood pressure measurement and does not include the apparatus in his list of instruments supplied to student in the article (1903) on the new installations in the McGill department of physiology. Nor does he mention arterial pressure in the clinical case reports of the patients he studied in relation to cardiac arrhythmias. (He discussed a total of 22 patients in six articles published in the years 1906 to 1918.) However, in the section on "Pulse" which he wrote for the *Reference Handbook of Medical Sciences*, he describes the methodology and clinical significance of arterial blood pressure measurement in excellent fashion (Segall, 1976).

None of Morrow's clinical notes related to his private practice are available, nor could I find a clue to the first time the Riva-Rocci cuff was introduced in the course on physiology. The measurement of arterial pressure, though a very simple procedure, only gradually became a regular routine procedure in the hospitals and in private practice. Because in North America the binaural stethoscope had completely replaced the primitive monaural instrument by the third quarter of the 19th century, the Korotkoff method was adopted more extensively and earlier in this part of the world than in areas where European influence made for continued use of the monaural stethoscope; these physicians were content with estimating systolic pressure by palpation of the radial pulse. The better-informed among them used a binaural stethoscope for measuring arterial pressure and found it at least as good, if not more efficient, for general clinical auscultation. Not until after World War II did the Europeans adopt the binaural stethoscope as the standard instrument. Some old die-hards remained convinced that the monaural stethoscope, made of a special kind of wood, was the superior instrument for detecting fine nuances of heart murmurs and of pulmonary rales. The preferred wood differed among different physicians.

CHAPTER SIX

Careers in Research

Louis Gross (5 May 1895 — 17 October 1937)
Harry Goldblatt (14 March 1891 — 6 January 1977)

McGill graduates Gross and Goldblatt both began their postgraduate careers in Montreal and then found good posts in the United States. Both achieved major accomplishments in work that began at McGill and the Royal Victoria Hospital. At graduation in 1916, Louis Gross, the youngest member of the class, ranked first in the aggregate marks for the five years of the course and received the Holmes Gold Medal, the highest award. He chose to embark on a career of research and teaching. A Douglas Memorial Fellowship provided a modest salary during the five years that he worked in the McGill Department of Pathology at the Royal Victoria Hospital, chiefly on arterial circulation related to the aging process.

In 1921, he published his classic monograph, *The Blood Supply to the Heart* (Gross, 1921). He injected the coronary arteries with a radio-opaque material, had stereoscopic X-ray films made, and studied the distribution of the arterial trees of the right and left coronary arteries. The method was his own invention. During the years 1921-1923, he held a Beit Memorial Fellowship and studied in Europe, beginning with biochemistry and physiology at University College, London and anthropology at the Royal College of Surgeons under Sir Arthur Keith. Following a tour of the continent, he settled in New York, first as pathologist of the Brownsville Hospital, then in 1926, in the very prestigious post of Director of Laboratories at the Mount Sinai Hospital. He represents the type of worker who studied disease by various available methods, bacteriological and immunological for the investigation of rheumatic fever, and employed physiological experimental techniques in search of a surgical procedure for the treatment of impaired coronary circulation.

In 1937, he decided to engage in clinical as well as experimental work. He was appointed to an appropriate post at the University of Southern California. He took the one-month course in clinical cardiology which Dr. Paul Dudley White was giving at that time, then visited his friends in Montreal before making the trip to California by air — at that time a novel and somewhat risky method of travel. En route he visited colleagues in Cleveland and Chicago. On the last leg of his journey, the airplane "Mainliner" crashed against Hayden's Peak on 17 October 1937. There were no survivors.

In that year, I was president of the Montreal Clinical Society which began to sponsor an annual Louis Gross Memorial Lecture. Harry Goldblatt delivered the first lecture (1938) in which he described his epoch-making experimental studies of hypertension. The forty-sixth lecture was delivered on 3 November 1983 by Professor Robert M. Zollinger on The Development and Current Concepts of the Gastrinoma Syndrome.

Harry Goldblatt and Louis Gross were close friends from the time they first met, when in 1912 Harry Goldblatt joined the class of Medicine 1916 at McGill. Louis Gross had entered in 1911 (a five-year course) directly from the Montreal High School, whereas Goldblatt had taken the B.A. course before beginning the study of medicine. Harry Goldblatt was a very highly respected and a most popular member in his class. Louis Gross was perhaps resented by some and regarded as conceited by others; of course, he had something about which to be conceited. I attended their graduation exercises, because during my freshman year (1915-1916) I enjoyed the friendship of both these men, also of two others who together made up a foursome of classmates, close friends, whose names began with the letter G, namely, Alton Goldbloom and E. S. (Si) Greenspon. They were dubbed *The Four G's* (Segall, 1982). At convocation, Goldbloom received a prize awarded by the McGill Medical Undergraduate Society for an essay. Goldblatt received a similar prize as well as the prize for having the highest marks in the final year; in addition, he delivered the valedictory address.

Goldblatt interned at the Royal Victoria Hospital. He had been born in Muscalin, Iowa, and in 1917, after the United States entered World War I, he enlisted in the American Army, and served overseas chiefly in orthopaedics. His first appointment after the War was as resident in neurosurgery under Harvey Cushing at the Peter Bent Brigham Hospital. At this stage, Louis Gross influenced him to devote himself to research in pathology and experimental medicine. After a year as resident in pathology at the Lakeside Hospital in Cleveland, he obtained a Beit Memorial Fellowship which made it possible for him to spend two years abroad (1921-1923) mainly at the Lister Institute and at University College in London.

During this phase of his career, he achieved valuable results in his studies of the effect of sunlight and of radiation from a mercury vapour quartz lamp on rickets. Soon after returning to Cleveland, he published a paper entitled *The Reaction of Blood Vessels to Ischaemia* (Heart, 1926, 12, 281).

By 1968, his bibliography listed 127 items on a wide variety of subjects. Dr. Goldblatt's name became a household word in medical circles throughout the world mainly because of his experimental work on hypertension, which began to appear in medical literature in 1934 (H. Goldblatt, J. Lynch, R. F. Hanzal and W. W. Summerville, "Studies on Experimental Hypertension, I. The Production of Persistent Elevation of Systolic Blood Pressure by Means of Renal Ischaemia," *J. Exp. Med.*, 1934, 59, 347).

In 1975, he wrote a short article telling how the idea for this work came to him (*Urologic Clinics of North America*, June 1975, 2, 219). The story begins with an event that occurred during his residency in surgery at the Royal Victoria Hospital in 1916-1917.

> As a medical student (1912-1916), I was taught that benign, so-called essential, human hypertension, is best defined as persistent elevation of blood pressure of unknown origin, unaccompanied by significant renal excretory, functional disturbance recognizeable by clinical and laboratory methods. Although it was known, even then, that intrarenal arterial and arteriolar sclerosis is a frequent finding at autopsy in human hypertensives, I was taught, and it is still being taught by some that the elevated blood pressure comes first and that the vascular sclerosis, including that of the kidney, is the result of persistently elevated blood pressure. It was known then that in some cases of human hypertension, impairment of renal excretory function eventually does develop and that fatal uraemia may occur.
>
> As a resident in surgery, in 1916, at the Royal Victoria Hospital, I witnessed a tragic event which made me realize, however, that uraemia alone is certainly not a sufficient condition for the elevation of the blood pressure. In a middle aged woman, a kidney was removed, presumably for a tumour. It proved to be a congenitally anomalous kidney; there was no tumour and unfortunately no other kidney. The patient survived six days and I had the opportunity to follow the fatal course. She died in profound uraemia, but at no time was there any elevation of blood pressure.
>
> In 1928, after I had been a pathologist for a number of years, and had performed autopsies on a large number of hypertensive

patients, I began to give serious thought to the problem of the origin of the elevated blood pressure. The striking thing to me was that, no matter what the mode of death (cardiac, cerebral, or obviously renal) almost invariably at autopsy some form of disease of the kidneys was present and most frequently, by far, obliterative bilateral, intrarenal arterial and arteriolar sclerosis. In most cases, of course, vascular sclerosis was also present in other parts of the body, so it was hazardous to incriminate the kidneys. I had, however, seen a number of cases of widespread arteriosclerosis with little or no involvement of the kidneys and no history of hypertension, as well as some with vascular sclerosis almost exclusively involving the kidneys with a definite history of persistent hypertension.

Contrary, therefore, to what I had been taught, I began to suspect that the vascular disease comes first and when it involves the kidneys, the resultant impairment of the renal circulation, probably, in some way, causes elevation of the blood pressure. The condition I assumed to be renal ischaemia, an idea which I considered to be amenable to experimental investigation. I reasoned that if the idea be correct, the production of variable degrees of bilateral renal ischaemia, by any means, should result in the development of elevated blood pressure, and at some degree of ischaemia, perhaps, without accompanying impairment of renal excretory function. This would satisfy the definition of benign essential human hypertension.

During the decade of 1934-1943, Goldblatt published twenty-one closely related articles on this subject. The world literature became suffused with studies by many research teams which confirmed Goldblatt's work and extended it. Of great importance is his article entitled "On the Purification of Renin," co-authored with Y. J. Katz (*J. Exp. Med.* 1943, 78, 67-74), for it is the first in a series of publications which clarified the close relation between renin and hypertension. The World Health Organization established the convention that the units of measurement of renin and of angiotensin be named Goldblatt. Renal artery stenosis with hypertension came to be known as the Goldblatt Syndrome. In many cases, it was effectively treated by surgical methods (by-pass of the obstruction, or nephrectomy).

In 1968, when I obtained his official curriculum vitae, it listed 15 awards beginning with the John Phillips Award of the American College of Physicians in 1936 to the American Heart Association's

Research Achievement Award in 1966, one of five he received in that year including the Stauffer Award which was accompanied by a cheque for $50,000. In 1962, when Dr. Goldblatt was 71 years old, the U.S. National Institutes of Health made a grant of $1,065,000 to the Beaumont Laboratories of the Mount Sinai Hospital of Cleveland for research on hypertension and cancer under his direction. In an editorial of the *Journal of the American Medical Association* (24 October, 1977), which is essentially an obituary, Dr. Leonard B. Berman wrote: "Goldblatt's original experiment might influence us to alter the Churchillian phrase to this: 'Seldom has so much been owed by so many to a single experiment by a single investigator'."

Dr. Goldblatt's career exemplifies the value of training in a broad spectrum of disciplines — clinical medicine and surgery biochemistry and morphological pathology. He focused his knowledge and skills of these specialties in scientific reasoning and in planning experiments requiring surgical skills and methods which he had learned. His thoughts on this subject are to be found in his article "The Clinical Pathologist as an Experimenter" (*Am. J. Clin. Path.*, 1943: 13, 329).

In 1978, the Harry Goldblatt Fellowship in Cardiovascular Research was established; it is administered by the Council for High Blood Pressure Research of the American Heart Association. Memorabilia collected by his younger sister, Mrs. Alta Kahn, some early reprints and correspondence with Harold Segall are preserved in the Osler Library at McGill.

CHAPTER SEVEN

The Electrocardiograph

The electrocardiograph evolved out of mankind's knowledge of electricity. The ancients had some primitive experience of electricity, such as that rubbing amber caused it to develop the property of attracting fragments of leaves, straw or feathers. The physician William Gilbert (1544-1603) laid the foundation for present knowledge of electrical phenomena, in his book *On the Magnet, Magnetic Bodies and the Great Magnet, The Earth*, published in 1600. For the lay person, the Encyclopaedia Britannica offers a good account of the evolution of scientific knowledge in this domain.

Electrocardiography began with Lippmann's electrometer. Gabriel Lippmann (1845-1921) was 27 years old when, while working on an engineering project related to the construction of an electric motor, he invented the electrometer. Geddes and Hoff (1961) have written an excellent historical essay about this instrument, the first to provide a method for graphic recording of bio-electric phenomena.

Gabriel Lippmann was born in Luxembourg, but lived in France most of his life. After attending l'Ecole Normale, with special interest in mathematics and physics, he studied physics with Helmholtz, that universal genius, then Professor of Physiology at Heidelberg and later Professor of Physics at Berlin (Koenigsberger, 1906). Lippmann began his long career in Paris at the Faculté des Sciences where he was promoted to Professor of Mathematical Physics in 1883. Some time later, he became Professor of Experimental Physics at the Sorbonne, a post he occupied during the remainder of his life. In 1908, he was awarded the Nobel Prize in Physics for work on colour photography which he published in 1891 (*Encyclopedia Judaica*, 1972).

The next step in the story of electrocardiography occurred in 1876, when Marey applied the Lippmann electrometer to the study of bio-electric phenomena. E. J. Marey (1876) pioneered in the development of graphic registration for experimental medicine, extending and expanding the method invented by Carl Ludwig. Two years later (1878), Burdon-Sanderson, professor of physiology at University College, London, recorded the first electrocardiogram. He used a frog's heart.

The recording of a human electrocardiogram occurred in 1887 when Augustus Désiré Waller (1887, 1888) also using the Lippmann electrometer, made this record in his London University laboratory. In the 1980s, when any one, even an illiterate person, can learn to record an electrocardiogram in minutes, it is interesting to read Waller's description of the technique in 1903 (Waller, 1922):

> Lippmann's Capillary Electrometer can be used:
> 1. as a refined instrument of research for the special purposes of electro-physiology, in which case its photographed indications must be mathematically analyzed; or
> 2. as an ordinary laboratory instrument for the summary inspection and the convenient demonstration of electrical changes that are too brief, or in too rapid succession to be readable by observing a galvanometer, e.g., the electrical changes accompanying the beat of the heart. By means of a very simple recording apparatus, the value of the electrometer as an ordinary instrument of inspection and demonstration is greatly enhanced. In this laboratory a capillary electrometer is currently used in place of a demonstrating galvanometer. The image of the capillary in the projection microscope, with 1/2 to 1/10 objective, is first thrown on a transparent screen where the movements of the column of mercury are shown. An opaque screen with a narrow vertical slit, behind which a vertical photographic plate travels horizontally, is then placed on the lecture table, so as to receive the image of the moving column of mercury, which is thus photographed. Lastly, the developed photograph is exhibited in the ordinary projection lantern. Thus, the record of movements that have just been seen is exhibited and examined.

Augustus Désiré Waller (1856-1922) was born in Paris, the son of a well-known physiologist, Augustus Volney Waller (1816-1870). After graduating in medicine at Edinburgh, he became a general practitioner in London. However, after a short time, he devoted himself entirely to physiologic research. He lectured in physiology at the London School of Medicine for Women at St. Mary's Hospital. In 1902 he was appointed director of the Physiological Laboratory of London University. He strongly favoured close communication between physiologist and clinician. From 1887 to 1917, he wrote 17 papers on eletrocardiography, including the Oliver-Sharpey Lectures in 1913 and the Harvey Lecture in New York in the same year. The eighteenth item is "Preliminary survey of 2000 electrocardiograms *(Proc. of the Physiological Society,* Vol. LI, 1917). He also wrote two books (1903 and 1922). In the book published in 1922, he reproduces the demonstration of electrocardiography he presented in 1889 at the first International Congress of Physiology. It makes interesting reading now, almost a century later.

Waller's slightly younger contemporary, Willem Einthoven (1860-1927) also used the Lippmann capillary electrometer and published his first study of the human electrocardiogram in 1894. This led him to invent a more efficient apparatus, the string galvanometer, for which he was awarded the Nobel Prize in 1924. Einthoven was born in Semarang, Dutch East Indies. His father, a military doctor and municipal health officer (Snellen, 1977) died when Willem was six. His mother returned to Holland with her six children and settled in Utrecht. During Einthoven's student years, he was very active in sports, especially rowing and fencing. At the University of Utrecht, he was greatly influenced by the anatomist, Koster, the physiologist Donders, and the eminent ophthalmologist, Snellen. At the age of 25, he was appointed Professor of Physiology.

Einthoven began to work with the Lippmann capillary electrometer in 1894. He identified the inadequacies of this instrument and proceeded to solve the problems by inventing a string galvanometer, which he described in a paper, "Un nouveau galvanomètre" in 1901. His classic article on electrocardiography appeared in 1903 but not much attention was given to it by his peers. Only after the publication of the next two papers did the medical profession begin to fully appreciate the importance of this new instrument. In 1906, an article on "Le Télécardiogramme" introduced clinical studies. The large, bulky, sensitive apparatus located in the physiological laboratory was connected to the hospital, 1.6 km distant from it, by a special cable strung on telegraph poles. Einthoven could then observe abnormal rhythms and telephone the clinician to inform him of the diagnosis. Dr. H. A. Snellen, referring to the biography of Einthoven by Hoogerwerf, mentions that this diagnostic pre-empting displeased the clinical establishment and the service was discontinued. The appearance of "Weiteres uber das Elektrokardiogramm" in 1908 initiated enthusiastic investigation of the mechanism of heart action by physiologists, and exploration of clinical diagnostic possibilities by clinicans. Edelmann and Sons Company of Munich manufactured the apparatus in continental Europe; the

Cambridge Instrument Company made it in England (Barron, 1952).

Apart from that by Einthoven, the earliest article on clinical electrocardiography, by Kraus and Nicolai of Berlin, appeared in 1907. Two years later, Nicolai and Simons described abnormalities of T waves produced by digitalis therapy. They used the Edelmann instrument. Thomas Lewis (1881-1945) was introduced to electrocardiography with the Lippmann electrometer by Waller in 1908 (Hollman, 1981). He acquired his first electrocardiograph, an Edelmann, in 1909, the year in which his first American pupil, Alfred E. Cohn brought the first electrocardiograph, also an Edelmann, to North America. It was installed at the Mount Sinai Hospital in New York (Burch, 1964).

The first electrocardiograph manufactured by the Cambridge Instrument Company was completed in 1911 and was supplied "on hire, with right to purchase," to Dr. Thomas Lewis. It was installed in a basement area in University College Hospital, London. Thirteen years later, in his Nobel Prize Lecture on 11 December 1924, Willem Einthoven declared:

> The insight and true nature of the deficiency [complete heart block] has been given to us by later investigators. Among them, the English investigator, Thomas Lewis, who has played a great part in the development of electrocardiography, deserves special mention. It is my conviction that the general interest in electrocardiography would certainly not have risen so high, nowadays, if we had had to do without his work, and I doubt whether without his valuable contributions I should have the privilege of standing before you today.

Lewis had started to study pulse waves in arterial tracings in 1906. He visited Einthoven in 1908 and acquired an Edelmann apparatus. He worked intensely, and by 1909 he elucidated the "irregular" heart and named it auricular fibrillation. In that year also, with the blessing of Sir James Mackenzie, he founded the journal *Heart*. Very soon, he attracted young men from both sides of the Atlantic Ocean who became pioneers of twentieth-century cardiology (Rautaharju, 1987).

CHAPTER EIGHT

Electrocardiography in Canada Phase I: 1914-1930

Julian Loudon (1881-1959)

The introduction of electrocardiography in Canada probably begins with the activities of Dr. Julian Loudon of Toronto, where his father was president of the University of Toronto. He graduated in medicine at this university in 1906, and immediately crossed the Atlantic to London for post-graduate work. He remained there from 1906-1911. On returning to Toronto, he joined the staff at St. Michael's Hospital and in 1913 he persuaded its board of management to purchase a Cambridge electrocardiograph. He did not pursue his career as electrocardiographer for a very long time, but he did publish an article on "Clinical Electrocardiography" in the July 1914 issue of the *Canadian Practitioner and Review*. This is the first clinical article on electrocardiography published in Canada.

Dr. John Oille (1878-1962) appears to have been one of the first Canadian physicians to develop a special interest in cardiovascular disease. He became a distinguished clinical cardiologist who contributed to the evolution of the specialty in Canada by his clinical work as an excellent diagnostician, a good doctor and, especially, a great clinical teacher who inspired many generations of students and interns at the Toronto General Hospital. Oille was born of a Quaker family on a farm near Sparta, Ontario. After graduation from the local public school he attended high school in St. Thomas. For several years he taught school, and worked on a farm during the summers, in order to earn the money he needed for attending medical school in Toronto. He graduated with the degree M.B. in 1903, winning the Gold Medal and also the George Brown Memorial Scholarship in Medical Science, which enabled him to devote the necessary time to a study in pathology that formed the subject for his doctoral thesis. After internship at the Toronto General Hospital he married Jennie Cole of Sparta and began to do general practice at Byng Inlet, a large lumbering settlement on Georgian Bay.

He developed a special interest in diseases of the heart and spent the year 1911 in London. The sparse biographical material available offers no clue to how his interest in heart disease came about nor how he spent that year in London. Sir James Mackenzie, the founder of modern British cardiology, was then in his prime and his polygraph was the dominant clinical cardiological instrument. Thomas Lewis, at University College, was at the beginning of his distinguished career as a pioneer in electrocardiography. Both Loudon and Oille surely learnt from these men as well as from their juniors, notably John Parkinson, who succeeded James Mackenzie at London Hospital. Early in 1912, Oille returned to his practice in Byng Inlet, but very soon afterward moved to Toronto to practise internal medicine with a special interest in heart disease. He obtained junior appointments to the staff of the Department of Medicine at the university and at the General Hospital.

The list of institutions and physicians who acquired Cambridge electrocardiographs between 1912 and 1915 contains the following Canadian names, presumably in chronological order (Barron, 1952): The University of Toronto; St. Michael's Hospital, Toronto; Drs. Dwyer and Loudon, Toronto; The Montreal General Hospital; Physiological Department of McGill University; Royal Victoria Hospital; Winnipeg General Hospital; Dr. E. Newton Drier, Vancouver, B.C.

It seems very likely that the arrival of Oille in Toronto coincided closely with that of a Cambridge electrocardiograph. Very wisely, Oille also continued using the Mackenzie polygraph. The electrocardiographic record consisted of the three standard leads, each of six seconds duration on a glass photographic plate. This severely limited the art and science of capturing and analyzing arrhythmias. The polygraph could record the venous, arterial, and hepatic pulses simultaneously on a continuously moving paper strip from an ample roll. An electrocardiograph, which had all these advantages of the polygraph and was also portable, was manufactured in Germany in 1911 by E. F. Huth with the cooperation of Professor E. Martins and Professor G. F. Nicolai of Berlin. However, its operation was at times very troublesome. If only its inventors had made it more foolproof, it might have greatly advanced the development of knowledge about the mechanism of the heart beat. It could record, simultaneously, the arterial pulse, the apex impulse, the heart sounds, and the electrocardiogram; it was far ahead of its time.

In 1915, together with Graham and Detweiler, Oille published an article on endocarditis. This was followed in 1924 by another reporting on patients with subacute bacterial endocarditis who had recovered and survived. Such cases were rare, and at the time, were a source of hope with which the physician could sustain the patient, the family and himself once the diagnosis was made. The advent of penicillin and the discovery of how it should be administered (Loewe, 1944) completely transformed the prognosis.

Dr. Oille was the second president of the Canadian Heart Association (in 1962, renamed the Canadian Cardiovascular Society). He served from 1949 to 1950. Both in chronological age and in experience, he was the senior cardiologist of Canada at that time. The fledgling society benefited greatly from his wise leadership.

A personal reminiscence seems appropriate here. The annual meeting of the society took place in Saskatoon in June, 1949. Harold Segall delivered a paper on "The Principal Patterns of Cardiac Pain Related to Arteriosclerotic Heart Disease" (Segall, 1950). In his brief discussion, Dr. Oille stressed the fact that a change in the pattern of symptoms in cases of angina pectoris was an ominous signal. Many years later, someone labelled this "unstable angina." Dr. Oille retired from teaching and routine hospital service in 1944 but continued in private practice until a few months before his death on 18 June 1962. A few weeks before, descending from an airplane after a fishing trip he fell and fractured his skull; he did not regain consciousness. One of his sons, William, carried on the legacy of internal medicine, but with a special interest in pulmonary diseases.

Dr. Thomas Forrest Cotton (1884-1965)

In the course of two and one half decades of friendship (1926-1951), my senior colleague, Dr. Cecil Birchard ("Birch") told me several times that our old Cambridge model electrocardiograph was the first one in Canada. In 1914 when Birch was an intern on the medical service, he had assisted Dr. Thomas Cotton in its installation and in overcoming early difficulties in making it function.

In 1955, I began to collect documentary material for composing a history of the introduction of electrocardiography in Canada (Segall, 1975, 1987). On 14 June of that year I wrote to Dr. Thomas Cotton in London to inquire about that period in his career. On 11 July, I received a friendly note dated 5 July together with three pages of his reminiscences which are quoted at length:

> The written story of the electrocardiograph in the Montreal General Hospital, and my identification with it, begins in a letter from Dr. H. A. Lafleur, always interested in my activities from

the days when I was his house physician. It was in the winter of 1912 that the letter reached me, at the Charité Hospital, Berlin, where I was working in the Clinic of Professor Friedrich Kraus, asking me to give the electrocardiograph some recognition before returning to Montreal. I wrote to Sir William Osler, at Oxford, to seek his advice, as I had been accustomed to do when in need of help. He replied that I must not begin the study of electrocardiography until I came to London, when he would arrange for me to work with Thomas Lewis, at University College Hospital, where he was forging a new world in the cardiovascular field of medicine. I acted on his advice, paid little attention to Nicolai, who was in charge of the electrocardiographic department [at the Charité Hospital] and making important contributions in this branch of medicine, and continued to do so until the 1914-1918 War, when for some unknown reason he faded out of the medical world. Later in the year (1912), I was with Professor Friedrich Muller at Munich, and Edens was responsible for the E.C.G.'s in the department.

The following winter I was in Paris (1913) with Widal, at the Cochin Hospital; Vaquez, at La Pitié Hospital, had commenced E.C.G. investigations, but I rarely visited his clinic for I was fully occupied with diseases of the kidney; it was the year that Widal gave his famous lectures on Chloride and Urea retention in renal diseases. I was in London in 1913, and that was the beginning of my active interest in the electrocardiograph. I arrived at the great European clinics armed with a letter from Sir William for the Professor, and the gates were opened wide for me to enter; a letter to Lewis from W. O. was all that was required to make life seem at its best. I was alone in the laboratory with Lewis for a considerable time and had plenty of work to do. There was the mechanism of the heart beat, as revealed by the E.C.G. and cardiorenal dysponea, in collaboration with Joseph Barcroft; they were great days, and I was sad when the time came for me to leave Lewis and University College Hospital. At the last weekend visit to "The Open Arms" [Sir William's home], Sir William told me he would use his influence to persuade the Governors of the M.G.H. through Dr. Shepherd to purchase an E.C.G. from the Cambridge Instrument Company, and would himself make a contribution.

Soon after my return to Montreal (1913), the outlook for the purchase of the E.C.G. seemed a dismal one until the Osler letter arrived, when the fog lifted and the Governors came forward with part of the $1,100 required for the Cambridge apparatus; the balance was found by Finley, Lafleur and others along with Osler's contribution. In due course the instrument was delivered at the hospital, early in 1914, and a place found for it in a suitable room on the fifth floor of the new building with use of the dark room in the X-ray department on the ground floor for developing and printing the E.C.G.S. My problems came after installing the instrument, from electrical interference which I could not get rid of for some weeks, and consequently there were no E.C.G.S. We had had similar trouble at U.C.H. which was dealt with on the advice of that great physicist, Sir William Bragg, by placing the instrument in a wire cage, a procedure which I wanted to avoid.

One evening, at 6 p.m., with patient connected and much interference, the whistle blew from the hospital laundry in a separate building, and there was no interference for the first time since the instrument had been in use. The source of the trouble was found to be a leaking dynamo, which until repaired, meant stopping the work of the laundry while recording E.C.G.S, a cumbersome procedure. At that time Birchard, House Physician to Dr. Finley, became interested in the apparatus and my troubles and was helpful, and I was grateful for his assistance from 1914-1915 when I left to join Lewis in London to investigate the Soldiers Heart for the War Office. During these years, 1914-1915, my official position was Clinical Assistant to Dr. Lafleur; I had the run of the medical wards for E.C.G. work, spent a good deal of time in the Pathological Department, dissecting and mounting hearts for museum purposes, and of course, no private practice.

Another interesting bit of apparatus which came with me from Paris was with me in London, and with which I was in daily contact in the M.G.H. laboratory, was an Yvon Ureameter, for estimating the blood urea by the hypobromite method. It has been useful at U.C.H. for study of cardiorenal dysponea, and a routine procedure in Widal's clinic, but not in London; so that the M.G.H. did not lag behind London in routine functional renal tests. Blood chlorides were estimated by the method employed at the Cochin Hospital. Thus the M.G.H. had two bits of apparatus which could easily call themselves the earliest pioneers in the virgin forests of the Canadian medical world of 1914.

I look back with some nostalgia at what seems to me a remote period of my life, for it is not without glamour that the M.G.H. should have been in the forefront in Canada with two valuable clinical methods of investigation.

Dr. Cotton was born into a medical family; his father, Dr. Cedric Cotton, practised in Cowansville, Quebec. For secondary education he attended the Montreal High School. Assuming that he was eighteen when he graduated from this school, and given that he graduated M.D., C.M. from the five-year course at McGill in 1909, there are two years to be accounted for. He did not have a B.A. degree; it therefore seems that he may have tried some other occupation before he started to study medicine. After two years of internship at the Montreal General Hospital, he engaged in general practice in Manchester, New Hampshire for a short time. He crossed the Atlantic in 1910 for postgraduate studies in Europe. In his reminiscences he does not mention which of the "great European clinics" he had visited. Dr. Alfred White Franklin mentions Munich and Vienna as centres which Cotton did visit, and in Vienna he worked with Professor Wenckebach (Franklin, 1965). After a sojourn in France he went to London and his initiation into twentieth-century cardiology.

In the history of the Montreal General Hospital, we find that with Osler's letter there came $25 in 1913, and that in 1914 Lafleur gave $50, Finley $100, and Cotton $100, to make up the $1100 needed to pay for the electrocardiograph. Once the apparatus functioned satisfactorily, requisitions for electrocardiograms came mainly from Finley and Lafleur, the two chiefs of medicine (MacDermot, 1950). Cotton also engaged in research on cardiac hypertrophy, extending work he had done with Lewis. On 9 July 1914 he delivered a paper on cardiac hypertrophy at the annual meeting of the Canadian Medical Association in Saint John, New Brunswick. He reviewed the history of the subject and briefly described the technique Lewis and he had used to weigh the entire heart and then each ventricle separately. He alluded to electrocardiography in the following two sentences:

> Lewis had observed in taking electrocardiographic records at the University College Hospital in London that many of the aortic and renal cases, where he had expected a left hypertrophy, showed a right predominance or no predominance. This suggested to him the exact weighing of the right and left ventricles and correlating these weights with clinical observations.

Lewis and Cotton had studied 100 cases, and in Montreal during that year (1913-1914) Cotton studied 50 cases. He was aware of left ventricular hypertrophy related to hypertension and to aortic valvular disease and right ventricular hypertrophy in mitral stenosis.

Another paper published in 1914 appeared in French in the *Archives des Maladies du Coeur.* It consists of a six-page review of the book *Clinical Electrocardiography* by Thomas Lewis (1913). Cotton cites examples of how useful the electrocardiograph can be in the study of both physiological and clinical problems related to the heart. This had yet to be learned at the Montreal General Hospital. The receipts for electrocardiography on private patients during the whole of 1915 was $16.

In 1915 Cotton enlisted in the army. A captain in the Canadian Army Medical Corps, he joined the team which Lewis was assembling for the study of the "Soldier's Heart syndrome." (The group is more fully described in the minibiography of J. C. Meakins, page 77.)

Papers recording the results of research appeared in the journal *Heart.* With J. G. Slade and Thomas Lewis, Cotton co-authored a paper in which they proved that capillaries can contract. This contributed significantly to the understanding of shock under war conditions (Cotton, 1917). In February 1918, Cotton was assigned to a forward depot in France for the treatment of cases of Soldier's Heart syndrome.

After the end of the war Cotton resumed his post in charge of electrocardiography at the Montreal General Hospital. However, in 1919 he returned to England to work as a research assistant to Lewis. His principal task was the follow-up study of the soldier-patients. In the course of this work he made the original observation of clubbed fingers as a clinical clue in cases of sub-acute bacterial endocarditis (Cotton, 1921-22). In 1920, he passed the M.R.C.P. exams and entered clinical practice in cardiology at 17 Wimpole Street, in the Harley Street district. In 1924, he was appointed physician to the National Heart Hospital.

> Cotton was a great doctor, rather than a great cardiologist. His patients enjoyed seeing him as much as he enjoyed seeing them, and his ebullient personality radiated cheerfulness even when the prospect was a fatal outcome. He had a way of getting the confidence of his patient and the family which was a source for them of great comfort, and this was always his first aim. Dr. K. Shirley-Smith recalls Cotton on hospital visits. "Freckled and

> with thinning reddish hair and debonair bearing, he entered the ward with an enigmatic smile and bringing with him an atmosphere of bay-rum and stylish elegance. He was a man of few words and those were spoken laconically. But like all communications that spring from understanding they carried great weight with patients and juniors alike. Rounds were conducted in a quiet vein and teaching was never didactic nor calculated to impress. Nevertheless, houseman and patient held his clinical judgments in high regard. On his departure after the ward round there would be a wave of the hand as he drove away in his white open sports car."
>
> Dr. Evan Bedford describes his characteristic attitude while lecturing, holding his glasses in one hand and speaking in a slow, deliberate drawl, without notes, much as if chatting to a few friends. His smile was famous. Never out of temper, he was ready and able to pour oil on troubled waters, but this does not mean that he lacked strong convictions. He certainly exerted an important and beneficial influence on cardiological affairs, as he did on his patients, one of whom could say "as long as I know where Dr. Cotton is I have no need to worry."
>
> A clubbable man with a fund of stories, he was a good companion, keeping his friendships in repair, and a good listener so that he was well informed on national as well as medical affairs (Franklin, 1965).

When Johns Hopkins Hospital began to admit patients in 1889, Osler, as the Chief of Medicine, had Henri A. Lafleur, a McGill graduate, as his resident. Twenty years later, Thomas Cotton began his pupil-teacher relationship with Lafleur, and William Osler became his lifelong hero. At the time of his death on 25 July 1965, Cotton's estate was large enough to provide for several rich endowments in the Royal College of Physicians, London, honouring Osler: namely an Osler Oration every two years, an Osler Room, and the Osler Club to occupy the Thomas Cotton Room, which is adorned with Osler relics. In addition, he endowed the Thomas Cotton Professorship in the History of Medicine at McGill.

In 1928, Cotton married Dr. Mary Marshall, a clinical assistant at the National Heart Hospital, who survived him in 1965.

Cotton was indeed the first Canadian to receive training in electrocardiography. He mentions that the apparatus came to the Montreal General Hospital early in 1914. It may have been the first in Canada, but only by a matter of days or weeks. Others also received their electrocardiographs in 1914: The Royal Victoria Hospital, Montreal, St. Michael's Hospital, Toronto, the University of Toronto, and the Toronto General Hospital, Dr. Burridge in Winnipeg, Dr. Newton Drier in Vancouver, and the Physiology Department of McGill University. The first electrocardiogram recorded at the Royal Victoria Hospital is dated July 1914.

Dr. George Ralph Mines (1885-1914)

In the fall of 1914, the McGill Faculty of Medicine was greatly enriched by the appointment of Dr. George Ralph Mines to the chair of physiology. As a youth in his native England, Mines looked forward to a career in music. When his family moved from Bath to Hereford, he came under the influence of Dr. O. M. Chapman, a general practitioner of the James Mackenzie type, who was studying heart rhythms with a polygraph. Mines began his university career at Cambridge. He chose to work as a biologist interested specially in the physiology of the heart. He used electrocardiography and cinematography in the study of the effects of electrolytes on myocardial function, and investigated muscular contraction in the light of the recent advances in colloid chemistry.

In 1913, he published an article entitled "Dynamic Equilibrium in the Heart." Early in the next year, he came to work as temporary assistant to Professor Brodie in the department of physiology at Toronto University. In that year, there appeared his classic article, "On circulating excitations in heart muscles and their possible relation to tachycardia and fibrillation," one of the strong pillars in support of the circus-movement theory.

On a Saturday afternoon, 7 November 1914, apparently in the course of performing an experiment on himself, he became very ill. Alone in his laboratory, he received help only when the watchman happened to make his rounds and had him transported in a moribund state to the Royal Victoria Hospital; he died at the age of 28 — a tragic event for his family and for the university (Rytand, 1966).

Jonathan Campbell Meakins (1882-1959)

Thomas Cotton was the first McGill graduate who sought and obtained training in electrocardiography. Jonathan Meakins, a close second, followed in his footsteps to Thomas Lewis at University College in London in the same year, 1913. Cotton settled in England after World War I and continued his special interest in cardiology. But Meakins, who had a distinguished and variegated career, favoured retaining his main interest in the general field of medicine, with cardiology only one part of it.

After attending Hamilton Collegiate, Meakins entered the study of medicine at McGill, graduating M.D. in 1904. Postgraduate education began with two years at the Royal Victoria Hospital, then a year in medicine at Johns Hopkins Hospital and three years in pathology at the New York Presbyterian Hospital. On returning to Montreal, he joined the staff of the Royal Victoria Hospital and the McGill Medical Faculty. In 1912, his seniors prophetically appointed him Director of Experimental Medicine. Soon after this event, he went to England to study cardiology with Sir James Mackenzie and with Thomas Lewis. As good luck would have it the other postgraduate student who had come to study with Lewis was Paul Dudley White of Boston. Their collaboration in research came to fruition in two publications, which they co-authored with Lewis (1914). On his return to Montreal as the first well-trained Canadian cardiologist, Meakins installed the Cambridge electrocardiograph which the Royal Victoria Hospital had bought in July, 1914.

At a medical board meeting in 1913 Charles F. Martin suggested that an electrocardiograph apparatus should be acquired by the hospital (Lewis, 1969, p. 144). In March, 1914, the purchase was authorized, and it was specified that the instrument would be for the use of Dr. Martin and Dr. Meakins. World War I for Canada began on 4 August 1914. Meakins promptly joined the Canadian Army Medical Corps and served until the end in 1918.

During the war he worked as team member of budding cardiologists associated with Thomas Lewis in the investigation of what eventually came to be known as neurocirculatory asthenia. It had other labels such as effort syndrome, soldier's heart, DaCosta syndrome, D.A.H. (disordered action of the heart). The committee consisted of Major J. C. Meakins C.A.M.C., Captain J. Parkinson, R.A.M.C., Captain E. B. Gunson, R.A.M.C., Captain T. F. Cotton, C.A.M.C., Lieutenant J. G. Slade, R.A.M.C., and Lieutenant A. N. Drury, R.A.M.C. and Thomas Lewis, M.D., the Director. Three distinguished senior consultants were associated with the committee; Sir Clifford Albutt, Sir James Mackenzie and Sir William Osler.

The work was carried on at University College Hospital until the end of 1915, when the group moved to a new unit at Mount Vernon. In September 1917, the group moved to the Sobraon Military Hospital, Colchester, and was joined by some American cardiologists, notably Samuel A. Levine, Frank N. Wilson, and William D. Stroud.

Full-time appointments in medicine began to be created after the war. Thus, Meakins became the first occupant of such a chair at Edinburgh where he remained a very effective and popular professor until 1924, when "Charlie" Martin, with considerable assistance from the Rockefeller Foundation, succeeded in creating the University Clinic with full time staff at the Royal Victoria Hospital and Meakins returned to Montreal in 1925 to be its first chief.

Dr. Charles Frederick Moffatt (1880-1954)

On Meakins' departure from Montreal in 1914, electrocardiography at the Royal Victoria Hospital became the responsibility of Dr. C. F. Moffatt. Moffatt, a well-trained internist with a special interest in cardio-renal diseases, belonged to the service of W. F. Hamilton in the manner in which Meakins belonged to that of C. F. Martin. Dr. Moffatt was born in Montreal and educated at the Montreal High School before entering McGill in 1900 and graduating in medicine in 1905. He interned at the Royal Victoria Hospital, pursued postgraduate studies in England and then joined the medical staff of the Royal Victoria Hospital and of the McGill Faculty. It was he who used the Mackenzie polygraph on the wards before the electrocardiograph was installed. He served in France in the Canadian Army Medical Corps. A few years after he became chief of electrocardiography, probably in 1925, he attended the two-week summer course in cardiology which Paul Dudley White initiated in 1924.

When I enquired about his career from his widow in 1968, fourteen years after his death, Mrs. Moffatt sent one of his reprints, an article entitled "The Electrocardiogram in prognosis," which appeared in the *Medical Clinics of North America* for May, 1924. Dr. Moffatt reported, in some detail, three cases in which the T waves of leads I and II were inverted as examples of 63 such cases. He noted a high mortality of 31% in two years in this group and mentions similar conclusions reached by Willius of the Mayo Clinic with respect to such T waves. The electrocardiograms are described in language designed for the uninitiated lay person. He quotes the experimental work of Fred M. Smith on ligature of the anterior descending branch of the left coronary artery in dogs, which results in T wave inversion. In the one case in which a post-mortem examination was made, the studies included visualization of the coronary arterial tree with the apparatus devised by Louis Gross (1921). It demonstrated the site of thrombotic arterial obstruction. Dr. Moffatt thanks the pathologist, Professor Oertel, for providing the picture and comments, "the injection method offers many possibilities of detecting blocks in the circulatory tree where routine sectioning would fail." This article reflects the thoughts of an able internist with a special interest in cardiovascular disease and electrocardiography in 1924.

Dr. Moffatt wrote a long editorial on the prevention of heart disease (Moffatt, 1923) in which he praised the work of the New York Association for the Prevention and Relief of Heart Disease. He dealt entirely with heart disease related to infection of one kind or another. He did not mention hypertension or coronary artery disease or arteriosclerosis. This editorial reflects the attitude of medical teachers and practising internists at that time, not only at McGill, but most likely everywhere. Nor could I find any trace of any effort he might have made to organize a Heart Association in Canada in emulation of the one in New York.

Dr. Moffatt initiated the Cardio-Renal Clinic at the Royal Victoria Hospital, probably in the early twenties, perhaps in 1920, and remained the chief of this clinic until his retirement. He was one of those who attended the meeting held in the physiology department of McGill on 25 September 1946 at which the Montreal Cardiac Society was organized and he was elected its first president. He also became a charter member of the Canadian Heart Association in 1947.

Dr. Ross Alex Jamieson (1883-1973)

In 1965 Dr. Jamieson was the oldest living cardiologist in Canada. His postgraduate studies began with internship at the Sick Children's Hospital (1910-11) followed by some months in 1912 at the Manhattan Maternity Hospital, New York. This was followed by internship at the Bellevue Hospital, 1912-14 and the Hospital of the Rockefeller Institute, 1914-15, working with the pioneer cardiologist, Alfred E. Cohn.

In 1916 to 1917, he worked in pathology and in 1917 to 1918, he was with Sir Thomas Lewis at the Colchester Military Hospital. After World War I, he was associated with the Toronto General Hospital (1919-1933) and Sunnybrook Hospital (1933-49) in the department of cardiology.

The following letter accompanied his curriculum vitae:

> I first considered cardiology as having a special interest for me when an intern at Bellevue Hospital [1912-1914] and had as my chief Dr. Van Horn Florrie. My interest in this line of work was naturally intensified by my appointment on the staff of the Hospital of the Rockefeller Institute and my association with Dr.

Alfred Cohn. Later during World War I, I had the opportunity of working for a year and a half with Dr. Thomas Lewis.

On returning to Canada, Toronto, where I had my early training, seemed the logical place for me to carry on. My hospital appointment gave me an opportunity to do some work in Cardiology, particularly electrocardiology.

I purchased my own electrocardiograph which was a Williams Model of the Hindle, in 1921.

Dr. Jamieson's reference to the electrocardiograph requires some clarification. Mr. Hindle, an expert electrician, was laboratory assistant to Professor Horatio B. Williams in the Department of Physiology at Columbia University. Williams accepted a commission from the Rockefeller Institute Hospital to build an Einthoven type of electrocardiograph. World War I was in progress and in 1914, when the Rockefeller Hospital expected to receive an apparatus from Germany, its delivery was delayed indefinitely by the war. Hindle assisted Williams to build a pair of electrocardiographs. One was delivered to the Rockefeller Hospital and the other was retained in the Department of Physiology at Columbia. Presently Williams was asked to build electrocardiographs for other institutions. He referred this work to Mr. Hindle, and the machines came to be known as Hindle electrocardiographs. Dr. Jamieson was one of the few who acquired such an apparatus as early as 1921.

Dr. Arthur Burridge (1875-1932)

Dr. Arthur Burridge died at the relatively early age of 57. He belongs in the story of cardiology in Canada, because he brought the first electrocardiographic apparatus to Manitoba. It was necessary to do some field research in order to obtain the little information about Dr. Burridge that we do have. In 1971, Dr. Robert Beamish visited Miss Connie Windatt, who was the first technician for electrocardiography in Manitoba. She recalled that Dr. Burridge bought the electrocardiograph with his own funds and installed it in the Winnipeg General Hospital. The appointment book for electrocardiograms showed that the first tracing was made in May, 1921.

The *Canadian Medical Association Journal* of May 1932 published the following obituary, which was composed by Dr. Ross Mitchell:

Dr. Arthur Burridge, Associate Professor of Medicine, University of Manitoba, died on March 15, 1932, at his home in Winnipeg, after a short illness. He was born at London, Ontario, on March 28, 1875, but the family moved to Winnipeg a year later. He was educated in the public schools of Winnipeg and Wesley College, where he graduated B.A. at the age of eighteen, and Manitoba Medical College, gaining his medical degree in 1897 at the age of twenty-two. Postgraduate work in London, Berlin, Vienna and the Johns Hopkins Hospital at Baltimore gave him a wide knowledge of medicine and in 1912 he was appointed lecturer in the Medical College. In 1919, he became Associate Professor of Medicine in the Faculty of Medicine, University of Manitoba. For many years he was a member of the Honorary Attending Staff of the Winnipeg General Hospital, where he was recognized as an expert in cardiac diseases and was widely consulted. He was a Fellow of the American College of Physicians, and also took a keen interest in the local medical societies. His widow and four sisters survive him. Thoroughly versed in internal medicine, possessed of authoritative knowledge on heart diseases, a loyal colleague, and a good companion, he will be greatly missed.

It is interesting to note that the post of Director of the Electrocardiography Laboratory at the Winnipeg General Hospital which became vacant on the death of Dr. Burridge, was filled by the appointment of Dr. John McEachern, a founding member of the Canadian Cardiovascular Society and its president during the years 1950 and 1951.

Dr. Beamish also interviewed Dr. Charles Walton to whom we are indebted for some interesting reminiscences about Dr. Burridge, his teacher during the undergraduate years and also during his internship. Dr. Walton wrote the following notes in 1972:

> I recall the late Dr. Burridge very well when I was a student and as an intern and resident. He was a wonderful clinician and teacher. He was a worthy member of the brilliant team of internists who taught us at that time. These included, of course, the late Dr. Charles Hunter, Dr. Fred Hart, Dr. J. D. Adamson, Dr. E. S. Moorhead and Dr. C. R. Gilmour.
>
> I am not sure of dates, but I was aware that Dr. Burridge had introduced the first electrocardiograph to this area and if my memory serves me correctly, this was in the Winnipeg General Hospital. It was an elaborate, bulky installation, but produced very nice tracings and, of course, involved a galvanometer string device. By the time I was an intern and resident, the instrument

had become considerably more sophisticated, but was still being used for the traditional three limb leads.

The late Dr. John McEachern was one of the earliest of the younger group of internists to take up cardiology and I had the good fortune to work with him for some time.

The late Miss Connie Windatt was, I believe, the original technician with Dr. Burridge and served with many subsequent heads of cardiography.

I doubt very much if Dr. Burridge was on the staff of Misericordia Hospital or that he introduced his electrocardiograph to that hospital. Dr. Burridge may have had admitting privileges at that hospital, as so many others did, although I do not recall this with any certainty. I would think that the introduction of a machine which was really an extension of physiology would not have occurred in Misericordia, but rather in the General.

It is my memory, although I have no documentary evidence, that the first instrument in Winnipeg was developed in the Winnipeg General Hospital and I would think it occurred some time in the early 20s although, again, I do not know for certain.

As an additional point of some personal interest, in the years 1935 to 1937, when I was working with Dr. McEachern, the new chest lead then called "Lead 4" was introduced. Little was known of it other than from the literature and, with Dr. McEachern's support, I undertook a study of the 4th lead at that time. The Great-West Life had introduced the 4th lead in their routine work under Dr. Mann and Dr. Olsen. The Great-West Life permitted me to review their records and Dr. McEachern and I felt that we were able to interpret the 4th lead with some insight although our studies were never put together formally or published.

Dr. Charles Walton also contributed some additional precious reminiscences about electrocardiography in the Canadian medical military service during World War II.

At the outbreak of World War II, on mobilization, I was appointed to No. 5 Canadian General Hospital as Officer-in-Charge, Division of Medicine, with the rank of lieutenant-colonel.

The hospital was moved to England in January, 1940. It did not function as a unit at first but its members were scattered into various other places until June of 1940, when a brand new hospital was constructed for it on the Astor estate at Cliveden. I believe the first patients were moved into that hospital in late June or early July, 1940. At the same time that we went overseas, or slightly later, No. 15 Canadian General Hospital from Toronto was sent to England and occupied buildings at Bramshott, in Hampshire. Our hospital was a 600-bed hospital. No. 15 Canadian General was a 1200-bed hospital.

Neither hospital was equipped with an electrocardiograph instrument and ... any patient who required electrocardiography was to be referred to Dr. Tom Cotton of London, in consultation. Dr. Cotton would do an electrocardiogram and send us a report. Needless to say, neither No. 15 General nor our hospital liked this idea very much.

Prior to the opening of our hospital I was posted to Middlesex Hospital in London, where it was my good fortune to develop considerable experience with the gastroscope.

As gastrointestinal problems were very common in the Army in those days, I recognized that gastroscopy should prove to be a useful aid ... having learned from the Army that it was impossible to obtain a gastroscope, [I] consulted Col. Neysmith, then Commissioner of the Canadian Red Cross in London, who authorized me to buy one at the expense of the Red Cross if I could find one in England.

I explored the surgical supply houses in London ... and one, the G. U. Manufacturing Company, which I believe was a German company originally, had one Schindler gastroscope which, fortunately, had not been taken over by the British authorities.

I was, of course, delighted with my find but, while I was there ... I discovered that they had a Cambridge electrocardiographic machine which used film and which was designed for the conventional three-limb leads. The manager of the shop told me that this was one machine which had not been taken over by the Government and that he could let me have it if I could get the money. I promptly returned to the Canadian Red Cross headquarters in the Sun Life Building on Trafalgar Square and told my story to Col. Neysmith and Major Scott, the Assistant Commissioner. They promptly decided that we should have the machine. Major Scott accompanied me by taxi back to the store and we took the Cambridge machine and the Schindler gastroscope in the taxi and took them to our hospital immediately.

This, of course, was a very thrilling event and from then

on we were able to carry out our own electrocardiographic examinations.

I may say, in passing, that the Army did not show any enthusiasm for the idea but they did allow me to keep the machine although I was told that this was a highly irregular procedure. Needless to say, No. 15 General Hospital was somewhat jealous of our find. They tried to find one and there were no more available in England, and requests to Canada for an instrument fell on deaf ears.

I was fortunate in having a highly intelligent ward master staff sergeant who was formerly a printer in Eaton's before the war. He was trained and became a very efficient cardiographer, and we carried out a great many cardiographic examinations.

Because the instrument used film it was easy for us to make prints of our tracings and to incorporate them into our records. Interestingly, the Record Department of the Army took a dim view of adding unauthorized material to Records, but it was allowed to continue.

As the war proceeded, of course, electrocardiography became standard in all general hospitals, but I think this was the first occasion on which an instrument was available to a hospital on active service, and as far as I could find out the British military hospitals were without the instrument too. However, when No. 5 Canadian General Hospital was sent to the Mediterranean in 1943 for the invasion of Sicily, we were not permitted to take our precious E.K.G. machine or gastroscope — of course, a beach landing behind assault troops hardly permitted such toys.

During a conversation I had at luncheon with the late Dr. Cecil Pace at Ottawa in May 1972, I enquired about the teaching of cardiology during his student days (1923-28). He recalled an event at the University of Manitoba Medical School. On Christmas Eve 1926, he joined a group of fellow students who made their way to the residence of "Daddy" Burridge, and standing in front of the house they sang Christmas carols. Presently the door opened, then Burridge appeared in nightcap and long dressing gown and said, "Not so loud, you'll wake up the cat. Come in and I'll give you another drink, then you must go home." Pace added, "they had a drink of good scotch with the Professor of Cardiology," who was very popular among the students.

Dr. Cecil Clifford Birchard (1886-1951)

When Birchard returned from the war, he changed the course of his career from gynaecology to internal medicine. He resumed his association with the Montreal General Hospital and McGill and also his post on the medical staff of the Sun Life Assurance Company. He trained Dr. C. R. Bourne, a general practitioner, in recording and reporting electrocardiograms. They had no technician until the 1930s. The glass plate negatives were developed and printed in the dark room of the X-ray department. Requisitions rarely called for a clinical cardiological opinion. Birchard's wartime experience included some months of work at the Heart Hospital in Colchester under the direction of Thomas Lewis, who was making a special study of so-called "disorderly action of the heart," which later came to be known as neurocirculatory asthenia. This stimulated Birchard's interest in cardiology.

In the early 1920s, he became aware of the existence of cardiac clinics in various North American medical centres, and tried to form one at the Montreal General Hospital. However, his seniors were disinclined to permit breaking up internal medicine into various sub-specialties. A few years later, when I returned from postgraduate studies in 1926, I prepared a brief on the need for such a clinic. It was presented to the medical board by the chief of medicine, Dr. Campbell Howard, who sponsored it and also my appointment to the Medical Staff. The board approved both. The personnel of the cardiac clinic consisted of Birchard as chief, Bourne and Segall. One morning per week, patients referred from other clinics were studied, case histories were recorded, and recommendations for treatment made. At first the patients were referred back to the clinic that sent them. Later, the cardiologist accepted the responsibility for therapy and long-term follow-up.

Birchard had many talents; he was good at mathematics and physics and had astronomy as a hobby. In 1930, he wrote an article on "Physics of Endocardial Murmurs" in which he applied Bernouilli's theorem to analysis of the dynamics of heart murmurs. It was not published; a copy which he gave me is in the archives of the Canadian Cardiovascular Society. Through his influence, in 1931, the Sun Life Assurance Company donated a new Cambridge Instrument Company two-string galvanometer for simultaneous recording of heart sounds and electrocardiogram on rolling photographic paper. This greatly improved the efficiency of studying arrhythmias and cardiovascular sounds.

When the Canadian Heart Association was formed in June 1947,

Birchard was elected its first president, an aspect of his activities more fully discussed in the chapter on Societies and Foundations. Perhaps the most important of Birchard's achievements is embodied in the present location of the Montreal General Hospital. When it was decided to move the hospital from Dorchester Street, where it had been since 1821, he played a leading role in determining its new site. The new building was opened in 1955, four years after his death at the age of 65.

The following comments in the obituary by Dr. H. E. MacDermot merit being quoted:

> Not many men had as diverse interests as Cecil Birchard, or 'Birch,' as he was always known to his friends, nor the mental power to pursue them so vigorously. Even if he had no particular knowledge of a given subject, he could always put difficult questions about it.

Dr. Charles Reginald Bourne (1880-1946)

The career of Charles R. Bourne also reveals a capacity to undertake new work. He was born in Florence, Ontario, and lived in British Columbia after the age of nine. He qualified as a pharmacist, and in association with his uncle, he managed a drug store at Atlin, B.C. in the northern frontier region, at the time of the gold rush.

In 1907, he entered the five-year course in medicine at McGill. Then he served internships for two years at the Montreal General Hospital until 1917, when he was appointed to the department of medicine and specialized in dermatology. In 1926, he changed his specialties and became a member of the Cardiac Clinic. He acquired a portable model of the Cambridge electrocardiograph in 1927; his son, Dr. Munro Bourne, has in his possession an electrocardiogram which his father had recorded in July 1927 with this apparatus. He published the report of a patient who had chronic auricular flutter in whom quinidine sulphate was effective in restoring sinus rhythm (Bourne, 1928).

Dr. John Hepburn (1888-1956)

At medical meetings such as the American College of Physicians, the American Heart Association, or the American Association of Physicians, one would regularly meet a familiar trio from Toronto: John Oille, John Hepburn and Ross Jamieson. Hepburn was somewhat taller than the others and walked with a military gait. As the trio approached, he was noticed first. His rather florid complexion and wiry constitution gave one the impression of a man with considerable physical and mental reserves. His presence at a meeting of the Executive or the Council of the Canadian Cardiovascular Society assured smooth course in the deliberation of controversial subjects. When he rose to speak to any subject on the program he was brief and to the point. He commanded the respect and friendship of all who came in contact with him.

When the group of men who met in Mexico City in October, 1946 organized the Inter-American Society of Cardiology, they chose John Hepburn as the representative from Canada although he was not present at the meeting. At the founding meeting of the Canadian Cardiovascular Society in Winnipeg on 24 June 1947, the cardiologists present chose him as a Member of Council, and in 1951 he was elected President of our Society and served for two years. After he died, his confrère and friend, Dr. Ray F. Farquharson, wrote a perceptive Appreciation. With the permission of the *Canadian Medical Association Journal* (1956: 74, 943) it is here reproduced:

> Dr. John Hepburn was admired, respected and loved by all who came under his influence and those who had even brief contact with him were always influenced by his great, strong, definite, sometimes a little frightening but always kindly personality. His life was an unusually interesting one and his whole being reflected his varied experiences.
>
> He was born in Glasgow on December 27, 1888 and grew up in the Orkney Islands where his father was principal of a high school.... Having a keen, clear mind, naturally strong and broad interests and great ability to concentrate and remember, he could not help being a good student. He entered the Edinburgh University Medical School at 16 years of age and began immediately the study of patients along with his premedical sciences. A misunderstanding with the famous Professor Cunningham and a subsequent heated discussion about it with his father led the impulsive high-spirited student to give up his medical course after the second year and come to Canada to make his own way, refusing help from home. One could tell of numerous interesting, amusing and exciting incidents as he went from job to job, always working well whether with a pick and shovel as the Canadian Northern Railway was being put through the mountains or as a teamster or in an explosives factory or in other occupations. He worked and played and read and discussed with zest. He was interested in the people and the places, the sport and

the natural phenomena and all the activities of his environment; and he always won the affection and respect of his associates. Once, in the depression of 1911, he walked the streets of Vancouver without food and slept in parks, seeking work and finding none for two days. On the morning of the third day he was beginning to feel that he would be obliged either to beg or to steal, each being about equally repulsive to him, when a man driving a wagon offered him a job as a teamster. He had never put harness on a horse before, yet within three months his employer offered to take him into partnership.

When war broke out in 1914 he joined the Seaforth Highlanders and served overseas till severely wounded early in 1918. He was sent back to Canada and discharged. Dr. Hermann Robertson, the medical officer who boarded him out of the Army in Toronto, suggested that he should resume his medical studies interrupted twelve years before. At first he would not consider it: he could not afford it; he was married. Couldn't his parents help him? Of course they could but he would not ask them. Dr. Robertson would ask them. He would not hear of that. But he finally agreed to accept the one year's vocational training offered by the Government and wrote about it to his father, who cabled back at once, offering the necessary funds. He began to review anatomy, physiology and biochemistry in the summer of 1918 and entered the University of Toronto class of 1921 in the same fall. He headed the year in the next final and all subsequent examinations and began a brilliant and colourful professional career.

After a year spent in physiology with Professor Macleod, while Banting and Best were working on insulin, he served a junior internship at the Toronto General Hospital. While on the medical wards he played an active part in early studies of the clinical use of insulin, frequently taking blood from patients for blood sugar determinations at one or two hour intervals day and night.

Professor Duncan Graham had early recognized his great qualities of mind and character and took him on the teaching staff in 1923, just two years after his graduation. Dr. Hepburn at once acquired a great reputation both as a lecturer and as a clinical teacher. He was clear and incisive, and he knew how to stress important factors and leave out details unnecessary for his students at their stage. His wit was as penetrating as his intellect and many students who tried to evade his very direct questions smarted under his quips. Those fortunate enough to be in his clinics often said that, even when he taught physical examination only, they learned more medicine from him than from any other teacher in the whole course.

He always remained conversant with the broad field of medicine and had an intensely practical knowledge of patients' symptoms and ills. As time went on, however, he paid greater attention to cardiology. Finally, he restricted his private practice (but never his interest and teaching) almost entirely to that field. He remained in the forefront of his growing specialty and became favourably known throughout our Western world as a leader in this work. He took part in many investigations of which the most noteworthy was the recognition, with his great friend, the late Dr. Harold Rykert, of the electrocardiographic changes indicative of severe left ventricular strain.

In dealing with sick people he had great ability to recognize essential factors quickly and to make up his mind at once on the proper action to be taken. No effort on his part was too great for the patient who needed help, and he instinctively knew how to give tremendous support.

He had a remarkably forceful personality which made him a dominant figure; he was vivid, virile, full of vigour and interest; he put his whole being into whatever he did whether it was studying the precise use of words, reading, playing bridge, golfing, fishing, or working. He made strong and enduring friendships. In particular, he was wonderfully fond of children, whether sick or well, and they all adored him.

He was steadily advanced in positions of influence and responsibility, becoming senior cardiologist to the Toronto General Hospital, Associate Professor of Medicine at the University of Toronto, President of the Canadian Heart Association, Canadian representative on the Inter-American Society of Cardiology and for two years President of the Royal College of Physicians and Surgeons of Canada.

In recent years his friends saw with regret that his health was failing. A severe gluteal intermittent claudication and a recurrently active thrombophlebitis forced him to give up the physical activities which he loved. His interest never flagged, however, and he continued to work although for shorter hours till the day before his death. He would read a book a day and, to the wonder of his friends, would remember well what he read. He continued to play bridge regularly and to take an active part in medical discussions. He carried on with heavy Royal College work while often tired out and when it was apparent that he was failing slowly.

On the day of his death, March 30, he began to suffer severe pain indicative to him of a perforating arteriosclerotic aneurysm. Knowing that his illness was serious, he went to the operating room for an attempted aorta transplant, apparently calm and joking about casual matters as he had always done. The haemorrhage was too extensive and he died before it was possible to help him.

His friends will always remember with admiration his great fortitude, his ability to endure quietly, his strong intellect and competence, his keen perception and robust humour, his great kindness and affection and his capability in all activities of life. They will remember his lack of vanity and arrogance, his hatred of sham and pomposity and humbug, and his pride of rectitude and fair dealing which would not let him stoop.

He is survived by his widow who had shared his trials and anxieties and joys from the days before the First World War, by his daughter, Mary (Mrs. John MacDougall), and by his year-old grandson, John Scott MacDougall, whose presence filled the last year of his life with interest and joy.

Dr. Ross Jamieson very probably had much influence in guiding Hepburn's training for cardiology. Dr. Hepburn's early publication on electrocardiography is co-authored with Dr. Jamieson, "The prognostic significance of several common electrocardiographic abnormalities" (*Am. Ht. J.*, 1926: 1, 23).

Dr. Kenneth Alexander Mackenzie (1880-1958)

> About 1910, largely due to the work of James Mackenzie with his polygraph, the nature of irregularities [of the pulse] became better understood and physicians were able to recognize with confidence, extrasystoles, sinus arrhythmias, heart block, and auricular fibrillation. The electrocardiogram was first used in Halifax in 1926.

These sentences appear in Dr. K. A. Mackenzie's 1953 article, "A Century of Medicine in Nova Scotia."

In 1971, I attended the annual meeting of the Canadian Medical Association, mainly as a private pilgrimage to celebrate the 50th anniversary of my first attendance at such a meeting. In 1921, Dr.

Maude Abbott, my chief, arranged for her two assistant curators, W. W. Beattie and Harold Segall, to participate in the scientific programme. One of the specimens which I demonstrated and discussed was a heart, with a syphilitic gumma in the region of the bundle of His, from a man who had had a very slow pulse and had died suddenly. During my 1971 visit to Halifax, I devoted most of the few days to collecting material for the archives of the Canadian Cardiovascular Society. Fortunately, I found Dr. W. A. Murray who was most helpful. He had begun as Dr. Kenneth Mackenzie's assistant and also married his daughter. Dr. and Mrs. Murray contributed much precious information, documents and photographs which are preserved in the archives of the Society. I also interviewed Dr. H. B. Atlee, a close friend and great admirer of Dr. Mackenzie. He recalled that he visited his namesake (Sir James Mackenzie), presumably in 1909, brought home a polygraph, and was the first to use this instrument in Halifax and most likely in all of the Maritimes. Dr. Murray recalled that the Cambridge type of electrocardiograph arrived from England in 1926 and was installed in the physiology laboratory of Dalhousie University Medical School. Dr. Cruikshank, the professor of physiology, was responsible for bringing the apparatus into his laboratory. Dr. Weld, who succeeded him, recalled that Dr. Kenneth Mackenzie sent his patients to the physiology lab for electrocardiograms which he interpreted himself. Then, some time in the 1930s, he bought a portable type of instrument, "manufactured by a New York firm" (Cambridge Instrument Co., Ossining, N.Y.), which he installed in his office. As it was portable, in two large boxes weighing about 50 pounds each, he also used it in patients' homes and travelled with it to various parts of the Maritimes where he was called in consultation.

Kenneth Alexander Mackenzie was born in Pictou, Nova Scotia on 3 August 1880. His parents, Annie Munro and Edward Mackenzie were descendants of the earliest Scottish emigrés to Pictou County. His father, an itinerant "mine-wright" (a carpenter) appears to have created circumstances that led Kenneth to grow up living with an uncle on a farm a few miles from the town of Pictou. One may imagine that the long walks to and from school made for fruitful reflections about his world and the world in general.

In "The Beginnings of Dalhousie Medical School," the first of two articles on the history of medicine in Nova Scotia, which were published in the June 1958 issue of the *Dalhousie Medical Journal,* a month after his death on 14 May 1958, Dr. Mackenzie relates how great obstacles were overcome during a number of years until due to the patient, persistent leadership of Dr. Charles Tupper, Joseph Howe, and their colleagues, the school came into existence in 1868. In the second article, "In Retrospect," he wrote of his personal experience as a medical student (1899-1903):

> When I decided to study medicine 60 years ago, I was a drug clerk in Springhill. My employers were physicians, two with degrees from McGill, and one from the College of Physicians and Surgeons in New York. I was strongly advised to go to McGill, but my decision to go to Dalhousie was made for economic reasons. I was encouraged by Dr. M. T. MacLean, Dalhousie 1899, who came to Springhill as a locum tenens. While Dalhousie was not as good as McGill, Toronto or some American schools, he felt that the training at Dalhousie was quite good for a general practitioner. I entered the medical school in the Fall of 1899 and joined a class of thirty: P.E.I. [Prince Edward Island], 3; N.B. [New Brunswick], 2; Nfld. [Newfoundland] 1; and N.S. [Nova Scotia], 25, the largest up to that year, and found that most of them had economic difficulties similar to mine. Only two students, ladies, had B.A. or M.A. degrees. All the others had certificates from Academy or High School — Grade 11 or 12. Of the class of thirty, twenty received their degrees in 1903. Four went to other schools, Toronto 2, McGill 1, and Bishop's 1. Three graduated from Dalhousie a year or two later and three retired from medicine.
>
> The main subject in the first year was anatomy and this kept most of the boys busy. I learned then and confirmed my opinion later that Dr. Lindsay taught his subject as well as teachers in the Old Country or American schools. He was assisted by a very capable Adjunct Professor, Dr. F. Uniacke Anderson, and two junior demonstrators, Dr. E. V. Hogan and Dr. J. A. Mackenzie. Our chemistry professor, Dr. Eben MacKay was excellent. We were fortunate in having a young Scot, Dr. Andrew Halliday teach zoology. He came from Shubenacadie twice a week. His lectures were wonderful and adjusted to the needs of medical students. He gave interesting lectures with blackboard drawings on embryology and on members of the zoological world which had a special interest to medical students. We had good lectures on malaria, and parasites. Histology was well taught by Dr. G. M. Campbell and Dr. H. D. Weacer who, by the way, was the first doctor to bring an X-ray machine to Halifax and he gave all the students the benefit of a demonstration in his office on Spring

Garden Road. We were instructed in microscopy in histology, zoology and botany. On the whole, our first year was satisfactory and no student could complain of having too little instruction.

In the second year the major subject was anatomy which was well taught. Organic chemistry was next in importance and was taught in a masterly manner by Dr. Eben MacKay. Materia medica was probably next in importance and was taught by didactic lectures with practical instruction in the Victoria General Hospital under Dr. Puttner. Physiology consisted in didactic lectures three times a week by Dr. Silver. There was still no laboratory instruction in physiology or pharmacology.

The third and fourth year was mainly clinical. Didactic lectures were given on all subjects of the curriculum, in clinic, ward, and theatre, were given daily in the Victoria General Hospital. Some of the teaching was excellent but there were some weak spots. It should be noted that all teaching was done without remuneration and the necessity to earn a living often kept teachers from keeping their appointments with their classes. An important advance was made in 1902 when a pathology wing was added to the Medical School building and Dr. Andrew Halliday was appointed full time director of pathology and bacteriology. The instruction on these subjects greatly improved under the supervision of Dr. Halliday, Dr. G. M. Campbell and Dr. W. H. Hattie. Halliday was a man of great promise but unfortunately died of tuberculosis at the age of 36, in 1903. His successor was Dr. L. M. Murray. The Halifax Dispensary was open to students and quite a lot of minor ailments were seen there.

It is of some interest today to note some of the conditions which existed in 1900. The wooden operating table was still in use. No rubber gloves were used. Sponges were the commercial sea-sponges which were sterilized and used over and over again. The complicated methods of sterilizing the hands in some instances caused a dermatitis which forced some surgeons to abandon surgery. The only private rooms in Halifax were five in the Victoria General Hospital and 30 in the Halifax Infirmary. Surgery was often done in the homes — kitchen surgery. Laboratory work in the V.G. [Victoria General] Hospital was done by the senior students and interns and included blood counts, urinary sediments and parasites. Chemical tests for albumen, sugar and blood in stools were routine. Sputum was examined for tubercle bacilli and other organisms. Anaesthetics were administered by senior students and interns, ether and chloroform by open method. There were no specialists in anaesthesia.

The X-ray had not yet come into use. Tuberculosis was recognized by a study of symptoms and signs and only diagnosed when in an advanced stage. Finding of tubercle [bacilli] was a step in advance but there was still no sign of a proper institution for tuberculosis. There was no blood chemistry yet, no blood pressure readings and no cystoscopy or other modern diagnostic aids.

It should be of some interest to the student of today to know what a medical education in Halifax cost in 1900. One hundred dollars paid for annual fees and twenty dollars paid for the required books. Most of the students "lodged," which meant that the landlady received one dollar and a half a week and prepared and served meals. In our house we purchased a winter's supply of potatoes from a schooner at the wharf for twenty-five cents a bushel. A barrel of apples could be bought for a dollar or sometimes a dollar and a half. Flour was bought by the barrel and baking was done by the landlady. The total cost of board varied from two dollars and a half to three dollars [per week] and caloric requirements were fully met. A few students boarded at three or four dollars a week. Re clothing — a custom made suit could be purchased at [six] dollars — shoes cost $1.00 or a little more a pair. The cap usually worn, seldom cost more than twenty-five cents. A peabouncer (bowler hat) was not allowed in college except by senior students. The total cost seldom exceeded three hundred dollars for those who were obligated to forego the luxuries.

At graduation Kenneth Mackenzie was the gold medallist. Then, guided by his mentor Dr. D. A. Morrison of Sydney, he entered general practice in Boularderie Island in the Bras d'Or Lakes region of Cape Breton; a few years later he settled in Halifax and in 1909 he went to England for postgraduate studies. He married Christine Morrison, the daughter of Dr. Morrison, and in 1913, accompanied by his wife, again spent some time in England. On this occasion he visited Oxford and came under the influence of Sir William Osler. He also visited Thomas Lewis and Sir James Mackenzie in London and spent some time in Edinburgh. Not long after his return to Halifax, World War I began and he enlisted in No. 7 Stationary Hospital of the Canadian Expeditionary Force (Dalhousie Unit) which was under the command of Lt. Col. John Stewart — the pioneer surgeon who had been Lister's assistant in 1877-1879. Among the memorabilia donated to our Archives by Dr. and Mrs. Murray, there is a picture of Kenneth Mackenzie with Sir William Osler (1913) and a picture of the officers of the No. 7 Stationary Hospital (1915). During his service in England he spent some time with Thomas Lewis at the special hospital for the study of neurocirculatory asthenia in Colchester. There he met pioneers of 20th century cardiology, Jonathan Meakins, Samuel Levine, Cecil Birchard and others. He returned to Halifax in 1919 to take part in the renaissance of the Dalhousie Medical School as the leading medical internist in the Maritimes.

Mackenzie refers to some "weak spots" in clinical teaching during his undergraduate years. These are more precisely described by Dr. H. B. Atlee, who entered the Halifax Medical College in 1907 and graduated in 1911. His article, which appeared in the same *Dalhousie Medical Journal* as the two mentioned above by Mackenzie bears the title "Dalhousie Medical School 1907-1957." The first paragraph contains a description of the meagre physical facilities of the school. The next three paragraphs described the academic features and are quoted here in full:

> I suppose that the next four years (1907-1911) constituted the absolute nadir of medical education here. The group of pioneers who had founded the Halifax College had lost their first fine careless rapture. They had no money aside from student fees and so could not afford to build the laboratories and other facilities that modern medical teaching was demanding. There was, for instance, no physiological laboratory — there was no real pathology laboratory. There were no full time teachers in the basic sciences. But, what was even worse, drink and dissension had destroyed a great deal of the teaching dynamic. Too many of the internists were the victims of alcohol and the surgeons of a disrupting emotional immaturity.
>
> Two quite able surgeons were available. One passed the school by like the Levite [Dr. John Stewart] as beneath his efforts; the other withdrew entirely from teaching in sheer pique. As a result we were left with only one good surgeon, Murdock Chisholm, to carry on the surgical teaching. In medicine, the situation was even worse. In my third year I would say that we lost three-quarters of our lectures through the inability of a man who was a very able teacher when sober to eschew the bottle. In practical obstetrics we were expected to witness only four

deliveries. Having witnessed two of these at the Poor House, conducted under a blanket by a dear old Victorian obstetrician who felt that it was a mortal sin to expose a female perineum, I finally saw a baby being born only because Dr. Kenneth Mackenzie kindly allowed me to deliver two of his Grafton St. patients, my equipment for this consisting of a pair of scissors, some string to tie the cord, a bottle of carbolic acid and some gauze.

The medical course lasted four years only. I entered it from high school and my high school marks were my matriculation. Chemistry, physics and biology were taught in the first two years along with anatomy and physiology. Since the non-medical subjects were handled by the regular university teachers, this instruction was up to par. Furthermore, we got a very fine course in anatomy from Dr. A. W. H. Lindsay; I doubt if many medical schools on this continent were giving better. But the physiology, which combined biochemistry and pharmacology, that of Edinburgh 1892, was practically a dead loss.

How could such teaching produce such able men as Hugh Schwartz, Kirk MacLellan, and the late Frank Davis and Dean Grant? Did these men excel in their fields despite the teaching, or could equally good men still be produced with less teaching than students now get? I ask this question — not that I yearn for the return of the bad old days of '07-11 — but because as a teacher it has troubled me of late years. Are we trying to cram too much into the modern medical student's head? Are we filling him so full of facts that his brain has no room for ideas? Is his nose being kept so close to the curricular grindstone that he has no time to look at the stars? I am convinced that this is a question for medical pedagogues to ponder — if they in turn can find time between practice, teaching and committee meetings for such a salutory meditation.

The Flexner report of 1910 rated the Dalhousie School "at the bottom of the heap." But as it was the only medical school in Eastern Canada and therefore had to be preserved, the Carnegie and Rockefeller Foundations undertook the necessary tasks. Thus in the 1920s and 30s, buildings and personnel were assembled to create a modern medical school, which continues to maintain its first class status. Atlee pays tribute to the men whose dedication to the interests of the school assured its progress. Of Kenneth Mackenzie he wrote:

> He did for the department of medicine what John George MacDougall did for surgery. A much more modest and less flashy man, he was an outstanding teacher and clinician. He achieved this through simplicity. It was a privilege to watch him make a diagnosis — not by some leap of intuition — but by steering by a few right stars. The ease with which, using his simple navigational aids, he arrived at a diagnostic port was amazing . . . He was a student whose mind ranged beyond medical texts and journals into the field of general culture.

Dr. William Murray was greatly impressed by his father-in-law's exceptionally good memory. This contributed significantly to his talent in acquiring knowledge in several specialties — neurology, psychiatry, gastro-enterology, cardiology — so that he fulfilled the role of a specialist in a variety of disciplines. He occupied the post of Professor of Medicine from 1921-1948 and Dalhousie University conferred the degree LL.D. on him in 1956. He served as president of the Nova Scotia Medical Association in 1933 and in 1938-39 he was president of the Canadian Medical Association. Especially in the last decade of his life he wrote about medical history in Nova Scotia. Reprints of a few of these articles were presented to the Archives of the Canadian Cardiovascular Society by Dr. and Mrs. W. A. Murray. There is also an undated manuscript entitled "Quinidine Sulphate" in which Mackenzie describes his experiences with this therapy in ten patients.

Dr. N. L. Scammell, a younger colleague, wrote of Dr. Mackenzie in 1971:

> He was sent a supply of Banting's insulin in 1922 for clinical trials at the Victoria General Hospital in Halifax. He stuck to Internal Medicine at a time when many were doing general practice as well . . . I knew Dr. Mackenzie well. I think he was as well informed in neurology as he was in cardiology . . . He was a big man physically, with a happy disposition and a splendid personality . . . He was beloved and respected by family and friends.

Dr. Maurice Aaron Pollock (1887-   )

Dr. Maurice Pollock belongs among the pioneers of cardiology because as a general practitioner who evolved into an internist without university affiliation, he began to record electrocardiograms in 1920. In 1965, he provided his curriculum vitae. The archivist wrote to him requesting reminiscences about the beginning of his special interest in cardiology and his early experiences as chief of medicine of Mount Sinai Hospital of Toronto. In 1968, the request was repeated and his son Ira wrote the following letter:

> My father, Dr. Maurice Aaron Pollock was born on June 9th, 1887. He attended public school to grade 8. He received private instruction in his high school subjects while working and received his matriculation in 1905 at which time he entered the University of Toronto in the B and P course. He received his B.A. in 1909 and his M.B. in 1911 and his M.D. in 1946. He received his certificate in Internal Medicine from the Royal College of Physicians and Surgeons in 1944.
>
> After graduation in 1911 he took a short internship (eight months) at McKellar General Hospital in Fort William, Ontario, followed by postgraduate studies in New York and Chicago (New York Post-Graduate Hospital, Chicago Children's Memorial Hospital). He had a general practice in Toronto until 1939 at which time he restricted his practice to internal medicine. During this early period he worked with Dr. Allan Brown, Chief of Paediatrics in well-baby clinics and was part-time physician with the Toronto Board of Education from 1912 to 1918. He first began to record electrocardiograms in 1920. He was Head of Medicine in Mount Sinai Hospital from its inception (1923), alternating with the late Drs. L. J. Solway and L. J. Breslin. During this period he taught the interns and held regular medical rounds for the staff. He is still associated with my brother, Dr. Oscar Pollock and myself in practice in Toronto, although he is away in the warmer climate during the winter months.

Dr. Charles Watson Hurlburt (1881-1944)

During the years of World War II, there were only two internists in Alberta who had a special interest in cardiology, Dr. Hurlburt and Dr. Scarlett, both veterans of World War I. The other thirteen Albertans who responded to the questionnaire all graduated during or after the 1940s. They found Canadian centres in which to train. Most began postgraduate education in these centres and then proceeded to the United States to acquire skills in cardiac catheterization and open heart surgery. Some capped this happy period of their lives by a sojourn across the Atlantic, beginning with London.

Dr. John W. Scott, former Dean at the University of Alberta Medical School, a McGill graduate of the class of 1922 and a founding member of our society, has been the only source of information about cardiology at the University of Alberta and in Edmonton during the three decades before World War II. He recalled that Dr. Charles Watson Hurlburt used a Mackenzie polygraph in the 1920s. He also used electrocardiography. The department of physiology at the University of Alberta had an electrocardiograph, probably a Cambridge model. Professor Downs cooperated with Dr. Hurlburt; he recorded the electrocardiograms on patients Hurlburt sent to the laboratory. Dr. Scott recalled that when clinical teaching was initiated at the University of Alberta in 1922, Dr. Hurlburt taught cardiology. At some time in the late 1920s or early 1930s, Dr. Hurlburt took the postgraduate course in cardiology given by Dr. Paul D. White at the Massachusetts General Hospital in Boston.

The obituary published in the *C.M.A.J.* (1944: 51, 592) provides the following information. Dr. Hurlburt was born in Mitchell, Ontario in 1881, and graduated in medicine at Toronto University in 1910. He opened an office in Coronation, Alberta in 1911. He served in the army medical corps during World War I, and while in England he had some postgraduate training in cardiology in London. When he returned to civilian life in 1919 he restricted his practice to internal medicine. At the University of Alberta, he was known as the "Cardiologist." He died suddenly while visiting Victoria, B.C. on 25 October 1944.

Dr. Ambrose Gerald McGhie (1893-1972)

Dr. McGhie's skill in administration played an important role in the creation of the Ontario Heart Foundation. Together with Dr. John Keith and Dr. John Hepburn, he belonged to a committee which received a research grant from the Ontario Department of Health through the Honourable Russell T. Kelley. He considered this method of obtaining grants-in-aid for research 'irregular' — he insisted that an organization be set up to avoid embarrassment to the committee or to the government. Out of this circumstance, the Ontario Heart Foundation was created. His curriculum vitae reveals him as a pioneer in the development of group practice in Canada. After visiting the Mayo Clinic in 1920 he decided to pursue this kind of practice and joined the McGregor Clinic in Hamilton, Ontario when it was organized in 1922. After spending some time studying under Dr. Richard C. Cabot at the Massachusetts General Hospital in Boston, he developed a special interest in cardiology and bought his first electrocardiograph apparatus, a Cambridge Instrument Company machine in 1927.

In answer to our request for more details about his career, he wrote as follows on 9 July, 1965:

> Yes, my first electrocardiograph machine was a Cambridge portable in two large boxes, and I think they weighed 40 to 60 lbs., but it was the first portable machine available, and I purchased it shortly after it came on the market.
>
> I am sorry that I have been very negligent in keeping a diary of any kind, and cannot remember dates and particularly circumstances as well as I should. I do not even know the auspices under which a group of cardiologists were meeting in Toronto at the time that the suggestion was made that it might be possible for us to get some Dominion funds through the Provincial Department of Health to help get some research work under way, nor can I remember the year, but Dr. Keith, Dr. Hepburn and I were nominated to make an appointment and consult with the Minister of Health at that time, Mr. Russell T. Kelley. I possibly was included because Russell T. Kelley was a Hamilton citizen, I knew him very well through the Rotary Club, being a fellow member, and because he had been a patient of mine. I volunteered to set up the appointment, and when I did so, it was in a personal conversation with Mr. Kelley, and I outlined to him exactly why I wished to see him. When the interview took place, Dr. Keith began to outline the situation to Mr. Kelley, when he interrupted him and said, "Yes, I know all about it and I am going to do what I can for you." Then for three years we received a grant of somewhere in the neighbourhood of $3,000.00, and the grant was in the name of the Committee. We all realized that this was very irregular, but after three years I felt that the Minister, his government and the profession might get into a political turmoil because of this irregularity, and so we insisted that some sort of organization, which could get this grant legally, must be set up, and this was proceeded with at this meeting.
>
> Soon after the organization was set up, Dr. Walmsley was employed by the organization for a short period of time. The records should show this, and that could fix the date very well.

In 1968, I wrote requesting reprints of his articles on medical history in Canada. Within a few days there arrived the *McGregor Clinic Bulletin* of September 1962, the fortieth anniversary addition, accompanied by a letter which is quoted in part:

Complying with your request I am sending you the Clinic Bulletin of September 1962 which contains four articles which I have written on historical subjects.

I retired from practice the first of January. Following this, the Hamilton Academy of Medicine appointed me official historian and at the present time I am going through old records, consulting the local library and hounding some of the older practitioners to try and piece together some of the data that is hard to find.

You are right. My first cardiograph machine was purchased in 1927. In 1930, I took my M.R.C.P. in Edinburgh with cardiology as my special subject and was the first cardiologist in Hamilton with any documents to back up my qualifications. The following year I became a charter member of the Royal College of Canada and following retirement of Dr. Howard Holbrook from the Board of Directors of that organization, I served on the Board for eight years.

I am now 75 years of age and for the last few years have given up attending medical conferences except that in 1966 I attended the International Conference in Cardiology in New Delhi and made it an excuse for a trip around the world and this spring I attended the Inter-American Conference in Lima, making it an excuse to see South America.

I have your letter before me and I just noticed now that you asked me if I had any documentation which would show the recording of the first electrocardiogram I took in 1927. Unfortunately, all of these documents were taken by the Trust Company when Dr. McGregor expired and I am not able to trace any of them.

The *Bulletin* contains three articles each by Dr. McGhie. Their titles are "Historical Notes on Medical Personalities in the Hamilton Area," "The Development of Medical Education in Canada," and "The Development of Group Practice." These articles will prove helpful in telling the story of medicine in Canada.

Through an obituary notice which appeared in the *Bulletin of the American College of Physicians* (July 1972), I became aware of the fact that Dr. McGhie died on 9 April 1972.

I recall a pleasant two hours I spent with Dr. McGhie in Hamilton, in March 1972. Among the places we visited was a room in the McGregor Clinic in which Dr. McGhie assembled documents and instruments related to the history of medicine. The exhibits included the first electrocardiograph, the "portable" model made by the Cambridge Instrument Company of New York in 1926 and bought by Dr. McGhie in 1927.

Dr. McGhie wrote in 1965:

> I have not published a lot of articles in national journals, and I have no record of the journals or dates of publication. I have published frequently in the *McGregor Clinic Bulletin.* The following is a list of articles which my secretary has been able to dig out.

The list of twelve items includes Pernicious Anaemia, Hypertension in Hyperthyroidism, Cardiac failure and its treatment, and Thromboangeitis Obliterans.

Dr. George Frederick Strong (1897-1957)

The committee that met in Winnipeg on 24 June 1947 to complete preparations for the meeting, later the same day, at which the Canadian Heart Association would be born, consisted of the following: John McEachern, who acted as chairman, David Baltzan, Francis Mathewson, George Strong, and Harold Segall. For these latter two, this was the first acquaintance in person.

I remember receiving a very nice letter from Strong in 1938 or 1939 congratulating me on having founded the Louis Gross Memorial Lecture. It now seems most likely that he met Louis Gross at the annual Canadian Medical Association meeting in Ottawa in 1937. Louis Gross mounted an exhibit on the anatomy and physiology of the coronary circulation at that meeting and won the first prize with it. Much later, in the spring of 1982, I realized that an article I coauthored with Paul White in 1923 referred to two publications that George Strong had written with a colleague during his stay in Boston, 1922-23. With Dr. Samuel A. Levine, he reported a case of ventricular paroxymal tachycardia characterized by a clinically detectable degree of arrhythmia (*Heart* 10: 125, 1923). With Dr. Albert Wilmaers, he had written about the potency of various preparations of digitalis and strophanthin that were being prescribed in Boston and vicinity in 1922 (*J.A.M.A.* 80: 1038, 1923). I did not remember these items in 1938 nor in 1947. They did become significant as I gathered the contents of George Strong's minibiography following his premature death in 1957. In retrospect, if there had been a local society of cardiologists in Boston such as a cardiac club, I would have met Strong in 1923 and would have enlisted his cooperation when I was trying to form a Canadian Heart Association in 1926. George Strong was very vigorous in his work on projects of this kind and it may be that with his support, this association might have been formed in 1926 instead of in 1947.

"Fritz" Strong was born in St. Paul, Minnesota, and had all his education there. He obtained the degree of Bachelor of Science in 1915 and M.D. in 1921 at the University of Minnesota. The "internship" he served at the University Hospital in 1921 probably occurred during his final year. He then served an internship at the Vancouver General Hospital in 1921-22. He obtained a National Research Council Fellowship and went to work at the Peter Bent Brigham Hospital in Boston in 1922. There he was associated largely with Dr. Samuel A. Levine. He was appointed to the staff of Vancouver General Hospital in 1926 and became director of the Heart Station in 1930. He rose to become Chief of Medicine at the hospital (1946-51) and Professor of Medicine at the University of British Columbia from 1951 until his death in 1957. He served as chairman of the Medical Board of the Vancouver General Hospital from 1954 to 1956. His keen and active interest in each organization to which he belonged was recognized and appreciated by his colleagues. He served as President of many organizations. The following is a partial list: Vancouver Medical Association (1929-30); The British Columbia Medical Association (1937-39); Canadian Medical Association (1954-55); American College of Physicians (1954-55); North Pacific Society of Internal Medicine, charter member and President; Canadian Heart Association, charter member and President (1955-56); National Heart Foundation of Canada, Founding President (1956-57); Family Welfare Bureau of Greater Vancouver, charter member and first President; B.C. Cancer Foundation, Founding President; B.C. Division of Canadian Cancer Society, Director; Western Society for Rehabilitation, Director and Vice-President; B.C. Medical Research Institute, Chairman of the Medical Board. After reading this list it seems remarkable that he was simply a member of the following: Pacific Inter-urban Clinical Club, B.C. Society of Internal Medicine, American Heart Association, International Heart Association, and the British Cardiac Society. Another measure of his significance to society in general and to medicine in particular are the following honours which were conferred upon him: D.Sc. (Hon.), University of British Columbia, 1954; LL.D., University of Toronto, 1955; Alumnus of the Year, University of Minnesota, 1955; Fellow Royal College of Physicians, London, 1955; Fellow Royal College of Physicians, Canada, 1948; Fellow of the American College of Physicians, 1937; D.Sc. (Hon.) Laval University, Quebec, 1966; Hon. F.R.A.C.P. (1956).

"Fritz" Strong played a leading role in the creation of the Canadian Heart Foundation. This facet of his career evolved against the background of growth in the functions of the New York Heart Association which stimulated similar growth of the American Heart Association (see chapter on Societies and Foundations.)

Dr. George Raymond Brow (1894-1985)

In the spring of 1926, Ray Brow, a graduate of the class of 1920, returned to Montreal after special training for a career in cardiology. He joined the University Clinic at the Royal Victoria Hospital on a part-time basis and opened his office for private practice in a suite of rooms in the Sherbrooke Apartments occupied by colleagues of the same hospital. His postgraduate education had started with one year's internship in urology, followed by a year in medicine at the Royal Victoria Hospital. He then enjoyed the great advantage of two years of research at the Rockefeller Institute, chiefly with Carl Binger on the human physiology of respiration. His final preparation consisted of almost two years with Sir Thomas Lewis at University College, London. At the Royal Victoria Hospital, he worked in the cardiorenal clinic and engaged in research for about three years in collaboration with C. N. H. Long, a biochemist, and John Beattie, the professor of anatomy at McGill University. In the course of his career, he developed a large private and also a consultant practice as a distinguished internist with a special interest in cardiology. He rose to the position of Chief of Medicine at the Royal Victoria Hospital and Professor of Medicine at McGill. He became Emeritus Professor in 1957 and retired from practice some years later when he was in his seventies. Perhaps it was Meakins' influence that led him to mould his career broadly as an internist rather than in the narrower field of cardiology. He played an active role in the Royal College of Physicians (Canada); he was present at the organizing meeting of the Montreal Cardiac Society on 25 September 1946, and was elected a member of the first council of the Canadian Heart Association in 1947. In 1929, he published an article on the observation of partial heart block in patients with typhoid fever and, in 1930, in collaboration with Long and Beattie, an important study of the relation between extrasystoles and the sympathetic nervous system.

*The biographical data about Dr. Brow are inadequate; he chose not to respond to the archivist's requests for information gathered by the questionnaire.

Dr. Albert de Guise (1894-1958)

The Class of Medicine of 1920 at the Université de Montréal had a student, Albert de Guise, who, after graduation would spend several years in Paris preparing for a career in cardiology. By happy coincidence, Albert de Guise and I first met in August 1919 when we happened to be paying guests in a farmer's home in the Laurentian Mountains. We were having a week or so of summer holiday before entering the final year of medical school in our respective universities. We soon discovered our common interests. One evening a little girl came to this farm house to request "the doctor" to go to attend her very sick grandmother. By the grapevine , the presence of de Guise had become known in the community. He invited me to join him. We found a somewhat obese, whitehaired, elderly woman sitting in a big chair in the kitchen. She presented obvious signs of marked generalized oedema. The skin over her shins was shiny and, where split, was weeping fluid. "Dr." de Guise prescribed tincture of digitalis and performed cupping on her chest and arms. I had heard about this latter form of therapy from my mother who grew up in a village in Romania. There the same person who performed as a barber also practised as a paramedic, known as a "felcher," and he carried out this procedure for a wide variety of both acute and chronic illnesses.

When I returned from studies abroad, I was delighted to learn that de Guise was already in practice as a cardiologist. Thus when I sought to initiate the organization of a Canadian Heart Association in 1926, I proposed the project to de Guise together with Birchard and Brow. What happened at this luncheon and afterward appears in the chapter which deals with the organization of the Montreal Cardiac Society in 1946.

As Dr. de Guise died on 22 November 1958, his minibiography had to be assembled from available sources. Thus, in 1965, Dr. Paul Bourgeois, then Deputy Administrator of the Notre Dame Hospital helped greatly. He searched the Archives of the institution and composed the following profile:

> In 1923, a cardiology laboratory under the direction of Dr. Albert de Guise was created and a year later the hospital received the gift of an electrocardiograph, an X-ray apparatus for fluoroscopy, and a basal metabolism apparatus. In 1931 or 1932, Dr. Gaetan Barry joined the staff and his activities led to the creation of a special heart clinic in the outpatient department in 1934, under the joint direction of Drs. de Guise and Barry.

Judging by the official positions to which Dr. de Guise was appointed, he functioned rather as an internist with special skills in electrocardiography and cardiovascular fluoroscopy. Thus in 1938 he became director of the General Medical Clinic in the Dispensary, and in 1939, the Associated Chief of the Department of Medicine. His university appointment in 1940 was "in charge of the course on Medical Pathology" and in 1942, Professor of Medical Pathology.

The obituary by Dr. Roger R. Dufresne (*Un. Méd. Can.*, 1959: 88, 367) provides a good profile of Dr. Albert de Guise (translation by Miss Marie Atkinson):

In Memoriam
Albert de Guise (1894-1958)

One of the dominant characteristics of the personality of Dr. Albert de Guise was that of 'discretion' [prudence, cautiousness]. Even his contemporary colleagues at the hospital and on the faculty scarcely knew the man, hidden behind the face of the doctor and professor.

I knew Doctor de Guise well in 1936 when I was a senior intern in medicine in the service of Professor Lesage. The team of Anselme Leger, Albert de Guise and Georges Hebert was responsible for half of this service. We worked on it three mornings a week starting at 8 a.m. After reading and considering the reports recorded by the junior intern we proceeded with objective discussion for treatment. For the examination of the heart Dr. de Guise always took precedence. There followed very precise auscultation often followed by a long discussion on the nature and timing of the murmurs and of the type of gallop. At the end of the morning Dr. de Guise put the bell of his stethoscope under running water. He continued this custom to the end of his years in practice, which had begun in 1923 when he returned from Paris and brought a Boullite Electrocardiograph for his office. He became Bachelor of Arts in 1915 and M.D. in 1920. He went to France immediately after graduation. It was the custom to do this at that time, since postgraduate studies were nonexistent here in the province of Quebec. For three years he worked in the field of internal medicine, specializing in cardiology with Vaquez and Laubry, the masters of that period. Dr. de Guise was the first French Canadian cardiologist and it was he who introduced specialization in pathological medicine at the Notre Dame Hospital.

In 1933 he became chief of the new department of cardiology

at the hospital. In 1939 he became assistant to the chief in the department of medicine, which position he occupied until his death. In 1929 he wrote a thesis on angina. He taught both pathology and clinical medicine from the time he returned from Europe. In 1942 he became professor of pathology. During this active decade he played an important role on the faculty, being secretary from 1944 to 1946.

At the University, as at the hospital, Dr. de Guise devoted twenty-five years of active participation and productivity. In the department of cardiology he contributed his experience, courtesy and 'discretion.' His younger colleagues always had in him a sympathetic and cautious advisor. The many positions which he held contributed to the scientific development at the institution. Each one contributes to the collective effort which could not progress without cooperation and ambition.

Dr. David Baltzan (1897-1983)

In 1971 the questionnaire was sent for the last time. Those who had not yet responded to two earlier requests in 1965 and 1968 were urged to do so. Those who had complied were asked to update their minibiographies. David Baltzan belonged in the latter group. He not only supplied new items for his curriculum vitae but, in answer to the special questions, he wrote a comprehensive essay in which he described the evolution of the practice of internal medicine and cardiology in Saskatoon during the 52 years since his graduation in 1920. Not only the facts belong here in the story of cardiology in Saskatchewan but also the special flavour imparted to the story by Baltzan, the pioneer in Western Canada. The essay is therefore presented in its entirety without editorial modification.

HISTORY OF CARDIOLOGY IN SASKATCHEWAN

Recording the emergence of cardiology as a specialty in this province is by one on the scene actively engaged in the practice of medicine for half a century. It is not a biography of individual participants or contributors except of the narrator's linkage in the chain of events.

The specialty did not exist in Western Canada 50 years ago. Those who concentrated on diagnosis and treatment of heart disease acquired the name "heart specialists." The subject matter was officially recognized as a subspecialty only, half way more or less between then and now. Organized postgraduate training was not a standard procedure. In the subspecialties there were few organized systematic courses offered in the Western world. One would obtain a post in the service of physicians of great repute who pioneered in special fields such as diseases of the heart, lungs, and other systems. In this period of the history of cardiology famous teachers, clinical investigators and/or innovators were the main attractions, not institutions.

In this province a trickling of physicians appeared on the scene who had U.K. fellowships in surgery, none in medicine at the start. Others later went overseas to acquire such fellowships in surgery. This specialty was then legitimately the big attraction. The aura carried over into the public arena. The greeting a physician received on returning after a period of study abroad or in the larger centres in the U.S.A. was "now you will be doing all your own surgery." When the answer was to the contrary, the retort invariably was "why did you go away?"

This narrator was no stranger in these parts or an exception to the rule. My parents were naturalized British subjects, homesteaders in the N.W.T. in that portion of Western Canada which was later incorporated as the province of Saskatchewan. All my preliminary schooling was obtained in this province, graduating in medicine from McGill, class of 1920. It was only natural to gravitate homeward to begin practice in the nearest little city, Saskatoon.

After five years as an assistant and later in private general practice, my senior colleagues in this small city observed an aptitude in medical diagnoses before my awareness, which destined my future course. In the quest embarked upon to acquire experiences, only that portion relevant to cardiology will be mentioned, adding that this was not my primary objective because that specialty was far from reaching the point of self-identity. The American College of Physicians was in its embryo state, and the Royal College of Physicians of Canada was incorporated in 1929, with four Saskatchewan physicians among its sponsors.

This peripatetic excursion started in the mid-twenties with no fixed plans except to see and learn about medicine, that ill-defined field which ultimately was labelled Internal Medicine in the Western hemisphere. Throughout this search, disparate experiences continually crowded in and side-tracked me, not to the exclusion of my primary pursuit.

This remote part of Canada strangely provided me the exception opportunity in the early years for practical experience, with daily access to the use of the most modern X-ray equipment obtainable anywhere in Canada. This exposure was without benefit of tutelage in the art because there was no fully trained roentgenologist at the time. Fluoroscopy was widely used because this presented an animated view of many anatomical structures. It saved the cost of film and processing. At present, it is a throwback to recall that the expense of a film or films were worth the effort only if positive pathology was found; otherwise it was a wasteful expenditure and a humiliating ego-buster experience for the examiner who felt his five senses, the standard bearers of clinical excellence, failed him. It is amusing, mentioning that later in my postgraduate perambulations a whole class of postgraduate students were called in to witness a newly installed metal frame X-ray apparatus in a top rate hospital medical school abroad. The room was dark, there was a patient behind a fluoroscopic screen. The question asked was what looked wrong on the screen. This innocent abroad shouted from the back of the room asking which way the patient faced. The patient was turned around and behold what was wrong was right — a dextrocardia! Therefore not as an alien in this field it was no wonder to find myself attracted to the work of Hugo Roesler in Vienna, who crystallized for me the phenomena of cardiac fluoroscopy and orthodiagraphy. This visual aid did more to remove the errors in diagnosing gross structural cardiopathies, in turn helping to explain some intrinsic derangements. It was a tremendous gain.

Simultaneously a more indirect impact was reading R. McNair Wilson's biography of *The Beloved Physician, Sir James Mackenzie*, published in 1926. This period seems to have initiated and/or accelerated instrument explorations in the recognition of heart disease, so it appears as the dates show below. Objective evidence was increasingly replacing conjectural explanations.

The third in order of attractions in the interest of cardiology was the emerging practical use of electrocardiography. At this time it is wonderful to recall that these attractions had occurred within the lifetime of the immortal contributors to medical science, Roentgen (1845-19<u>23</u>), Einthoven (1860-19<u>27</u>), Mackenzie (1853-19<u>25</u>). The underlined figures are years pertinent to this story. The first E.C.G. I owned was a Victor string galvanometer model serial 574-200 — which I brought to Saskatoon in late 1928 or early 1929. This was a sturdy, bulky, portable apparatus which remained in use for some time after the V4 lead only was introduced.

My first encounter abroad with the electrocardiograph was disheartening, not because of the apparatus. It occurred the first morning of bedside "cardiac" ward rounds when the instructor asked me to feel the pulse of the patient. It was too fast to count or be sure of any irregularity. This aroused my curiosity and like a freshman I asked if an electrocardiogram had been taken and if it had been examined. The answer was "yes" for the first part and "no" for the second part. Later, wandering into the developing room the wet film was shown to me, and assuredly it had been examined before demonstrating the patient. The graphic illustration of a very fast irregular heart beat which eluded detection by this novice was an exciting moment. The teacher's denial of help from another source was shockingly immoral. Time tempered the tempest, the lesson was worthwhile.

This interim concentration on cardiology paved the course of cardiology for Saskatchewan. None of these bits of trends started during my absence. Before returning home I sidetracked for a family reunion in Edmonton. During this short visit I stopped in the University of Alberta College of Medicine where I had been a pre-med student. Unexpectedly, an offer was made by Professor Pope, head of the department of Medicine, to join his department. It was a most attractive offer. Near the end of these arrangements a telegram came from colleagues in Saskatoon which read, "Hear you are back, letter en route, make no decisions, see us first." In discussions in both cities it is important to record there was no talk at all about cardiology! This shows the low estate of cardiology at this juncture. The status of what was to be known as Internal Medicine is illustrated on recall by the greeting of our family physician whose remark is indelible: "What is this nonsense I hear about your plan not to do any surgery and how can you expect a livelihood without an occasional appendectomy, hemorrhoidectomy, etc. etc.?" In retrospect, it is most gratifying to have shared in the transition and transformation, promoting the diagnosis and treatment of heart disease in my province.

The practice of internal medicine was my arena and cardiology a fascination. The biggest surprise to me was the frequency of having to undiagnose what was termed a big heart, a weak heart, a heart murmur and to alter emphatic prognoses which were the physician's biggest gamble of the age! A compelling, voluntary undertaking to review digitalis preparations prescribed and dispensed in the cat and frog unit era, led me to the first (1933) publication in the realm of cardiology and a total production of ten papers in a decade in the cardiovascular field.

In the first demonstration of my electrocardiograph, transported for presentation to the medical staff of the Saskatoon City Hospital, I emphasized what this apparatus cannot be expected to do. The repercussions were in the reverse order. Patients were sent for an electrocardiographic diagnosis of heart disease. My part was to interpret the electrocardiogram and that was relayed by the referring physician to his patient as my diagnosis of the heart ailment. With due appreciation for this patronage I had to disassociate myself from this ventriloquism. As a consequence patients were directed to a separate room where the technician produced the E.C.G. out of my sight and the report was telephoned and/or mailed to the attending physician. There was no malice on either side, it was an inoffensive way to come to terms about an important distinction.

A contemporary highly rated colleague in another large centre in the province telephoned me about coming for a few days to learn electrocardiographic interpretations. I explained he would be welcomed but cautioned him I did not yet feel qualified to act as instructor.

The first to follow in my footsteps was Dr. Harold Sugarman, who joined me in 1933 as an apprentice in the old-fashioned, traditional manner following a year's internship in the Saskatoon City Hospital. He received his total experience with me except for World War II services overseas in the R.C.A.M.C. He returned to resume his association with me which is now in its 39th year. My lamented colleague and friend, Dr. Lloyd Anderson, pursued an interest in cardiology a bit later. His brother, Dr. Jack Anderson, will best remember whether Lloyd preceded Dr. Sugarman's participation in the field, not that this matters — only that the wrong impression is not to be conveyed, and to establish when the second E.C.G. came to Saskatoon, brought by the late Lloyd Anderson — the second in Saskatchewan. Other participants and their activities and their contributions will no doubt come from members on the roster of the Canadian Cardiovascular Society. A distinguished confrère was Dr. Max Israels of Regina who speaks of himself as a "pioneer in cardiology beginning in 1938 and grew up with the specialty." To which I add, "in the venerable prairie style."

Referring to Dr. John Fiddes, professor of physiology in the University of Saskatchewan because of his former association with MacWilliams of Aberdeen, it is speculated, "he would have acquired this apparatus (E.C.G.) when he began to teach in Saskatchewan in 1930 — or perhaps his predecessor, Professor Scott, would have acquired the apparatus . . ." Both references are erroneous. My friend Fiddes wanted me, if not more my E.C.G., to help him in some of his experimental work on animals. That project was overruled by two penny-pinching overlords (both of whom I knew well) on grounds that the two-year premedical college could not undertake this expansionist posture.

To my knowledge no other medical publications originated in this province or appeared in the literature for many years. Professor Rudolph Altschul, who came to the University of Saskatchewan in 1945, published 71 papers and one classic book on arteriosclerosis. The work of Professor Louis Jacques, an authority on heparin, is included in this era. They were respectively professor of anatomy and professor of physiology in the two-year premedical course in the Faculty of Medicine in the University of Saskatchewan.

A new horizon appeared on the completion of the University Hospital in 1955 and completion of the full course leading to the M.D. degree in 1957. Preceding this joint leap forward, clinical research on an individual, privately financed basis is on record. During this time, Saskatchewan made its mark in research and experimentation on the provision of health services. The pioneer work of Dr. George Ferguson under the auspices of the Saskatchewan Anti-Tuberculosis League was widely acclaimed. Other enduring innovations like the universal hospitalization scheme, the basic medical science courses, and bedside hospital teaching, belonged to that period, and further back, *circa* 1926, when our first hospital internship commenced. Also to the credit of those living or who survived there are published reports on brucellosis in Saskatchewan, the second in Canada, bronchomoniliasis, the first in Canada, human equine encephalitis by Dr. John Fulton at the University of Saskatchewan, who was Professor and Director of the Animal Diseases Laboratory and also a Professor in the College of Agriculture.

The development of a cardiological unit in the University Hospital took on the leading role. One noteworthy aspect was the town-and-gown alliance of full-time and part-time teaching personnel and agreement to avoid duplications of specific projects and costly expenditures.

The foregoing information concerns this province not isolated from the course of events in this country. The third meeting of the Canadian Heart Association preceding the new title, the Canadian Cardiovascular Society, was held in Saskatoon in 1949. A founding member of council in the formation of the Canadian Heart Association was this Saskatchewan representative, who was for a long time vice-president and continues as a director of the Saskatchewan Heart Foundation.

To complete the questionnaire circulated collecting data for this history would take up more space than one wishes to occupy. Memory is long and time is short.

Continuing along this crimson circulatory path, mention of the role or influence of attending national and international Heart Association meetings is a must. One can only tell what these have meant in his own life. It was for me a necessity in these formative years. The first and nearest were the American Heart Association meetings. For me, attending was imperative. The Inter-American Heart Congress, the World Heart Congress and other National Heart Association meetings were added spices. (Amongst many more I choose to mention attending a South African Heart Association meeting [1968]; the attraction was to observe the background of experiences which led to the first heart transplant. This epochal event was definitely not a freak accident.) Each meeting has a flavour all its own, in the setting but also in essence. Presenting a paper at the First World Heart Congress in Paris in 1950 and no less our own Canadian Heart Association meeting in 1949 seem more spectacular later on, when the occasions prove to have become milestones. These excursions are in the end valuable investments in terms of stimulating multidimensional education of a type long before what is currently in vogue. The Canadian Medical Association tried hard for a long time to make that point with our government. The final frugal travel tax exemptions came far past half-way after my many excursions. This lack of needed support must not be a barrier in the future to meet these educational advancements.

In this province there are no accredited cardiologists as formalized by the more recent innovation of certification by examination under the aegis of the Royal College of Physicians. The exceptions are cardiothoracic surgeons. In all of Canada there is only a sprinkling of the new breed. Many co-workers in Canada have been invited and have accepted chartered memberships as Fellows of the American College of Cardiology as was this person — who regretfully was at the time too involved, delaying acceptance of this distinction in the allotted time. Fulfilling the requirements for acceptance as a Fellow of the American College of Cardiology is a more liberal recognition than our restrictive examinations might allow. Contemporary frustrations are proof that overly severe restrictions in human affairs operate in the reverse order.

In retrospect, the past 50-year period was not a primitive type of practice in cardiology. The practice proceeded on a staircase course. As knowledge was gained and facilities increased, new conditions were met. On recall, in my experience, the first big bother mentioned at the start was concern with the quality of digitalis preparations and the guesstimated prescriptions. It is still a bother. In earlier times the results usually were short of the potential benefits because of the uncertain standardization of available products. Oddly, with the correction of these shortcomings, insidious intoxications were rarely recognized soon enough, even in modern times. We may only now be on the threshold of properly managing the foxglove before it victimizes patients when blood plasma quantitative analysis proves its worth. This alone may not fill the bill. Digitalis preparations alone did not meet all expectations. In due time the xanthines helped remove barriers, the potent saluretics made the big leap forward, and electrolyte policing was a big boon. Ouabain had a short run as a cardiotonic and may be coming back.

The point of these several reminders is that astute clinical recognitions fostered development of many reliable technological aids which rationalized suppositions, exemplifying "the thought is father of the deed." Who can forget the incongruous anasarcas, the salt-depletion syndrome and other ambiguities, relics of the past conceived at the bedside and later confirmed by laboratory methods. In this respect the combined art and science of modern practice extended lives and increased the comforts of countless cardiopaths. Progress may seem to have been slow but it was sure and the foundations were sound.

Twentieth-century cardiology entered Saskatchewan, as in other parts of North America, riding on electrocardiography. The physician who practised internal medicine became a heart specialist to the patient with a cardiovascular problem, as he was a lung specialist to the patient with pulmonary disease and a stomach specialist for the person with peptic ulcer. He became a cardiologist when he devoted himself entirely or almost entirely to the cardiovascular system in his practice, teaching and research. The generation which followed that of Dr. David Baltzan when cardiac catheterization and open heart surgery came into being included such physicians.

Dr. Baltzan's bibliography reflects his keen interest in many aspects of the human condition. With regard to cardiology, in 1933, he published the interesting observation related to smoking, that during the acute illness of myocardial infarction the appetite for smoking disappears for some days and even weeks, only to recur when convalescence begins. In 1950 he published an article on a peculiar type of familial methaemaglobinaemia that caused cyanosis. He has written about medical education and about the administration of medical services to the community. He was co-founder of the first prepaid medical services organization in Saskatoon.

Dr. Max Israels (1906-)

Although Max Israels graduated M.D. from the University of Manitoba nine years after David Baltzan, they should be considered contemporary pioneers. He began as a general practitioner presumably performing some surgery. His natural inclination toward internal medicine led him to attend postgraduate courses including some in cardiology, notably with George Fahr of Minnesota and Frank N. Wilson of Ann Arbor, Michigan, both great pioneers of electrocardiography. He also attended such courses at Harvard Medical School. As the city of Regina grew in size and physicians and their patients became aware of progress in cardiology, the demand for his services grew and he could omit surgery and obstetrics and concentrate his postgraduate, ongoing education and his practice on subjects related to internal medicine. His progress brought him one step further than his colleague, David Baltzan, for Max Israels performed the first catheterization in Regina in 1952.

Following is his letter in response to the four special questions in June 1965:

> As a pioneer in cardiology in Saskatchewan, I may say that I began in 1938 and grew up with the specialty as it became one of the most important disciplines in Internal Medicine. The advances of the past twenty-seven years have made it one of the most rewarding fields in medicine, both from the standpoint of

diagnosis and therapy. I was influenced by attending the clinics of George Fahr of the University of Minnesota (who worked with Einthoven) and Frank Wilson of Ann Arbor, Michigan. Most of my P.G. work was done intermittently during active practice here and attending meetings of the American Heart Association. The chief obstacle was the demands on my time away from practice and working in a small city (at that time population 65,000). With increasing population, and referrals from rural Saskatchewan and from North Dakota and Montana, I had a wealth of material in this field. I chose this city because I have lived here for many years and an opening presented itself. At that time specialization in restricted fields was in its infancy and certification in the specialties only beginning. I purchased my first EKG machine in 1938. Later I was the first to use the cathode-ray oscillograph (condemned at that time by reputed cardiologists), a copy of the original made by Siemens of Germany. I did the first cardiac catherization in this city (possibly in the province) in 1952. Dr. David Stein, now a cardiologist in Winnipeg, was my resident at the Regina General Hospital. He later worked with Hans Hecht at Salt Lake City. I 'lugged' my portable EKG machine to numerous towns in southern Saskatchewan and even to Montana. At that time no EKG machines were in either hospital in this city. Despite the work of Herrick of Chicago as early as 1912, coronary thrombosis was still an uncommon diagnosis even in the 30s.

Dr. Earle Parkhill Scarlett (1896-1982)

Before he settled in Calgary in 1930, Dr. Scarlett devoted six years to postgraduate education. He went to several medical centres in the eastern United States, he served a longish time in Detroit at the Henry Ford Hospital (1924-26) and he crossed the Atlantic to London and Edinburgh. In 1930, he was Associate Professor of Medicine at the University of Iowa.

During these years, he worked with the Cambridge electrocardiograph and similar types of apparatus. He purchased an electrocardiograph in 1930, the first to be installed in Calgary. This represents the introduction of twentieth-century cardiology into the Calgary region of Alberta. In 1938, he engaged in postgraduate studies in London at the National Heart Hospital and the Hospital for Nervous Diseases; in Edinburgh he worked as a visiting resident. In 1965 Dr. Scarlett wrote:

It is impossible for me to write an *Apologia pro vita sua in Cardiologia* because, due to various circumstances, my interest in cardiology and in matters cardiovascular was fostered and continued within the framework of Internal Medicine. In particular, due to the size of the city of Calgary prior to the Age of Devonian* (and American) oil, it was possible to practise only as an internist with an interest in cardiology, thus producing that grotesque medical creature who was at once a specialist and a sub-specialist. In time I found that the public accepted me readily as 'a heart specialist,' but found it quite impossible to understand what 'an internist' was, which, I suspect, they regarded as something akin to that mythical creature, the unicorn. So to save embarrassment I went along under the title of 'heart specialist' which in strict reality I never really was. However, the cardiological were generous enough to accept my dubious passport. Now that Calgary has become Baghdad-on-the-Bow it is quite possible to be respectable and to feed one's family as a cardiologist, pure and simple.

But I should add that in both spheres — Internal Medicine and Cardiology — I never attained too much knowledge; but I did, I think, attain ignorance, which, possibly, in the result, may be much the same thing.

To return to the rubric which you have set down:

A. The decision to specialize in Cardiology. I should say that my interest in this field was stimulated by the example, the clinical skill and the friendship of three men. The first, Dr. F. Janney Smith of the Henry Ford Hospital, Detroit, whose quiet urbanity and incarnation of the spirit of the Johns Hopkins School, left a deep impression on a whole generation of students. The second, Dr. Fred M. Smith, Professor of Medicine, University of Iowa, who did much of the early experimental work on coronary heart disease, and who continued in that tradition when he moved into clinical circles. The third, Dr. James B. Herrick of Chicago, one of the medical elect in this century of medicine in America.

B. Initial planning and influences in adopting Cardiology. As I have intimated, Cardiology came as a sort of grace that was

*Age of Devonian, a geological name for a system of rocks lying below the carboniferous and above the Silverian formations. The erudite Dr. Scarlett thus alludes to Alberta's rich sources of oil.

added during my painful progress as an internist. Having in the twenties worked on experimental models of the electrocardiograph (some of them as large and as elaborate as a satellite of today), with much satisfaction I purchased my first machine in 1930, the first of its kind to be used in Calgary.

C. The role of the Canadian Cardiovascular Society. The Society played a distinct part, as it provided a rallying point for one's interest in matters of cardiovascular disease, and symbolized the growing maturity of Canadian medicine.

D. Extracurricular decorative activities. It is apparent from what has been said above that mine is a limited mind with an ingrained promiscuous habit, thus making it possible for me to present a respectable front to the world. I have always been busily engaged in doing many things not recognized in the dogmatic formularies of medical custom and practice.

To put it shortly, I am a polymath, and in consequence, looked on with a curious reserve if not suspicion by my medical brethren. To persist in this uncanonical bent in younger life, I found, entailed a certain loneliness, and later, a growing defiance and courage, both of which were happily fortified with age.

Since I no longer have to answer the demands of patients or of teaching, I conduct a regular column or section in three medical journals — *The Archives of Internal Medicine* where I appear under the title of 'Doctor Out of Zebulun;' *Group Practice*, the journal of the American Association of Medical Clinics, where I answer to the title 'The Medical Jackdaw;' and *The Alberta Medical Bulletin*, the journal of the Alberta Division of the C.M.A., where I am the conductor of a more sober causerie under the masthead of 'A Doctor's Notebook.' In this fashion I have set up a little booth in the medical market place filled with austere clinical shop-fronts where I am engaged in rescuing from the turmoil of our chaotic age some of those old truths which we are wise to remember, but which in the midst of countless distractions we are apt to forget.

Finally, may I add that, whether at a Cardiological Assize such as yours, or, in the last day, at the bar of times, the individual's best recommendation for mercy surely resides in the words: *Quia multum amavit.*

After receiving this illuminating and charming comment on Dr. Scarlett's contributions to cardiology in particular and to life in general I wrote to him requesting a copy of his bibliography. My object was to learn more about his contributions and about him as his talents and personality are reflected in his writings. When it arrived, the bibliography (in 1965) contained 276 items published between 1928 and 1964. A supplementary list which I received in November 1967 brought the growing bibliography to 375 items on a very wide variety of subjects. The first publication appeared as a brochure on the history of the College of Medicine of the State University of Iowa. It was prepared for the occasion of the opening of the New General Hospital and Medical Laboratories Building in November 1928. The second item is on "The Significance of High-Grade Anaemia in Chronic Nephritis," published in the *American Journal of Medical Sciences*, August 1929. The fifth is on "Jean Paul Marat: The Physician as Revolutionist" *(Annals of Medical History*, January 1930). The eighth is one of three medical articles he published in 1932 in the *Journal of the Canadian Medical Association*, its title, "The Significance of Infection in Cardiovascular Disease."

The eleventh item is "Realms of Gold: A Study of John Keats. An address to the University Women's Club of Calgary, January 22, 1935. Privately Circulated." The fourteenth marks the beginning of his project, the publication of the *Historical Bulletin (Calgary Associate Clinic)* — "The Odyssey of Medicine" in Volume 1, No.1, Page 2, May 1936. With this Dr. Scarlett began a long series of articles on a very wide range of subjects related to human behaviour and the search for understanding the world in which we live and die. The impact of this *Historical Bulletin* may be judged by reading some portions of what he wrote in the last number, February 1958, under the title "Vale."

> With this issue the Bulletin comes to an end after twenty-two years of continuous publication. No journal of its kind has attained such an age in this country. In some eighty-eight issues with the enthusiasm of the amateur and innocent of the more severe disciplines of history, we have dealt with all phases of medical history and have ranged widely into para-medical channels of past and contemporary thought and opinion.
>
> In the first number of the *Bulletin* (May, 1936) we set out certain ideas — our apologia for adding still another publication to the shelves of a profession which at times threatens to be drowned in its own secretions. Our aims were to secure some sort of perspective in the steadily increasing complexity of medicine, to assist in correcting the tendency for medicine to be rich in facts and poor in principle, to present medical history as a

rallying point for an intelligible knowledge of man as an individual. And we added, "Medicine, for all its scientific categories, is still primarily an art, and must retain and incorporate traditions of proven value and good report ... For this reason medical history and commentary, besides being a corrective to the exuberant science-mongering of our time, should express and illuminate the deepest realities of medicine" ...

... To some members of the medical tribes what has been written in these pages has been foolishness, and to others "a stumbling-block." To still others, it may even have caused an acute fibrillation of the ligament of Treitz. Nevertheless once again — and as a valedictory act — we stubbornly but with entire good nature assert these values, and hope that they may continue to be expressed through some medium in Canadian medicine. Such medical commentary and discussion are vital in providing a matrix and framework for the daily business of medicine, and in developing and deepening insights and judgements. Not that we are too fearful of the future. Medicine through the centuries has been able to provide its own saving graces and disciplines. And what we might call 'the humanities' in medicine will not disappear as long as there is one physician left who has not bowed the knee to Baal or who continues to hold the ramparts against the Philistines.

These few quotations reflect the superb humanist well endowed with that rare talent of writing about his thoughts and sentiments, lucidly, brightly, in an eminently readable style. His erudition is infectious. Reading any one of his articles requires looking up an unusual word, a story indirectly mentioned by introducing a biblical name or the name of a Greek hero which calls for learning about an ancient myth. A large dictionary, the *Encyclopedia Britannica,* the Bible including the Apocrypha, Crudden's *Complete Concordance of the Bible* and Garrison's *History of Medicine* are some of the reference books I have found useful in the pleasant and fruitful exercise of reading Dr. Scarlett's essays.

In 1972 I made the following addendum in Dr. Scarlett's minibiography:

Dr. Scarlett has made some good recoveries from some important illnesses related to the cardiovascular system. He continues to enjoy his hobbies which include horticulture as well as scholarly interests. In 1971 he had the pleasure of attending the opening of the E. P. Scarlett High School in Calgary and he has been visiting it to mingle with its students. During this year he was also made a charter member of the American Osler Society, another recognition of his scholarly contributions.

Dr. Atholl Munro McNabb (1898-1962)

Dr. McNabb joined the class of McGill 1920 together with me in October 1915 and we were assigned together with H. E. Gillanders and Charles Shapiro to a cadaver for anatomical dissection. We worked together during our freshman year. McNabb joined the army after his 18th birthday in 1916 and served in a machine gun battalion. He was decorated with the Military Cross and according to Dr. J. David Roger, his pupil and colleague, it was for exceptional bravery at the Battle of Passchendaele. In December 1986 Dr. Roger wrote me:

> I joined [McNabb] in April 1946, shortly after I returned from the war of 1939-1945. He had given up all his private practice of internal medicine on the first of January 1946, except a few special patients whom he carried on. One of these was Colonel, I think Lieutenant-Colonel Franklin, who was Gentleman-Usher of the Black Rod in the House of Commons. I knew that he had a warm feeling for him and one time Dr. McNabb told me that in the war of 1914-18 his commanding officer volunteered him for some extremely hazardous scouting which would almost certainly have been lethal and that Colonel Franklin talked the commanding officer out of it, saving McNabb's life.

In 1918, he resumed his medical studies at McGill University and graduated in 1922 at head of his class for which he received the Holmes Gold Medal.

He settled in Ottawa, practising as an internist, who was a skilful, well-informed radiologist, and equally skilled and informed in electrocardiography and clinical cardiology. He devoted himself to teaching these skills to interns and members of the staff of the Ottawa Civic Hospital. His junior partners, Dr. J. David Roger and Dr. John T. M. Fraser also received the major elements of their training from him. He instituted formal courses in electrocardiography and clinical cardiology for interns and residents at the Ottawa Civic Hospital as early as 1940. He was a very early pioneer of modern cardiology in Ottawa.

Dr. John M. McEachern (1896-1954)

Dr. John M. McEachern who served as President of the Society during the year 1950-1951, died on 20 March, 1954 in his 58th year. He was born in Elmvale, Ontario and educated at St. Andrew's College and the University of Toronto (M.D., 1923). During World War I he served in the Queen's Own Cameron Highlanders of Winnipeg, a regiment founded by his father and friends. In 1953 Dr. McEachern was appointed Honorary Lieutenant-Colonel of the regiment. Among the positions that he held were: Associate Professor of Medicine, University of Manitoba, Physician of the Winnipeg General Hospital, Director of its electrocardiograph laboratory, and a member of the Manitoba Clinic. He was a Fellow of the Royal College of Physicians of Canada and of the American College of Physicians. He served as the cardiologist of the Misericordia Hospital and of the Children's Hospital in Winnipeg. In June 1947 he was the host of the Steering Committee which was concerned with organizing the Canadian Heart Association. Thus he was among the founders and the charter members of the Association which later (1962) changed its name to the Canadian Cardiovascular Society.

Dr. Gaetan Barry (1899-1954)

Dr. Barry was more a true specialist in cardiology than his senior colleague, de Guise. After graduating from the Collège Ste Marie, he studied medicine at the University of Montreal and obtained his M.D. degree in 1926. He served his internship at the Notre Dame Hospital until 1928 when he went to Paris for postgraduate studies. There he worked chiefly with Professor Antonin Clerc for four years. On his return to Montreal he was appointed to the medical staff of the Notre Dame Hospital and restricted his activities to cardiology, both in his clinical work and as an instructor on the staff of the University of Montreal. Dr. Barry acquired knowledge and skills related to electronics which led him to create a laboratory in the basement of his home. He constructed an electrophonocardiograph and published articles on studies of cardiovascular sound. He was a "quiet," gentle type of person and an assiduous worker. His untimely death was due to complications associated with severe hypertension. He was greatly respected and appreciated by his peers and his students. In 1963, the newly equipped haemodynamics laboratory at the Notre Dame Hospital was named in his honour.

Dr. Harold N. Segall (1897-   )

Harold N. Segall graduated M.D. at McGill in 1920. In May of that year he was appointed Assistant Curator of the McGill Medical Museum; Dr. Maude E. Abbott was the Curator. The following year he worked as a Research Fellow in the McGill Department of Pathology. Professor Horst Oertel arranged for him to work at the Royal Victoria Hospital and to use the apparatus designed by Louis Gross. With this injection technique he studied the blood vessels and the bile channels within the liver. He demonstrated the very rich anastamoses between the right and left branches of the hepatic artery through a profuse network of large arterioles under Glisson's capsule. The following year he chose to do some clinical work. Dr. Charles F. Martin introduced him to the Chief of Medicine at the Massachusetts General Hospital, Dr. David Edsall, who appointed him the Henry P. Walcott Fellow of Harvard University to assist Dr. J. H. Means in the recently created Thyroid Clinic. During this year the treatment of thyrotoxicosis by subtotal thyroidectomy and by administering iodine were studied and reported. In the year 1923-34 he was granted a Dalton Scholarship and served as Resident in Dr. Paul Dudley White's Cardiac Clinic. He studied the efficiency of calcium chloride as a diuretic.

In the next two years he enjoyed the support of a Libman Scholarship and worked at University College, London in Professor Starling's laboratory, mainly with G. V. Anrep on regulation of coronary circulation. In the autumn of 1925 and early winter of 1926 he was in Vienna working principally at Professor Rudolph Kaufmann's Herzstazion and at the Wenckebach Clinic. In the winter and spring of 1926 he visited several hospitals in Paris to observe the work of the French cardiologists Prof. Henri Vaquez and Prof. Antonin Clerc.

In April 1926 he returned to North America to find a suitable place in which to settle. Eventually he chose Montreal and again Dr. Charles F. Martin arranged for him to meet with the Chief of Medicine at the Montreal General Hospital, Dr. Campbell P. Howard. An attempt to create a cardiac clinic in this hospital had not succeeded because the internists on the Medical Board objected to fragmenting their specialty. Segall undertook to prepare a memorandum which would change their minds. In this essay he traced the development of new techniques and directions of research from the middle of the nineteenth century to 1926. Dr. Howard presented the brief to the Medical Board and at the same meeting recommended the appointment of Segall as a Junior Assistant in his department.

Both the Clinic and the appointment were approved. Dr. Cecil C. Birchard was named Chief of the Cardiac Clinic with C. R. Bourne and H. N. Segall as assistants. The clinic had no budget, and as in other clinics, the physicians' services were without salary. To be a member of the hospital staff was a special privilege. Those above the level of junior could admit and treat their private patients. Segall was also appointed Assistant Demonstrator on the McGill teaching staff. In addition, he was accorded the privilege of working in the department of physiology to continue experimental investigation of the regulation of coronary circulation. In 1927 he opened a cardiac clinic in the Herzl Dispensary and the following year another such clinic in the newly built Women's General Hospital which was later named the Herbert L. Reddy Memorial Hospital.

A few years later the demands of clinical work left too little time for physiological experiments and he adopted the study of cardiovascular sound as the field of research. When the Jewish General Hospital was opened, he was appointed Chief of Cardiology and also one of four senior physicians in charge of the Department of Medicine. Two years later, he and Dr. David Mendel shared the work by alternating on duty every six months.

The development of private practice, the only source of income, was particularly slow because colleagues had to be taught what a cardiologist could contribute in the care of patients, and when this problem began to be solved, the Great Depression deprived professionals of clients and physicians suffered from a shortage of paying patients while people did not receive the medical services they needed. Through a fortunate circumstance, Segall was appointed consultant physician to the newly opened Medical Clinic of the Canadian National Railways in 1928. His duties included serving as physician to the president, Sir Henry Thornton. The annual salary of $2,400 provided for the basic expenses of maintaining an office and a car which was essential for house calls; the patients were treated mainly at home. A portable electrocardiograph acquired in 1927 (the first in Montreal and probably in Canada), proved to be a great advantage in educating both physicians and lay people about the usefulness of a cardiologist.

A physician's reputation becomes greatly enhanced when famous people or the very rich choose him. In 1940 the Baron Alphonse de Rothschild developed a myocardial infarct when he was in Montreal en route to the Laurentian Mountains for a holiday. His New York physician, Dr. David Scherf, gave him Segall's address to be used if a physician were needed. The Baron suffered severe complications, including pulmonary infarction and pneumonia. Eventually he recovered and returned to New York. This experience enhanced the growth of Segall's private practice.

In the course of preparing the memorandum in favour of having a cardiac clinic, Segall consulted some books which were written at about the time when James Mackenzie was studying cardiac rhythm and pioneering cardiology. In *Diseases of the Heart and Aorta* by Byrom Bramwell, he found symbols for heart sounds which he modified to develop a method of writing quantitative symbols for heart sounds and murmurs. At the end of about ten years of clinical work he embarked on a project to analyze the records he had amassed. He used an 80-column Hollerith punch card for the statistical analysis of more than 11,000 observations on over 6,000 patients, an early use of I.B.M. sorting machines to study clinical observations made mainly in the course of private practice. He discussed this work in the 1967 Annual Lecture of the Canadian Cardiovascular Society, "On Learning About Cardiovascular Sound" (Segall, 1968). Because Sir James Mackenzie taught that sounds and murmurs are chiefly of academic interest and only the subjective symptoms were significant signals of cardiac malfunction, Segall's careful auscultation with the new type of stethoscope, the Sprague Model, of combined bell and diaphragm, tended to identify him as a studious cardiologist who concerned himself with impractical matters.

As soon as the amplifier type of electrocardiograph became available in 1935, Segall bought one. Whereas the Cambridge portable he had since 1927 was housed in two large boxes, each weighing about 50 pounds, this new model weighed only 28 pounds. At the Jewish General Hospital, Segall taught interns and residents how to record electrocardiograms and also how to read them. He initiated a weekly seminar on electrocardiography at which hospital resident staff and practising physicians were welcome. Out of this grew the first postgraduate course in cardiology in 1938. The number of persons interested in attending two sessions per week from 8-10 a.m. gradually increased. In 1949, Segall and Albert Lapin, who resumed his training in 1946 on returning from war service, gave a special course of 80 hours (two hours twice a week) which included new developments in electrocardiography introduced by Frank Wilson. In 1950, they gave their first two-week course on all aspects of cardiology for physicians outside of Montreal. In the early thirties, clinical experiences with patients who dared to disobey the orders for absolute bed rest for six weeks in the treatment of acute myocardial infarction gradually convinced Segall that fear of cardiac rupture was excessive and not rational. His analysis of clinicopathological studies of cardiac rupture led him to the following conclusion expressed in his article on this subject (Segall, 1945):

> Cardiac rupture occurs relatively rarely. The determining factor is probably the plane in which tearing of infarcted necrotic muscle is initiated, a purely accidental element, and not related to ordinary exertion. Absolute rest does not prevent cardiac rupture. The general policy of treatment of coronary disease with myocardial infarction should not be determined by the fear of cardiac rupture, but rather by the probability that cardiac rupture will not occur.

During the 1930s he had begun to recommend early ambulation and ordinary bathroom privileges early in the illness. This made treatment of the patient at home less stressful to all concerned.

In the course of the years 1926 to 1960, when he retired, his status at the Montreal General Hospital rose to Associate Physician and at McGill to Assistant Professor.

In 1923 Segall attended meetings of the recently founded New England Heart Association and following year he witnessed Dr. Paul Dudley White's activities related to the formation of the American Heart Association. When he began to work in Montreal in 1926, he attempted to bring about the creation of similar societies in Montreal. This aspect of his career is dealt with in the chapter on Societies and Foundations.*

*Segall's 50-page miniautobiography is in the Archives of the Society; it describes in some detail opportunities for training in cardiology that could be found in Vienna, London, Paris, Munich and Boston in the early 1920s.

CHAPTER NINE

Electrocardiography in Canada Phase II, 1930-1970

The minibiographies that follow are presented in groups according to the provinces from east to west and in each group according to year of M.D. graduation.

Newfoundland

Dr. James Baggs Roberts, 27 November 1917, St. John's, Newfoundland; Queen's University, 39; University of Toronto, M.D. 42; F.R.C.P.(C) 52.

Following graduation and military service in World War II, Dr. Roberts began postgraduate studies with six months at the Beth Israel Hospital in Boston (1948), where he was exposed to Herman Blumgart and Louis Wolff, important pioneers of modern cardiology. He served internships and residencies at Sunnybrook Hospital (1951-52) and the Toronto General Hospital (1952-53). At the time he submitted the questionnaire in 1965, he was Senior Physician at the St. John's General Hospital, Consultant Physician to the St. Clare's Mercy Hospital, Chief of Medical Service at the D.V.A. Newfoundland District Hospital, and Chief Physician at the Grace Hospital.

In commenting on the four questions, he stated:

> I am not a cardiologist, rather an internist with a major interest in cardiology and rheumatology. I became interested in cardiology in particular because after the war there was no one in Newfoundland with any training or interest in cardiac disease.

Dr. Roberts is the pioneer of cardiology in Canada's newest province.

Dr. Ian Edwin Lawman Hollands Rusted, 12 July, 1921, Newfoundland; University of Toronto, B.A. 43; Dalhousie, M.D., C.M. 48; McGill, M.Sc., 49; Mayo Clinic, University of Minnesota, Graduate School 49-52; F.R.C.P.(C): F.R.C.P.S.(C).

Dr. Rusted began his postgraduate training with studies leading to the M.Sc. degree at McGill University. He then joined the three-year course in the Graduate School of the University of Minnesota, which was associated with the Mayo Clinic (1949-1952). Dr. Rusted wrote, in reply to the questionnaire:

The major research project for my M.Sc. thesis at McGill University was entitled "Cardiac Catheterization Studies of Induced Asthma-like Attacks in Man." Because these studies were carried out in 1948 and 1949, it was necessary for me to review the entire literature of cardiac catheterization up to that point. Following my two years at McGill University, my first experience at the Mayo was with the Cardiology Section. This contact with their cardiologists and cardiac pathologists (notably Dr. Jesse Edwards) led to several cardiac research projects, especially studies of the mitral valve—a timely topic in those early days of mitral valve surgery.

Upon my return to Newfoundland late in 1952, as medical consultant to the Newfoundland Department of Health, I found that, since I was the first formally trained internist to practise in the province, it was impossible to develop singlehandedly a Cardiac Catheterization Unit. Indeed, there were only two or three electrocardiographs in the entire province at that time. However, one of the major challenges was to cooperate with doctors throughout the province in beginning an index of patients with congenital and acquired heart diseases.

Membership in the Canadian Cardiovascular Society made it easier for me to consult with cardiologists from various parts of Canada with respect to mutual problems. I was able to convene the first meeting at which the Newfoundland branch of the Canadian Heart Foundation was formed.

Dr. Rusted's bibliography begins in 1950 with his M.Sc. thesis, followed by articles related to the same subject co-authored with Dr. J. A. Fownes and Dr. B. Rose in 1950 and 1951. Then follows a series of articles on the mitral valve with members of the Mayo Clinic staff. The last article on a medical, technical subject was entitled "Hemorrhagic and interstitial pneumonitis with nephritis" (with T. W. Parkin, H. B. Burchell and J. E. Edwards, *Am. J. Med.*, 1955, 18, 220-235).

The preparation for a medical career which Dr. Rusted initiated by his postgraduate training would justify the assumption that he became associated with a well-equipped university clinic and continued to work in developing knowledge and in teaching the new generations. However, he chose another course: to pioneer the creation and development of modern medical facilities in the new Canadian province, his native Newfoundland, where he introduced modern cardiology and internal medicine. This required a good deal of person-to-person teaching among his colleagues. His first publication following his return to Newfoundland was entitled "The Case for a Medical School in Newfoundland" (*NMA Newsletter,* Vol. VI, No. IV, November 1964).

It is clear that Rusted has played a major role in promoting the creation and the staffing of the Health Sciences Centre of Memorial University. In 1972 he was Dean of the Faculty of Medicine and almost totally immersed in promoting the growth of this new and very promising medical school.

Dr. Albert Reginald Cox, 18 April 1928, Victoria, B.C.; University of British Columbia, B.A. 50; M.D. 54; F.R.C.P.(C) 59; F.A.C.C. 67; F.A.C.P. 68; F.A.H.A. 67.

Dr. Cox began his postgraduate training with internships and residencies at the Vancouver General Hospital for four years (1955-59).

During this period, he integrated one year, 1956-57, as British Council Scholar on the London Postgraduate Medical Program Hammersmith and at the National Heart Hospital. These four years prepared him for working as a Fellow in Cardiology at the Washington University Hospital in Seattle (1959-1961).

In 1962, he began his career in Vancouver, and rose to the rank of Associate Professor of Medicine. In 1965, he spent some time with the teacher-training program at the University of Illinois. He made an excellent preparation for the major responsibilities he assumed in 1969 as Professor and Chairman of the Department of Medicine at Memorial University, St. John's.

Dr. Roland Clifton Kean Way, 10 April 1934, Flower's Cove, Newfoundland; Bishop's University, B.A. 53; McGill, M.D., C.M. 58; F.R.C.P.(C) 66; Cert. Ped. R.C.P.(C) 65; F.A.A.P.; F.A.C.C.

After graduation, Dr. Way had two years of internship and residency in internal medicine at the Montreal General Hospital (1958-1960), two years in paediatrics at the Montreal Children's Hospital and one year of paediatric cardiology in the same hospital. This was followed by two years as Fellow in Paediatric Cardiology at Oregon University Medical School (1965-1967).

In 1972, when Way submitted his curriculum vitae, he held the following posts: Assistant Professor of Medicine at Memorial University, physician in charge of internal medicine and paediatrics at the Grenfell Mission Hospital, Paediatric Consultant to the Charles A. Janeway Child Health Centre, and a member of the consultant staff of the General Hospital, the Grace General Hospital and the St. Clare's Mercy Hospital in St. John's.

Dr. Way wrote an informative summary of his career in education and training for a career in paediatric cardiology, which is here quoted in full:

> Following early childhood in a small fishing outport in Newfoundland, moved to St. Anthony, Newfoundland, under the supervision of the Grenfell Mission to continue high school education. Was orphaned at age of 11 through TB in mother and a brain tumour in father, both of whom died at age 29. Following completion of high school, was then sponsored for higher education by the Grenfell Mission. Was sent to Sherbrooke, Quebec, to do a year of high school for grounding in science subjects and then went on to Bishop's University graduating in 1953 with a B.A. degree. Then worked fifteen months in the paper mill at Windsor Mills, Quebec, to obtain sufficient funds to enter medical school. Graduated M.D., C.M. from McGill in 1958, and then proceeded to do postgraduate training in Montreal, Vancouver and Portland, Oregon. Returned to St. Anthony for one year (1964-65) to serve with the Grenfell Mission as physician in charge of the medical and paediatric services. Then went to Portland, Oregon to complete training in paediatric cardiology. In 1967, returned to St. John's, Newfoundland to join the staff of the newly opened Dr. Charles A. Janeway Child Health Centre in order to utilize specialty training in paediatric cardiology and assist with development of paediatric consultant facilities for the entire province. Served as Acting Chief of Paediatrics for eight months during the interim period before organization of the Faculty of Medicine at Memorial University and appointment as Professor of Paediatrics. Assisted with early organizational aspects of Faculty of Medicine, Department of Paediatrics, at Memorial University in April, 1969. At present working as Principal Administrative Assistant to the Professor of Paediatrics at Memorial University, retaining major responsibilities for Interns and Residents training in paediatrics, and supervision of the Faculty of Medicine 4th year (clerkship) program in paediatrics. Also continuing work as Principal Consultant in paediatric cardiology at the Janeway Child Health Centre and assisting with development of open-heart surgery in Newfoundland.
>
> Main extracurricular activities include The Newfoundland Medical Association, Newfoundland Division of the Canadian

Heart Foundation, and young people's work at a local church. Main hobby is classical music and building of high-fi stereo equipment.

Between 1958 and 1969, Way's bibliography grew to ten items. He wrote the first item when a student, entitled "The Role of Steroid Hormones in the Treatment of Collagen Diseases" (*McGill Med. J.*, 1958). The tenth item is an address he delivered in 1969 before the Canadian Tuberculosis and Respiratory Association on "Ventilation-Perfusion Relationships in Health and Disease."

Nova Scotia

Dr. Clyde W. Holland, 27 April 1896, Halifax – 22 April 1971, Halifax; Dalhousie, M.D. 1923; F.R.C.B.(C); F.A.C.P., LL.D.

A younger contemporary of Kenneth MacKenzie who enjoyed the privileges and opportunities of postgraduate training provided by a Rockefeller Scholarship, Dr. Holland was a charter member of the Canadian Cardiovascular Society. He did not respond to the request of the archivist, but a brief sketch of his career appeared in an obituary written by Dr. Lea Steeves.

Dr. Holland was born in Halifax on 27 April 1896. He entered Dalhousie University Arts Course in 1912, enlisted in the army and served overseas 1915-1919. He graduated M.D. in 1923 as Gold Medallist and in 1928 received a Rockefeller Fellowship for Internal Medicine and studied at the Peter Bent Brigham Hospital. On returning to Halifax, he became Assistant Professor of Medicine and entered private practice. In 1945 he became the first full-time Professor of Medicine at Dalhousie. His interest in cardiology was that of a specialist in internal medicine.

Dr. Lea Chapman Steeves, 4 November 1915, New Westminster, B.C.; Mount Allison University, B.A. 36, McGill, M.D., C.M. 40; F.R.C.P.(C), F.A.C.P., Mount Allison, LL.D. 69.

Early in his career, indeed as a third-year medical student, Dr. Lea C. Steeves was aware of a preference for cardiology in choosing his specialty. He discussed his ideas with Professor J. S. L. Brown, who expressed the opinion that during the next few decades principal progress would be made in the domain of heart-muscle metabolism. As luck would have it, his actual career moved along entirely different lines. Trained in internal medicine with emphasis on cardiology, his activities at Dalhousie University have been concerned with medical education both undergraduate and postgraduate, and particularly continuing medical education throughout the four Atlantic provinces. In this he has been a leader in North America, and his bibliography reflects these interests. Between 1940 and 1944, he wrote on technical matters related to diagnosis and therapy of cardiovascular conditions. Subsequently, his contributions to medical literature have been related principally to problems of medical education.

Dr. Srul Tul Laufer, 30 June 1903, Seletin, Roumania; University of Naples, Italy, M.D. 30; F.A.C.P. 48; F.A.C.C. 58; F.R.C.P.(C) 44.

The European political and social turbulence of the 1930s and 1940s spun off survivors who migrated in all directions throughout the world. Among the relatively few whom the shortsighted Government of Canada allowed to enter as immigrants was Dr. Srul Tul Laufer. He had escaped from the enemies of civilized humanity by taking refuge with his wife's family in Switzerland in 1939, and later in that year he came to Canada. In Toronto he sought advice from Sir Frederick Banting, who strongly favoured Halifax as a city in which Laufer should establish himself. In Montreal he visited me and I, independently, chose Halifax for him. A significant advantage was that the laws of Nova Scotia made it possible for him to obtain, with no delay, an enabling certificate which gave him the right to take the Dominion Council Examinations and thus obtain the necessary licence to practise medicine. In the province of Quebec he would have had to wait five years for Canadian citizenship before he could apply for a licence.

Dr. Laufer was then already a well-trained cardiologist who had published original work related to electrocardiography and clinical cardiology. Soon after his graduation in 1930 he went to Vienna where he obtained training in cardiology at the "Herzstation," one of the first special heart hospitals in the world. That institution had developed from the creation of a heart hospital for the Austrian army during World War I under the direction of Professor Rudolph Kaufmann. The group of lively, bright, young men who gathered around Kaufmann ultimately became noted contributors to the progressive evolution of modern cardiology. Of importance among these were Dr. Emil Kauf who wrote a classic monograph on the heart related to sports, Dr. Hugo Roesler who pioneered the new techniques of radiology related to the study of the cardiovascular system, and

Dr. H. Dressler, now well known for his delineation of the post-infarction syndrome.

Dr. Laufer chose to specialize in cardiology, devoting about equal time to laboratory research, clinical cardiology, and teaching. Thus when he came to Halifax he was the first modern-trained specialist in cardiology to settle there. Patients very soon appreciated his clinical skills; somewhat later, members of the medical profession began to welcome him in their midst. He participated in teaching undergraduate students and nurses, served a term as president of the Nova Scotia Heart Society, and participated in the postgraduate courses offered by Dalhousie University Medical School. He published the results of clinical studies related to electrocardiography, cardiovascular sound, and therapeutic trials with new drugs. His keen interest in and special knowledge of music led him to be associated with initiatives for the creation of the Halifax Symphony Society; he served as its president for several years. He was a founding member of the Nova Scotia Operatic Society, and in addition, served as a member of the Board of Directors of the Nova Scotia College of Art and also of the Nova Scotia Boy Scouts Association. Canada's restrictive policies with respect to refugees from Hitlerism reduced to a minimum the gains it could have enjoyed from receiving such immigrants as Dr. Laufer.

Prince Edward Island

In 1968, the Canadian Cardiovascular Society had only one member in Prince Edward Island, namely John Bell Downing who had been practising internal medicine in Summerside since 1951. Of the several physicians from whom the archivist sought information about the introduction of cardiology in Prince Edward Island, he is the only one who responded. In 1971 he wrote:

> I believe electrocardiography was begun in Prince Edward Island by Dr. Wendell Mackenzie of Charlottetown, now deceased. Dr. Henry Moyse first introduced electrocardiography in Summerside in 1939, following courses at the Cook County Hospital at Chicago. The first electrocardiograph machines produced records on clear film, then on photographic paper, and finally the direct writers came into use. Dr. Moyse is still active in practice.

Regrettably, no information could be elicited from Dr. Moyse. In a book entitled *The History of the Practice of Medicine in Prince*

Edward Island, 1700 to 1950, its author, Dr. R. G. Lea, mentions neither Dr. Wendell Mackenzie nor Dr. Moyse nor cardiology and electrocardiography.

Together with Dr. John Beattie, Professor of Anatomy at McGill University, I formed a team of "barnstorming" teachers who delivered lectures in several of the larger cities of the Maritime Provinces during the summer of 1930. We visited Charlottetown where the audience consisted of about 15 to 20 physicians. Beattie's subject was neurology, and mine, cardiology, especially clinical auscultation, cardiac arrhythmias, and coronary artery disease. The chairman of the meeting was Dr. W. J. P. MacMillan, a graduate of McGill who spoke of his having been in the audience when Dr. Osler delivered a lecture at the Royal Victoria Hospital during a visit to Montreal in April 1905. MacMillan was active in provincial politics; in 1931 he led the Conservative Party to victory and was Premier for four years. I remember that he complimented me on my resemblance to Osler; this amused me for I never had a moustache, and Osler's pictures from at least 1871 onward show him with a quite luxuriant moustache. In 1930, I had not met anyone in Charlottetown or Summerside who had a special interest in cardiovascular disease.

Dr. John Bell Downing, 19 July 1920, Summerside, P.E.I.; Dalhousie, M.D., C.M., 43, C.R.C.P.(C), F.A.C.P.

Dr. Downing served his internship and residency at the Montreal General Hospital from 1948 to 1951, and then settled in his native city to practise internal medicine. In 1968 he held the post of Chief of Medicine at the Prince County Hospital.

In commenting on the questionnaire, Downing pointed out that as he was the only internist in a region with quite a large population, he could not restrict himself to cardiology. He purchased his first electrocardiograph in 1951. He appreciated the training he had in cardiology as part of his education in internal medicine at the Montreal General Hospital.

New Brunswick

Dr. Hugh A. Farris, 1881-1953; F.R.C.P.(C), F.A.C.P.

Dr. Farris practised in Saint John as a specialist in heart and lung diseases. He was born at White's Cove, had primary education in Gagetown Grammar School, secondary schooling at Fredericton High and pre-medical education at Acadia University. He graduated

M.D., C.M., McGill, 1907. He was Director of the Saint John Tuberculosis Hospital from 1915 to 1930. No other information about him could be gathered.

Dr. Robert D. Roach, 1898, Tatamagouche, Nova Scotia - 8 July 1952, Moncton, N.B.; McGill, M.D., C.M., 25; F.R.C.P. London, F.A.C.P., F.R.C.P.(C).

Soon after graduation Dr. Roach did general practice in Hillsborough and Dorchester. He interrupted his work to do postgraduate studies in England. He practised in Moncton from 1932 to 1952 as an internist. His office was equipped with an X-ray apparatus and an electrocardiograph which he bought in 1932, most likely the first in Moncton. After his death, this apparatus was donated to the Physics Department of the University of New Brunswick.

Dr. Hector McKinnon, 20 June 1915, Upper Musquodoboit, N.S.; University of New Brunswick, B.A. 36; University of Toronto, M.D. 41; McGill, Tropical Medicine 44; F.R.C.P.(C) 53, F.A.C.P. 59.

Dr. McKinnon did not mention any postgraduate education immediately after graduation. One may assume he entered general practice. Three years later he took the McGill course in Tropical Medicine, and in 1946-47 he worked in the Medical Division of Sunnybrook Hospital in Toronto. Soon after, he was the first to introduce electrocardiography in Fredericton. He practised internal medicine with a special interest in cardiology. In 1949 he published an article on "Post-partum Heart Disease" in the *C.M.A.J.* and in 1959 he published "Pre-operative Assessment" in the *Nova Scotia Medical Bulletin*.

Dr. Garfield MacLeod Moffat, 25 March 1921, Sydney, N.S.; Mount Allison University, B.A. 42; Dalhousie, M.D., C.M. 47.

The route by which Dr. Moffatt became a member of the Canadian Cardiovascular Society was that of pragmatic adjustments to immediate needs. He found that as his work changed from that of general practice to internal medicine, a considerable portion of his patients demanded skills related to the diagnosis and treatment of cardiovascular disease. He applied himself to improving his ability to analyze heart sounds and murmurs and to record and interpret electrocardiograms, and kept himself well informed about progress in medical and surgical therapy. He bought his first electrocardiograph ten years after graduation. His senior colleague, Dr. Hector

McKinnon, helped him in this learning process. When Dr. McKinnon went to Halifax in 1965 for a sabbatical year, the city of Fredericton continued to have in Moffat the services of a good internist with special knowledge of and skills in cardiology.

Dr. Moffat's career reflects the dedicated physician who feels the need for and devotes time and effort to continuing education. Such men provide their patients with the best of medical care.

In responding to the special questions he wrote in 1965:

> Actually, I never did arrive at the decision to specialize in cardiology. Once in practice, particularly in Fredericton, I realized that a large part of the practice of internal medicine was that of cardiology. My interests were mainly in arthritis, metabolism, and neurology. However, to do the work of an internist, I was obliged to become more and more involved in cardiology. I found the interpretation of murmurs and cardiac arrhythmias on an electrocardiogram most difficult. I still consider them my *bête noire.* My associate, Dr. H. H. McKinnon, finds cardiology his forte. He has been most kind in assisting me over these hurdles.
>
> Earlier in cardiology, approximately 1956, I found my main problem was interpreting the various causes of chest pain. I am always concerned that I will consider chest pain in young men to be that of coronary artery disease, whereas it may be skeletal. This diagnosis has bothered me a great deal. However, as my training increases and my interest in cardiology improves, I am able to sort out these various causes of chest pain. I believe that in more recent years my assessment of chest pain is correct on most occasions.
>
> With cardiac surgery playing an important part in valvular disease and congenital heart disease, my problem is one of interpreting heart murmurs. I am sure that I will never become competent in this field.
>
> I bought my first electrocardiogram machine in 1957. I recently bought a new one in 1963.

In 1965, he practised as a member of a group of 22 physicians and surgeons which included Dr. McKinnon.

Dr. Edouard S. Eddie, 27 January 1927, Lebanon; American University Beirut, B.A. 46, Université de Paris, France, M.D., 53; F.C.C.P.; F.I.C.A.; F.A.C.C.

Dr. Eddie established himself in Bathurst after an excellent course of postgraduate training in Soissons, France; in Houston, Texas

(1954), and during three years at the Institute of Cardiology in Montreal (1954-57). He did not comment on the four questions.

In 1968 he was consultant in cardiology to hospitals in Bathurst, Dalhousie, Tracadie and Caraquet in addition to holding the post of Chief of Medicine at Hôtel Dieu in Bathurst. His bibliography includes an article co-authored with Drs. Paul David and Osman Gialloreto, entitled "Les thromboses auriculaires massives," *Congrès Français de Médecins,* xxxe Session — Alger 1955. He wrote three articles as sole author, the most recent, "Etude electrocardiographique de 150 cas de stenose mitrale avant et aprés commissureotomy" *(Un. Méd. Can.,*1958: 88).

Quebec

Dr. Samuel Eidlow (1889-1962)

The postgraduate course in cardiology which Dr. Paul Dudley White began to provide for general practitioners and internists in 1924 created a special type of pioneer in so-called primary medicine. The acquisition of special knowledge and skills related to eliciting a good clinical history, and fine-tuning of clinical methods including auscultation and the acquisition of skill in electrocardiography, made for a physician who could recognize and treat cardiovascular disease quite as well as a cardiologist. An early pioneer in this category, who is mentioned here as an example, is Dr. Samuel Eidlow of Montreal. He also has special merit in that he was the first to report a case of aberrant coronary artery from the pulmonary artery diagnosed clinically and confirmed at autopsy (1946).

Born in Roumania, he emigrated with his family in 1903 to New York. He was then fourteen years old. In the next seven years he completed high school education by earning his living during the day and attending school at night. He completed the course in medicine at New York University by attending school during the day and working at night. Usually young men in this category of the social structure did not serve internships; they hung a shingle and proceeded to do general practice immediately after graduation. But Eidlow served internships for two and one-half years after graduation in 1910. He recalled with great pleasure the year and a half that he spent at the Hospital of the Yale Medical School with Professor George Blumer as his teacher.

During this period he had an unusual experience which he recalled when a similar event occurred at the Jewish General Hospital (about 1947) in Montreal. A patient was declared dead at about 4 a.m.; when the orderly came to bring the corpse to the Department of Pathology about an hour later, he found the patient still alive. Dr. Eidlow recalled that in New Haven a patient had already been placed in the morgue of the hospital when it was discovered that he was alive. Both these patients died some hours later. These experiences underlined the importance of great care in making final decisions.

Eidlow came to settle in Montreal in 1913, when established general practitioners in this area were not inclined to give such competitors a warm and friendly reception. His small stature and slender build did not give him an imposing presence. He had served internships in obstetrics and paediatrics, so it was not very long before a growing number of people discovered his dedication as a good physician with better training than most of his competitors. He developed a very large general practice which threatened to prevent him from devoting time to continuing education. He enjoyed the advantage of a low-man-on-the-totem-pole appointment at the Royal Victoria Hospital, where he worked diligently in the outpatient department and took advantage of attending ward rounds and clinical-pathological conferences. In 1933 he went to Boston for the two-week intensive course in cardiology given by Paul D. White and his associates at the Massachusetts General Hospital under the auspices of the Harvard Medical School. He bought a Sanborn string galvanometer and thus added electrocardiography to his diagnostic skills. In this regard he was a pioneer for he was the first general practitioner of Montreal to acquire special training in cardiology in this manner.

By eliminating obstetrics and minor surgery from his activities he became an internist. He did not entirely discontinue treating infants and children; a considerable number of people in the city regarded him as an eminent paediatrician. He concentrated his continuing education in the domain of cardiology. When the Jewish General Hospital was opened in 1934, he was welcomed as a member of the Department of Cardiology and of the medical team headed by Segall. He continued his association with the Royal Victoria Hospital, and thus carried the load of public clinic service at two institutions — and he met all his commitments in full. At the Jewish General Hospital he served one morning a week in the general medicine clinic and one morning in the cardiac clinic. Later, he devoted two mornings a week to the cardiac clinic. For six months of the year he made ward rounds on the medical service seven days a week, which was the habit of my team. All of this work was voluntary. He earned a little income as one of four members of the Department of Cardiology who were the official readers of electrocardiograms for the hospital. At that time the number of records made was relatively small, averaging eight per day, which included the records of two or three private patients, the only ones who provided some remuneration.

In 1946, a young mother came to Eidlow with her sick baby. Her paediatrician was experiencing difficulty in managing the illness, which seemed to be due to allergy with bronchial spasm. Eidlow had been the general practitioner in her family when the mother was born, and he had delivered her. His expertise as a paediatrician led him to suspect congenital heart disease and thus he recorded an electrocardiogram. In reflecting about the case, he remembered a reference to aberrant left coronary artery from the pulmonary artery at a conference of the cardiology department. He reviewed the available literature and made the diagnosis of this condition antemortem. His case report, published in 1946 in association with the pathologist, Dr. E. R. Mackenzie, is the first record of this condition in which an ante-mortem diagnosis was confirmed by autopsy (Eidlow and Mackenzie, 1946).

Eidlow's career exemplifies the manner in which the rapid progress in cardiology was applied in the management of patients by general practitioners who chose to concentrate their continuing education in this field. They were usually good students who, as they reached their late forties, sought to practise internal medicine with a particular interest in one specialty.

Eidlow was not a religious man in the formal sense. A few days before he died, realizing that he was not going to recover, he asked the nurse to take some dictation which he wished to serve as his own obituary. He instructed her to give it to his daughter who would release it, should the press ask for an obituary. There is no better way of completing this story than by quoting it:

> Dr. Samuel Eidlow, a staff member of the Jewish General Hospital, the Royal Victoria Hospital and the Jewish Hospital of Hope, died in the Jewish General Hospital after a short illness. Dr. Eidlow, who was born in Roumania, went to New York University Medical School and graduated in medicine in 1910. He interned in several hospitals in the United States. Dr. Eidlow came to Montreal in 1913 and engaged in general practice for fifteen years, after which he entered practice in internal medicine and cardiology. He was a member of the Canadian Heart Associa-

tion, the Montreal Cardiac Society, the Montreal Clinical Society. The deceased is survived by his wife Sadie, and three daughters, Mrs. Leona Schriber, of Los Angeles; Bernice Palye, of Ottawa; Sonia Castle, Los Angeles; and four grandchildren.

Dr. Samuel Eidlow died on 20 September 1962. The following physician's prayer, attributed to Maimonides, may not have been known to Dr. Eidlow, but he translated it into action in the course of his entire career: "May there never develop in me a notion that my education is complete, but give me strength and leisure and zeal continually to enlarge my knowledge" (Kagan, 1938).

Dr. John H. Palmer (1896-1958)

At the time when Dr. Palmer's mini-biography was needed for the Archives of the Canadian Cardiovascular Society, fourteen years had elapsed since his death. Efforts to obtain more information than is available in the obituary that appeared in the *Canadian Medical Association Journal* (Sept. 15, 1958) were not fruitful. The obituary is here quoted in full:

> Dr. John Palmer, 62, died at the Royal Victoria Hospital, Montreal, on August 9. He was born in Bedeque, P.E.I., and received his early education at Gagetown, N.B. and Mount Allison University. He entered McGill University in 1913, but interrupted his medical studies to serve in the First World War. He went overseas with the No. 3 Canadian General Hospital (McGill) and was later transferred to the No. 2 Canadian Field Ambulance. He then became surgeon probationer to the RCNVR, where he served until the end of the war. In 1921, Dr. Palmer graduated in medicine from McGill University, interned at the Royal Victoria Hospital, and then went to Trail, B.C., where he practised for a number of years. He did postgraduate work in London and Vienna in 1930-31. From 1934-36, he worked with Sir John Parkinson in cardiology, and was appointed to the attending staff of the Royal Victoria Hospital, Montreal. In 1940, he went overseas with the Canadian General Hospital as a major. He was promoted later to lieutenant-colonel and served in the Italian campaign. After some months, he was promoted to colonel and appointed consultant for the Canadian Corps in Italy. He returned to England in 1945. After the war, he returned to his post at the Royal Victoria Hospital, Montreal, where he remained as head of the department of cardiology until his death.
>
> Dr. Palmer is survived by his widow and three daughters.

I recall other details. We first met in 1921 when he was in his final year of the five-year course in medicine and I was demonstrating pathological specimens to a group of students in which he found himself during a session at the McGill Medical Museum. About fifteen years later I met him again and became aware of the book he wrote together with Sir John Parkinson on cardiac hypertrophy, which represented several years of hard work correlating clinical, radiographic, and electrocardiographic observations with pathological studies. Only a patient, persistent, and hard worker could have accomplished this task.

Before World War II Palmer was working at three hospitals; the Royal Victoria Hospital was his main base, but he was also consultant in cardiology at the Montreal Children's Hospital and at the Reddy Memorial Hospital. In his style of general behaviour he seemed to have the talent for emphasizing what is currently accepted as 'very, very British' — an apparently unflappable mood, cool to cold in a crisis, deliberate in his speech, and answering questions after considerable pause. In a small group he would talk less than most others. On some rare occasions, usually when he was indignant, he would speak rapidly.

Palmer was enthusiastic about the formation of the Montreal Cardiac Society, which was founded on September 25, 1946. He was the ablest representative of the Royal Victoria Hospital in this effort. He volunteered for any kind of task that needed to be done. He gathered together the eleven men in Ottawa who represented medicine in all parts of Canada and who agreed that a Canadian Heart Association should be formed. This led to the next step in June 1947, when the Association (now the Canadian Cardiovascular Society) came into existence.

Palmer willingly and enthusiastically accepted tasks related to the creation of the Quebec Heart Foundation. A very important contribution was his discovery that Mr. J. Bruce Brown, an influential industrialist, might accept the initiative to establish the Foundation, which had been refused by several prominent Montrealers. The committee which undertook to find such a leader was already at its wits' end because of the repeated refusals. Then Mr. Lazarus Phillips, one man who had refused the task but recognized its importance, suggested that we approach Brown and I spoke of this to Palmer, who was his friend.

The story of Brown's contribution to the Canadian effort for the prevention and relief of heart disease is a subject in itself. Here only a brief allusion can be made. Brown laid substantial foundations which are still the basis for the Quebec Heart Foundation in the 1980s. He served as secretary-treasurer and did everybody's work, filling the gap that existed when there was no executive secretary. In this he was ably assisted by Miss Marie Atkinson, the secretary in his business office. At the time of his death, Palmer was the senior medical person on the Board of Directors of the National Heart Foundation, where he held the position of vice-president. His loss was acutely felt by all of us when he died of carcinoma of the lung.

Dr. Adélard Tétrault, 26 February 1901, Ste-Madeleine Co., St. Hyacinthe, Québec; Université de Montréal, B.Sc. 25, M.D. 25, R.C.P.(C) Cert. Int. Med.; C.S.P.Q. Int. Med. and Cardiol.

As might be expected, the earliest innovations of cardiology occurred in the university centres. The introduction of electrocardiography in towns or cities at a considerable distance from the university depended upon the presence of an energetic, enthusiastic physician who practised internal medicine with a special interest in cardiology. The city of Trois Rivières was blessed with such a man in the person of Adélard Tétrault.

After two years of internship at the Saint Joseph Hospital in Trois Rivières, he began private practice in that city. Tétrault became interested in cardiology and went to Paris in 1930, where he spent about two years studying mainly with Professors Antonin Clerc and Charles Laubry. In 1937, he introduced electrocardiography in Trois Rivières. The bibliography which he listed in 1965 begins with an article on "Angina Pectoris and Its Treatment" published in the *Union Médical du Canada,* 1932. Following that are articles principally on topics related to clinical cardiology. Tétrault was a charter member of the Canadian Heart Association and served as president of the Quebec Division of the Canadian Medical Association.

Dr. Kenneth Ivan Melville, 5 July 1902, Kingston, Jamaica; McGill University, B.Sc., M.D., C.M. 1926.

When Dr. Kenneth Melville graduated in medicine at McGill University in May 1926, he was awarded the Holmes Gold Medal for the highest aggregate standing throughout the entire course. He chose to devote himself to research and teaching and attained the post of Professor of Pharmacology at McGill. He began with a subject that is very close to one of the principal achievements of therapy for congestive heart failure that was initiated in the twentieth century. His first publication (1927) was on the diuresis produced by Novasurol. Not long afterwards, he began to study coronary circulation. His first paper in this sphere, "The Influence of the Heart Beat Upon the Flow of Blood Into the Coronary Arteries" in 1932, was followed by a large number of publications which represent intense and extensive work designed to clarify the physiology and pharmacology of the coronary circulation. Melville neatly summarized this aspect of his achievements in the following sentence: "My career has been a continuous struggle with the problem of the physiology and pharmacology of the coronary circulation." In 1965, item number 132 of his bibliography was a chapter for *Drill's Textbook of Pharmacology* on "Nitrites, Nitrates and Miscellaneous Drugs."

Dr. Paul Morin, 13 May 1902, Montreal; Université de Montréal, M.D. 28; C.P.S.Q. Med. 52; C.P.S.Q. Cardiol., 52, F.R.C.P.(C).

For postgraduate training in cardiology, Dr. Paul Morin went to Paris and "followed" Professors Antonin Clerc, Henri Vaquez and E. Bordet during the years 1929-1931. He joined the staff of the Hôpital St-Luc and the Université de Montréal in 1931 and was active in private practice in 1965 when he responded to the questionnaire. However, the archivist failed to obtain comments on the special questions and a bibliography. Morin was probably the first cardiologist associated with the Hôpital St-Luc in Montreal.

Dr. Rodrigue Lefebvre, 12 August 1902, Montreal; Université de Montréal, M.D. 1929; C.P.S.Q. Int. Med. and Cardiol. 52.

Dr. Rodrigue Lefebvre was a pioneer in developing cardiology in the francophone sector of Montreal. He served on the first council of the Montreal Cardiac Society and the Canadian Cardiovascular Society. As an enthusiastic teacher of many generations of students of the Université de Montréal and resident staff of the Hôtel-Dieu, his contributions have indeed been large.

In 1965 he wrote about his beginnings in cardiology:

> I was attracted to cardiology and endocrinology. However, I did not make my decision until the years of my senior internship in the service of the late Professor Albert Lesage at the Nôtre Dame Hospital. He knew my aptitudes, could judge my talents. His advice led me to choose cardiology. The only obstacle in the way of studying abroad was the lack of money. Fortunately, I obtained a scholarship from the Quebec Government which

permitted me to spend the years 1931-1934 in Paris and 1934-1935 in Boston. I went to France first because my native language being French, I knew I could study more conveniently to obtain the essential knowledge of the specialty. The second reason stemmed from the fact that I had met most of the physicians who were my teachers in Paris when they came to Montreal to deliver lectures. After three years in the French capital, I went to the clinic of Dr. Paul White in Boston. His worldwide reputation had already been established and I felt sure that I would complete and extend my knowledge of cardiology under his influence. This proved to be correct.

Dr. Lefebvre published on a variety of subjects within the fields of internal medicine and cardiology. His articles in collaboration with others have appeared in the *Archives des Maladies du Coeur* (septembre 1934), *le Journal Médical Français* (décembre 1934), *le Journal de l'Hôtel-Dieu* (1935 à 1942) and *l'Union Médicale du Canada* (1940 à 1965). He did not provide a detailed bibliography.

He bought his first electrocardiograph in 1940.

Dr. Richard Lessard, 4 July 1905, Quebec City; Laval, B.A. 24, M.D. 29, M.D. Paris 33; F.R.C.P.(C) 37; F.A.C.P. 48; C.P.S.Q. Int. Med. and Cardiol. F.R.C.P.(C) 44.

Dr. Lessard brought cardiology from Paris to Quebec City in 1933. He chose to introduce it gradually, functioning as an internist with a special fondness for matters cardiological.

Dr. Lessard served his internship at the Hôtel-Dieu in 1928-1929 and residency in 1929-1930. He then went to Paris, where he became Assistant Etranger de la Faculté de Médecine and studied cardiology mainly with Professor Camille Lian. On his return home, he joined the staff of the Hôtel-Dieu and Laval University.

In a charming brief essay on "The Beginnings of Cardiology in Quebec," employing the editorial "we," he wrote as follows:

> When in 1933 we started to practice our specialty, we must say we were well received, everybody recognized we were trying to fill a gap. Far from wishing to upset everything we willingly accepted the old established norms. In short, we were mainly specialists in internal medicine with what might be termed a predilection for cardiology. That is to say, we had to modify the strongly entrenched traditions with much prudence and patience. The task of pioneers is far from always being easy. A new

> expression which is much in use at present [1982] and is very popular in our region summarizes the situation very well. We had to proceed *par étapisme* [step by step] (Lessard, 1982).

He relates, among other things, that in 1933, there were only two mercury manometers for measuring arterial pressure in the hospital. The one on the male ward, he noted, could measure up to 300 mm and that on the female ward only up to 260 mm. In accordance with traditions of medical practice in France, the nurse who accompanied the staff on ward rounds had a thin towel available for use in practising direct auscultation. The physician spread the towel on the surface of the chest where he was to listen and then applied his ear directly over the area. The rigid monaural stethoscope was being used only for listening to fetal sounds. In the department of medicine, the binaural stethoscope was already in general use.

As to the introduction of electrocardiography, he relates the following story:

> Dr. Jean-Baptiste Lacroix was studying surgery in France when he became sick and had to follow a rest cure. When he was declared to be cured his physicians advised him to change his orientation and he chose to become a physiologist. He became the first full-time professor in the Faculty of Medicine at Laval. Among the instruments he acquired there was a Boulitte electrocardiograph. It would appear that this instrument was not used very often.
>
> In 1933, as I entered the career of Cardiology, Dr. Romeo Blanchet, who had succeeded Dr. Lacroix as professor of physiology, was good enough to offer to lend me, for use in the Hôtel-Dieu, the Boulitte apparatus which rested quietly in a corner of his laboratory. Its unemployed state came to an end and it soon became very active.

Lessard's bibliography reveals a keen interest in clinical cardiology both in his publication of original observations and in addresses he delivered to medical societies in and around Quebec City. However, he also wrote on other subjects, e.g., purpura, acute nephritis, Hippocratic fingers in cases of pulmonary suppuration, calcification of the nucleus pulposus. He is well known for his erudition in the history of medicine. Several items in his bibliography deal with subjects related to life-insurance medicine.

Dr. Hans Selye, 26 January 1907, Vienna; German University of Prague, M.D. 29; Ph.D. 31; D.Sc. McGill 42; F.R.S.(C); F.R.S. Med. (Eng.); LL.D. (14 Honorary Degrees).

In 1972, in response to our third and final request, Dr. Hans Selye responded with the following notes in addition to his curriculum vitae:

> Hans Selye, Professor and Director of the Institute of Experimental Medicine and Surgery in the University of Montreal, was born on January 26, 1907, in Vienna. He is mainly interested in correlations and the holistic approach to medical research. His major contributions were the description of the general adaptation or 'stress' syndrome, anaphylactoid oedema, calciphylaxis, calcergy, and steroid anaesthesia. At present [1965], most of his research is concerned with the prophylaxis of cardiovascular disease and a group of hormones which he calls 'catatoxic steroids.'

Selye is the author of twenty-six books and more than 1400 publications in technical journals. He holds earned doctorates in medicine, philosophy and science, as well as fourteen honorary degrees conferred on him by universities in Argentina, Austria, Canada, Chile, Czechoslovakia, Germany, Guatemala, Italy, Japan, Uruguay and the U.S.A. He is a Fellow of the Royal Society of Canada and an Honorary Fellow of 42 other scientific societies throughout the world. A recipient of numerous medals and honorary citizenships, he has been made a Companion of the Order of Canada, the highest decoration awarded by his country.

Dr. Selye did not include his bibliography, which is an unusually large one. His books and articles both technical and popular on stress are numerous; some have been translated into several languages and are widely distributed. Dr. Selye's work on stress is world renowned.

Dr. Guy Drouin, 19 November 1908, Quebec; Laval, M.D. 32; F.A.C.C., F.A.C.P., C.P.S.Q. Int. Med. and Cardiol. R.C.P.(C) Cert. Int. Med.

Dr. Drouin, a pioneer of cardiology in Quebec City, has the special distinction of having pursued postgraduate studies not only in Paris but also in London, England. His studies abroad began in November 1936, four years after graduation from the Medical School of Laval University. He went first to London, where he spent four months at the National Heart Hospital with Dr. Paul Wood. He then worked in

Paris until July 1938, mostly with Professors Emile Sergent and Antonin Clerc. On returning to Quebec City, he practised and taught internal medicine with a special interest in cardiology. From 1957-1964 he served as chief of the medical service at the Institute of Cardiology while remaining a member of the department of medicine at the St. Sacrament Hospital, of which he became chief in 1965. In that year also, he was appointed full-time professor of medicine and in 1970 became the Professeur Titulaire at Laval University.

Drouin provided his curriculum vitae but not his bibliography.

Dr. Hyman Shister, 21 January 1906, Russia; McGill, M.D., C.M. 32, F.A.C.C., C.P.S.Q. Cardiol. and Int. Med. 50, R.C.P.(C) Cert. Int. Med. 45.

The career of Dr. Hyman Shister includes clinical cardiology and experimental research in the pharmacology laboratory of McGill University along with Professor K. I. Melville. This career has been exceptional because he did not enjoy the privilege of a fellowship or scholarship with opportunities for learning experimental techniques. He was educated by "working on the job." He learned clinical cardiology by attending the cardiac clinic at the Montreal General Hospital as an observer and by joining the staff of the Herbert Reddy Memorial Hospital, where he worked with me. This hospital did not own an electrocardiograph until after 1936. (I had initiated the Cardiac Clinic in 1928, using my own portable Cambridge machine, the first of its kind in Montreal.)

In 1936, Dr. Shister took full charge of the Cardiac Clinic when I resigned to devote myself to the recently opened Jewish General Hospital. The Reddy Memorial Hospital acquired both its own electrocardiograph and a new consultant, Dr. John Palmer, whose influence on Shister's education was keenly appreciated.

To pursue his taste for basic research, Shister associated himself with Professor Kenneth I. Melville and worked in the Department of Pharmacology at McGill University. His bibliography reflects his interest in medical history as well as in clinical cardiology and pharmacology.

In 1965, Dr. Shister's bibliography consisted of seven items. With Dr. E. Gubbay he co-authored "Paraxysmal tachycardia during therapy with L-Noradrenaline" (*C.M.A.J.* 1959; 81, 560); with Dr. Melville he co-authored "Cardiac responses to epinephrine and nor-epinephrine during prolonged cholesterol and high-fat feeding in rabbits" (*Am. J. Cardiol.* 1959; 4, 391); and with Melville and Dr. S. Hug he co-authored "Improveratril; experimental data on coronary dilatation and antiarrhythmic action" (*C.M.A.J.* 1964; 90, 76).

Dr. Jacques Genest, 29 May 1919, Montreal; Collège Jean de Brébeuf, B.A. 37; Université de Montréal, M.D. 42; Hon. LL.D. Queen's University, 66; Hon. LL.D. University of Toronto 70; F.A.C.P. 49; F.R.C.P.(C) 47; F.R.S.C. 65; Cert. Spec. Coll. of Phys. & Surg. P.Q. 55; Companion Order of Can.; A.C.F.A.S.(C) 65; C.S.C.I.

Dr. Genest began his ten-year postgraduate training with residency in medicine at the Hôtel-Dieu de Montréal (1942-1944). Then followed residency in pathology at the same hospital (1944-1945). During the next three years (1945-1948) he worked at Johns Hopkins Hospital in research on renal physiology related to sodium metabolism. In 1948 he took a course in organic chemistry at Harvard University and during the years 1948-1951 he engaged in research at the Rockefeller Institute in New York City. On his return to Montreal he became Director of the Department of Clinical Research at the Hôtel-Dieu. Since 1963 he has been Canadian Professor, Department of Medicine, Université de Montréal. In 1964 he became Director of the Clinical Research Institute of Montreal. He has been Chief of the Nephrology and Hypertension Service at the Hôtel-Dieu since 1963.

In 1968 he wrote the following comments on the special questions:

> This question applies to me only slightly, that is, because though my activities have in large part been centred on the mechanism and the treatment of hypertension, my approach has been entirely hormonal and metabolic. Apart from hypertension I am really not to be considered as a cardiologist according to the current meaning of this term.
>
> The problem of hypertension to which I have devoted twenty years of my life attracted me because of my interest in nephrology and particularly in the mechanism of sodium regulation and the oedemas. It was my reading about the metabolism of sodium which engaged my interest more and more in the problem of hypertension. I became convinced that sodium plays a fundamental role in the pathology of arterial hypertension in humans. This conviction has been at the basis of all the hypotheses which guided our work. My long periods of study at Johns Hopkins and at the Rockefeller University had the purpose of familiarizing me with the method of renal clearance and the factors which

modify tubal reabsorption of sodium, and also of studying the corticosteroid hormones which play a major role in this tubular reabsorption of sodium and which also are involved in both experimental and human hypertension.

My extracurricular activities have been concerned with service to university life as Governor of the University of Montreal, and the study of the French fact in America as Vice-President of the Lionel Groulx Foundation. One of my continuing interests since graduation has been the reading and intensive study about the social problems related to medical care in various parts of the western world. Recently as a guest of the Academy of Sciences of the U.S.S.R. I had the opportunity to study the Russian system personally.

During the past fifteen years I have been intensely interested in the promotion of clinical research in Canada. I was one of the three men who founded the Canadian Society of Clinical Research, was its first President, and then was re-elected in 1958. During the past twelve years I have served on a variety of committees of the Medical Research Council of Canada. Since 1964 I have been the President of the Medical Research Council of Quebec. During the past fifteen years I have been a member of various committees of the Royal College of Physicians and Surgeons of Canada and since 1959 I have been a member of its Council.

In 1968 Dr. Genest's bibliography contained 175 items. The first item, in 1943, dealt with the treatment of tetanus, and the second, in 1944, with the diagnosis and semiology of rheumatism. The third item, in 1947, marks the beginning of his major subject of continuing research, renal physiology. Early in his career he manifested active concern about the social structure as related to medicine. Thus in 1948 he wrote on "L'Avenir de la médecine Canadienne Française" (*Un. Méd. Can.*, 1948: 77, 1187). He created and developed a great school of clinical research at the Hôtel-Dieu and the Institute which is closely allied to it. The bibliography reveals that he had 79 different persons as co-authors; these have been trainees, pupils and associates.

A world-renowned scientist, Genest has had many honours and rewards bestowed on him; a few which appeared in his curriculum vitae of 1971, are the Gairdner Award (Toronto, 1963); the Archambeault Medal, A.C.F.A.S. (Canada) 1965; the Stauffer Award, 1969; and Sims Commonwealth Travelling Professor, 1970.

Dr. Maurice McGregor, 26 March 1920, South Africa; University of Witwatersrand, Johannesburg, M.B., B.Ch. 42; C.P.S.Q. Cardiol. F.R.C.P. (London) C.S.C.I.: A.S.C.I.

In 1971 Dr. McGregor submitted the following succinct sketch of his career:

> Dr. Maurice McGregor is a product of a basic medical education in South Africa, followed by military service in the Mediterranean theatre of the Second World War, a cardiology training in London and sabbatical year in physiology in Boston. His career as a teacher, researcher and practitioner of cardiothoracic disease has been carried out at the University of the Witwatersrand in Johannesburg and at McGill University in Montreal. His extensive research contributions have been in the field of cardiorespiratory function and disease and have been characterised by the application of physiological methods to the study of problems encountered in his observation of disease in man. He is currently a Professor of Clinical and Experimental Medicine and Dean of the Faculty of Medicine of McGill University.

In 1971, Dr. McGregor was Professor of Medicine, McGill Research Director of the Joint Cardio-respiratory Service of the Royal Victoria Hospital and the Montreal Children's Hospital, and Physician-in-chief of the Royal Victoria Hospital. Between 1946 and 1965, Dr. McGregor's bibliography grew to 76 items. Of these he was co-author in 67 and there are 69 colleagues associated with him in the wide range of works which these articles represent. This is a measure of the influence he has exerted in the education of candidates for leadership in the study of the cardiovascular system. He has left his mark literally all over the world as he has worked in South Africa, England, the United States and Canada.

Dr. Michael Gold, 22 November 1919, Montreal; McGill, B.Sc. 40, M.D., C.M. 43; M.Sc. 45, C.P.S.Q. Int. Med. and Cardiol. 53; F.R.C.P.(C).

Dr. Gold is one of a very few who chose to specialize in cardiology because a loved one (his father) suffered from heart disease and died of it. After good training and the commencement of work in the Cardiac Clinic at the Jewish General Hospital, he developed a special interest in hypertension. He studied its problems with biochemical methods and was thus led to create and direct a department of nephrology at the hospital. Dr. Gold did not provide his bibliography.

Dr. Ronald Leland Stanford, 7 February 1914, Montreal; Loyola College, B.A. 36; McGill, M.D., C.M. 43, C.P.S.Q. Int. Med. and Cardiol.; F.R.C.P.(C).

Dr. Stanford's brief comments about the four questions written in 1965 indicate that he was attracted to cardiology while working with Dr. Neil Feeney at the Montreal General Hospital in his final undergraduate year. His postgraduate studies began with internship at the Montreal General Hospital (1943-44) followed by military service (1944-46). After the war he resumed internships at the Queen Mary Veterans Hospital (1946-48) and the Royal Victoria Hospital (1948-50). He spent part of the year 1950 at the National Heart Hospital, London and in 1952 he studied cardiology at the Peter Bent Brigham Hospital, Boston. When he submitted the questionnaire in 1972, Stanford was Lecturer in the McGill Faculty of Medicine and Director of the Division of Cardiology of St. Mary's Hospital. He did not provide his bibliography.

Dr. Pierre Marion, 7 March 1917, Montreal; Collège Ste-Marie, B.A. 37; Université de Montréal; M.D. 43, C.P.S.Q. Internal Med. 52, Cardiol. 52, F.A.H.A., F.A.C.C.

Dr. Marion is one of the early pioneers of modern paediatric, as well as adult, cardiology in the francophone milieu of Montreal. He tells a very interesting story of postgraduate education in his comments on the special questions:

> In answer to your first question — as you know my father has practised general and obstetrical medicine most of his life. I saw him leave at all hours of the day and night for emergency cases, medical, surgical and obstetrical. I often observed how helpless a physician could be in the treatment of cardiac patients whether it was rheumatic heart disease, coronary or atherosclerotic. This gave me the idea to specialize in cardiology because at this time in my studies the future importance of cardiology was already apparent. More and more physiologists began to penetrate the interesting mysteries surrounding the problems of heart disease. It was during my internship at Hôtel-Dieu that I came to this decision.
>
> There were, however, many obstacles in my way. The war was not over, and there were few opportunities in both France and the United States for a residency in cardiology. Because my knowledge of English was so limited, I felt I must first improve and attempt to master it. And so during my holidays, I became

interested in the Society for Crippled Children whose directors and benefactors were mostly English. Whenever English-speaking visitors came to the camp I had to deliver a little speech and of course because most of the children were English, communication with them was only in English too. Once I felt that I had mastered the language sufficiently, I decided to attend the cardiology clinic at the Royal Victoria Hospital, directed by Dr. G. R. Brow, who welcomed me most graciously and allowed me to go on rounds two or three times a week. In this way, I spent at least a year attending the cardiology service at the Royal Victoria Hospital. At the end of that year, I applied to the Massachusetts General Hospital in Boston for a residency so that I might study under Dr. Paul White. The provincial government provided me with a bursary and so I went to Boston. But when I came back to Montreal, realizing that I would be teaching in a francophone medical school, I decided it would be useful to become well acquainted with French clinical methods. For nearly a year, I worked with Professor Gaston Giraud in Montpellier. Returning from Montpellier, I joined the staff at the Hôtel-Dieu as well as that of St. Justine Hospital in the Department of Cardiology. At that time there was no cardiologist at St. Justine Hospital and I felt that there was great opportunity there since the era of congenital heart disease and heart surgery was in its infancy. I became the Director of Cardiology Service at St. Justine Hospital. This introduced me to new studies with Dr. Richard Bing at Johns Hopkins.

Unfortunately, because of lack of funds, St. Justine Hospital could not organize a Department of Physiology and I could only practise paediatric clinical cardiology. Several years later the Department of Cardiovascular Physiology was established.

Marion had good cause to be very pleased with the progress made in paediatric cardiology at the St. Justine Hospital where he sowed the first seeds of its growth. He has been active in local, provincial and national cardiology organizations. He and Drs. Rodrigue Lefebvre and Georges Garneau were the only three francophone cardiologists who came to the meeting in the McGill Department of Physiology at which the Montreal Cardiac Society was organized on 25 September 1946.

At the time he responded to the questionnaire in 1968, Marion held the position of Assistant Professor of Medicine at the Université de Montréal, Chief of Cardiology at the St. Justine Hospital and Assistant in the Cardiology service at the Hôtel-Dieu.

Marion's bibliography lists 43 items, including both published articles and unpublished addresses. As early as 1948, he delivered a paper on the rehabilitation of cardiacs at the annual meeting of l'Association de Médecins de Langue Française de l'Amerique du Nord, and on the same occasion, he presented a paper on the surgical treatment of congenital cardiac abnormalities.

In 1949, Marion wrote a series of papers which were published in the *Fichier Médical*, Montpellier, on subjects which were new to postwar French cardiology, namely modern diagnostic methods for congenital heart disease and the surgical treatment of congenital heart disease. In 1946, he delivered a paper on precordial leads of the electrocardiogram at the Hôpital St-Eloi, in Montpellier. Before the war, francophone physicians went from Canada to France for postgraduate education; in 1946, Dr. Marion was bringing new knowledge from North America to France.

Dr. Paul Pierre David, 25 December 1919, Montreal; Université de Paris, B.A. 39; Université de Montréal, M.D. 44; Cert. Int. Med. and Cardiol., C.P.S.Q., 52; O.C.; F.A.H.A.; F.A.C.C.

Dr. David's postgraduate education began at the Notre Dame Hospital, where he was exposed to internal medicine, surgery and radiology. This experience led him to make the positive decision that he preferred a career in internal medicine. During his senior internship it was suggested to him that he should specialize in cardiology in order to bring some new strength to the department at the Notre Dame Hospital. Dr. Albert de Guise was at that time Chief and Dr. Gaetan Barry his first assistant in cardiology. David had the opportunity of working with these two men for a short period of time and recognized that this department was indeed in need of re-organization. He planned his postgraduate education in cardiology to begin with study under Dr. Paul Dudley White (Paul, 1986), a choice arising directly from the experience of reading White's classic textbook on cardiology. It required more than usual courage and initiative for him to seek training at the Massachusetts General Hospital because at that time he could not speak English for all practical purposes. His education had been restricted to French schools in France and the French medical school in Montreal.

During the year 1945-46 which he spent with White he learnt to speak English fluently, and of course to read and write it. Moreover, his studies assured him that he had made a good choice, both as to a specialty and in the selection of his teacher, for White became for him an inspiring influence. The year 1946-47, David spent as a pupil of Professors Pierre Soulié and Jean Lenègre. These leaders of French cardiology each had a service of 100 beds for cardiac patients at the Hôpital Lariboisière. David's experience at the Massachusetts General Hospital prepared him very well to make the most of the excellent opportunities for studying patients and for appreciating the special advantages offered by the teaching in progress in the French school.

On his return from Paris to the staff of the Notre Dame Hospital, he soon discovered he had a battle on his hands if he was to effectively contribute towards the re-organization of the Department of Cardiology. He soon succeeded in asserting his influence with the members of the institution and with his seniors to the extent of improving the equipment of the department. A portable Sanborn electrocardiograph and a new fluoroscope apparatus were installed. A technician, who also functioned as a secretary of the department, was added to the staff. David instituted the system of having the technician record the electrocardiogram and having the report dictated to and typed by the secretary. The portable electrocardiograph made it possible to record electrocardiograms on the wards and in the outpatients' department whereas previously records were made in a dark room which was usually locked when not in use. Electrocardiography at this hospital was now deprived of its mystery and was being taught to the younger men.

During his career in Notre Dame Hospital (1947-53) David established an outpatients' cardiac clinic which attracted an increasing number of patients, so that the clinic had to be held on two days a week. Several of the interns and residents, aware of this new force in the hospital, were inspired to become cardiologists. They started their education with David and then did as he had done, namely, continued their education in the United States or in France, or in both.

In 1950 David and his contemporary in surgery, Dr. Edouard Gagnon, joined to develop cardiac surgery. Together they pioneered the surgical treatment of mitral stenosis and were most likely the first to perform this operation in Canada. They went to Philadelphia to observe the work of Dr. Charles Bailey, who had introduced the operation for commissureotomy. After spending two weeks in Philadelphia they returned to Montreal, and Gagnon perfected his technique by animal experimentation and, whenever the opportunity presented itself, on human postmortem specimens. Shortly before their departure for Philadelphia, David had already selected the first patient whom they would treat — a boy of about 17 who had lived in an orphanage until shortly before his admission to the Notre Dame Hospital for haemoptysis. This was shown to be due to very severe mitral stenosis, and thus the boy was an ideal case for treatment with commissureotomy. He had no known relatives and lived in the hospital for several months until Gagnon and David felt that they were ready to perform the operation. David invited me to examine the patient and to express my opinion about the advisability of surgical treatment. I remember with great pleasure the admiration I felt for these two young men who were pioneering surgical treatment of heart disease. My feelings were particularly warm because some months previously I had spoken at a staff meeting of the Montreal General Hospital urging that the surgeons should undertake to perform commissureotomy in suitable cases. I demonstrated four patients with mitral stenosis to draw attention to the difference between those who are good candidates for the operation and those who are not. The Chief Surgeon at the hospital at that time declared that the operation would prove to be ineffectual and that in his opinion it should not be done. Another six or seven years were to elapse before cardiac surgery of this type was undertaken at the Montreal General Hospital. By that time it had already been given worldwide acceptance.

At the Royal Victoria Hospital there was a surgeon, Dr. Arthur Vineberg, eager to perform the operation, but the medical staff were less enthusiastic than he, and it was several years after 1950 that the first commissureotomy was performed there.

David's career at the Notre Dame Hospital was progressing very satisfactorily and he had no intention of interrupting it, when a special event initiated the second phase of his career in Montreal. In 1953 he was the youngest and also the most progressive and best trained cardiologist in the francophone community. He had very early demonstrated his talent for organization and for initiative. It is, therefore, not surprising that when the Order of Grey Nuns was seeking a chief of cardiology for the new hospital they were to build, they invited David to take this post. With great wisdom he looked upon this opportunity as the occasion for examining the future of cardiology in Montreal, and how he could contribute towards furthering its progress in the right direction. Thus he developed the idea of creating an Institute of Cardiology which would fulfil the functions of giving expert treatment to cardiac patients, training new cardiologists, teaching practising physicians the new knowledge in this specialty, and providing facilities for research by competent workers. His first goal was to raise the level of quality to the highest that already existed in North America and later to move forward from this level by way of research to leadership in the field. This would mean a serious change in his own way of life; he would become a full-time employee of the Institute of Cardiology instead of working as a private practitioner. He would face important problems of organization, bringing together the necessary personnel, and attracting money to pay for equipment and to support research. When he made his conditions for accepting the post at the new hospital he expected that he would be rejected because they required a great deal of the new institute. However, negotiations with the Order resulted in the creation of the Institute of Cardiology in 1952, and the Institute began to function in January 1954. The Institute was lodged in a wing of the hospital, where it occupied two stories. There were 45 beds, adequate space for research laboratories, and an assembly room for teaching which provided space for about 100 people. Thus the Montreal Institute of Cardiology started its career. Its many peaks and very few valleys come into view as Paul David's story is told in his biography by Alain Jacques.*

Not surprisingly, in the light of proven skills as an administrator, Paul David served as secretary-treasurer, then as President of the Montreal Cardiac Society, as President of the Canadian Cardiovascular Society, Vice-President of the Canadian Heart Foundation, and President of the Inter-American Society of Cardiology when it met in Montreal in 1964. He was associated with Dr. Paul Dudley White in managing the International Society of Cardiology.

The first item of Dr. David's bibliography which in 1972 numbered more than one hundred articles is unique. No other bibliography which accompanied a questionnaire contains such an article as this first item. It is a letter to the editor entitled "Chez P. D. White et Ch. Laubry" (*Un. Méd. Can.* 1947: 76, 870). Paul David introduced his letter to the editor of the journal with the following comment:

> This title fits precisely the inspiring thought contained in this letter. It places the reader before two men, already illustrious representatives of contemporary cardiology. It describes two typical clinics, one American, the other French. Attending these two special centres makes for clear impressions. I want to describe them to you simply.

**Docteur Paul David, Institut de Cardiologie de Montréal,* 1986; Laporte & Cie (Editeurs) Inc., Case Postale 248, Succursale "C," Montréal, Québec. H2L 4K1. Dr. David himself submitted an excellent 45-page miniautobiography, updated to 1971, for the Archives of the Society.

The letter is in three parts — the first describes what went on in the Department of Cardiology at the Massachusetts General Hospital and the second deals with l'Hôpital de Lariboisière in Paris. Finally, four short paragraphs reflect David's view of what each of these two can contribute to the education of a cardiologist. This letter reflects Dr. David's concern about the process of education. Early in his career he looked for the methods, the technique by which he could communicate what he had learned to those with whom he would be working in Montreal.

The second item of his bibliography is based on work which he did during the year that he spent with Dr. Paul White, "Dissecting Aneurysm of the Aorta" (Paul David, Edgar M. McPeak, Enrique Vivassalas and Paul D. White, *Ann. In. Med.;* 1948: 27, 149). Of the first ten articles which he published after his return to Montreal three are co-authored, the remainder are by him alone. All deal with the diagnosis and management of acquired valvular disease, with the exception of the third item, a case report about complete A-V dissociation in an infant aged five months. In 1948 he wrote item number five, "Les Coeurs Chirurgicaux" (*Un. Méd. Can.* 1948: 77, 954) and in 1950 there appeared the article on mitral commissureotomy which described the first operation of this kind in Canada, "Traitement Chirurgical de la Sténose Mitrale; Commissurotomie" (E. G. Gagnon, Paul David, *Un. Méd. Can.* 1950: 79, 1142.

In 1959 the journal *Union Médicale du Canada* devoted the entire number for the month of November to the publication of original work achieved at the Institute of Cardiology. Dr. David and his colleagues published twelve articles on a wide variety of subjects related to both congenital and acquired heart disease. One team of men wrote a seventeen-page article on open heart surgery giving the results of two series of cases. The earlier one concerned nineteen patients on whom the operations were performed between June 1958 and march 1959. The second series was about thirty-one patients who had their operations between March 1959 and September 1959. This series of articles demonstrated how effectively Paul David gave leadership to the modernization of cardiology in Quebec.

His bibliography includes articles which he published with nearly all those who have worked in the Institute. No less important are those which represent his philosophy as a physician and teacher, for example, item number 63, "La Nécessité de la Recherche dans un Hôpital d'Enseignement" (*Un. Méd. Can.* 1962: 9, 656).

Dr. Gerard Boudreault, 29 May 1914, St-Jérôme, Québec; Laval, M.D. 44; C.P.S.Q. Int. Med. 52 and Card. 53; F.A.C.C.P.

Dr. Boudreault did not mention any details about his postgraduate training. When he submitted his curriculum vitae in 1965 he was associated with Hôtel-Dieu St. Valier de Chicoutimi, and in 1971 when he updated his c.v., he was Chief of Medicine in this hospital and also Assistant Universitaire since he began to serve on its staff.

In his comments on the special questions, Dr. Gerard Boudreault states that he chose to specialize in internal medicine with emphasis on cardiology on the advice of Dr. Napoléon Larochelle of Quebec, because there was no cardiologist in Chicoutimi in the mid-1940s. He bought his first electrocardiograph in 1946. As his parents pioneered in developing a new region of the province, he pioneered in bringing modern medicine, cardiology, to his home city.

Dr. Jean-R. Marcoux, 30 August 1915, St. Cuthbert; Université de Montréal, M.D. 1944; C.P.S.Q. Cardiology 58.

In relatively brief comments on the special questions, Dr. Jean-R. Marcoux tells the story of how a general practitioner obtained the necessary training to practise cardiology in a non-university town. Three times a week, for five years, he travelled from Sorel to Montreal to observe cardiologists at work at the Hôtel-Dieu with adult patients, and at the St. Justine Hospital with children. During the next five years, he made this journey once a week. Then he devoted one year to the Harvard Cardiology course at the Massachusetts General Hospital in Boston. During the subsequent six months he worked in the cardiology department of the Hôtel-Dieu of Montreal. In 1958, he passed the examinations for certification in cardiology in the province of Quebec. He then bought his first electrocardiograph and practised cardiology in Sorel. Regular attendance at meetings of the Canadian Cardiovascular Society made for keeping up-to-date in knowledge.

Dr. Hubert Saint-Pierre, 2 November 1922, Victoriaville, Quebec; Université de Montréal, M.D. 50; F.R.C.P.(C).

Dr. Saint-Pierre chose to practise in Drummondville, population approximately 3,500. Knowing that this city and its region had no cardiologist, he sought thorough training in this specialty and brought modern cardiology to a non-university centre.

After a year of senior internship at the Hôpital Notre Dame in Montreal, he spent three years at the Cleveland Clinic. He co-authored one article with A. C. Corcoran, R.D. Taylor, and H. P. Dustan, "On Relief of Hypertensive Headache by Intravenous Injection of Thiocyanate" (*J.A.M.A.* 1953: 152, 493-495).

Dr. Georges Saulnier, 3 June 1919, Chicoutimi, Quebec; Laval, M.D. 44; C.P.S.Q. Int. Med. 52, Cardiol. 53.

Dr. Georges Saulnier was one of the Province of Quebec's early post-war pupils of Professor Lenègre in Paris.

On returning to civilian life after service in the army (1944-46) he had two years of internship at the Hôtel-Dieu de Québec. During this period, his chief, Dr. Richard Lessard, inspired him to specialize in cardiology. He chose to begin his training in France.

During the two years 1948-1950, he observed the work of Professor Lenègre and his staff. He did much reading culminating in the composition of a thesis on the incidence of pain in myocardial infarction. With this thesis he earned the title *Assistant-étranger des Hopitaux de Paris.* During the following year, he worked on the medical service of Dr. Ray Farquharson at the Toronto General Hospital. Immediately after this, in 1951, he joined the medical department of the Hôtel-Dieu de Québec. In 1965 when he filled in the questionnaire, he was Professeur Agrégé at Laval University and Chief of Cardiology at the Hôtel-Dieu de Québec.

Dr. Gilles Leduc, 14 October 1923, Montreal; University of Ottawa, B.A. 44; Université de Montréal, M.D. 59; C.P.S.Q. Cardiol. and Int. Med 55; F.A.C.C. 66.

Dr. Gilles Leduc, a pioneer of post-World War II cardiology developed his career as a member of the medical staff of the Hôtel-Dieu de Montréal. In 1965, he wrote about his choice of cardiology and training:

> I decided to specialize in cardiology in 1952 while I was a resident in internal medicine at the Hôtel-Dieu. I came to this decision especially because there was at this time much interesting progress in the advancement of heart surgery. Many physicians and surgeons were particularly concerned with the introduction of heart surgery. But, of course, the personal influence of my Chief, Dr. Rodrigue Lefebvre was an important factor. The devotion to his patients, his love of medicine and his competence influenced me greatly and made the practice of cardiology

most attractive. Besides which, the fact that one could make a complete examination, including an electrocardiogram and a fluoroscopic and then arrive at a precise diagnosis was for me a most attractive aspect. Is there any other 'discipline' in which one can make a relatively precise diagnosis so readily?

I went to the United States and France for my special studies in cardiology. It was by my own initiative that I obtained the opportunities to study cardiology as a specialty. I was fortunate in getting a bursary in the U.S.A. and to work for two years in the cardiopulmonary laboratory at St. Luke's Hospital, New York City. My Chief at that time, Dr. Cathcart, was a great inspiration for me. The extensive study of cardiac and pulmonary physiology was a turning point in my career and I must say I still feel the influence of those two years.

Shortly after, I continued my studies in France with Professor Lenègre. He too played an important role in my medical education and it was with his book on electrocardiology that I was able to synthesize my knowledge of this subject. My clinical training was greatly enhanced by this great French cardiologist.

When I came back to Montreal, Dr. Lefebvre invited me to join the staff of cardiologists at the Hôtel-Dieu: he realized at that time that there should be in the Department a cardiologist knowledgeable about the more recent advances in cardiology.

In 1971, when Dr. Leduc updated his curriculum vitae, he was director of the Hypertension Clinic at the Montreal Institute for Clinical Research and Professeur Agrégé at the Université de Montréal.

Dr. Leduc's bibliography of 10 items deals with quite a wide variety of subjects. The first is "Peripheral Assimilation of Fructose in Man" (*Proc. Soc. Exp. Biol. Med.* 1953). The fourth is "Pericardite Chronique constrictive Post Traumatique" (*C.M.A.J.* 1962). The tenth is "Evaluation de l'Aptine, un Nouveau Beta-Bloqueur dans le Traitment de l'Angine de Poitrine" (*Un. Méd. Can.*, juin 1971).

Dr. Yves Desrochers, 8 February 1927, Montreal; Université de Paris, B.A. 45; Université de Montréal, M.D. 51; C.P.S.Q. Cardiologie 57; F.A.C.C.; F.A.C.C.P.

Dr. Yves Desrochers' postgraduate education began with medical internship and residency in cardiology at the Notre Dame Hospital in Montreal (1951-1953), followed by residency at the Montreal Institute of Cardiology (1954). After this, he had a year at the Massachusetts General Hospital Cardiology Department on the Harvard Medical School postgraduate education program. He capped these formative years with a year in Paris at the Hôpital Lariboisière (1955-1956). He then joined the staff of the Institute of Cardiology and took a special interest in electrocardiography and vectocardiography. In 1964, he became chief of cardiology at the Hôpital Maisonneuve.

In his brief comments on the special questions, Dr. Desrochers tells how he was influenced to choose a career in cardiology.

> I seriously considered specializing in cardiology at the time of my internship at the Notre Dame Hospital, 1950-1951, when the first mitral commissureotomy in Canada was performed by Dr. Edouard Gagnon. During service in cardiology I became a close friend of Dr. Osman Gialloreto who had just come from Europe after having learned the technique of cardiac catheterization in Professor Lenègre's clinic in Paris. Dr. Gialloreto taught me the basic concepts of electrocardiography and haemodynamics. Thus I participated in the first cardiac catheterization and angiocardiography studies at the Notre Dame Hospital. Having become familiar with pre-operative studies of cardiac patients and post-operative complications of cardiac surgery I became especially interested in the practice of cardiology in the course of the two years of internship.

Dr. James Eastwood Gibbons, 22 February 1926, Smiths Falls, Ontario; Queen's University, M.D., C.M. 50, F.A.A.P.; F.A.C.C.; C.P.S.Q. Cardiol. 58.

Dr. Gibbons belongs to the pioneers of paediatric cardiology. He trained for this specialty and developed his career at the Montreal Children's Hospital. He commented in 1972:

> I seriously became interested in specializing in cardiology working with Drs. A. L. Johnson and Charlotte Ferencz in 1954 following training in Internal Medicine at the Royal Victoria Hospital. Dr. J. S. L. Browne and Dr. Richard Murphy (deceased) assisted me in obtaining the appointment as Fellow in Cardiology and Instructor in Medicine in Duke University for two years, 1954-1956. The sub-specialty of Paediatric Cardiology was advancing rapidly in 1956 and I was fortunate enough to join an active and progressive department at the Montreal Children's Hospital with Dr. Arnold L. Johnson.

When Dr. Gibbons updated his curriculum vitae in 1972, he was Associate Professor in the McGill Medical Faculty, Director of the

Department of Cardiology at the Montreal Children's Hospital and Consultant in Cardiology at the Royal Victoria Hospital.

Between 1955 and 1972, Dr. Gibbons' bibliography grew to thirteen items, all on subjects related to the cardiovascular system. The last item is a chapter in *Conn's Current Therapy* (1973) on "Congenital Malformations of the Heart."

Dr. Emile Marcotte, 18 November 1932; St. Basile, Quebec; Laval, M.D. 58; C.P.S.Q. Méd. Int. 62; C.P.S.Q. Cardiologie 63; F.R.C.P.(C) 63; F.A.C.C.

After graduation in 1958, Dr. Emile Marcotte spent the next five years on postgraduate training in Montreal, at Hôpital Maisonneuve, Queen Mary Veterans Hospital, The Institute of Cardiology and at the Hôtel-Dieu de Montréal where he worked with Dr. Jacques Genest.

In 1963, he joined the staff of the Hôtel-Dieu de Montréal. He exemplifies the generation of physicians who could obtain excellent training in cardiology in Canada, once those who had gone abroad returned to establish centres of research and teaching.

In 1965, when he filled in the questionnaire he commented briefly on the special questions. He decided to specialize in cardiology in 1957 during his junior internship year at the Maisonneuve Hospital in which the Montreal Institute of Cardiology was situated at that time.

In 1965, he was Moniteur at the Université de Montréal and was a consultant in cardiology at the Lakeshore Hospital.

Dr. Robert Francis Patrick Cronin, 1 September 1926, London, England; Princeton 49; McGill, M.D. 53; M.Sc. (Med) 60; M.R.C.P. (London) 55; F.R.C.P.(C) 58; F.A.C.P., F.A.H.A., F.A.C.C., C.S.C.I., A.O.A.

Dr. R. F. P. (Pat) Cronin began postgraduate work at McGill and continued to study at London Postgraduate Hospital, the Brompton Chest Hospital in England, and at the Massachusetts Memorial Hospital in Boston. When he filled in the questionnaire in 1965 he was Assistant Professor of Medicine and Physiology at McGill and Assistant Physician and Assistant Cardiologist at the Montreal General Hospital. He did not make any comments on the special questions. His career is unique in that he devoted himself equally to physiology and to clinical medicine and restricted his activities within the academic sphere. In 1972, he was Dean of the Faculty of Medicine, a post he held for five years.

Between 1958 and 1965, Dr. Cronin's bibliography grew to eight items which deal with both clinical and experimental work. The first item is on "Venous Pressure and Venous Pulse in Clinical Examination" (*C.M.A.J.*, 1958: 78, 337). The fourth item, co-authored with J. B. Calatayud, is "Haemodynamic effects of synchronous arterio-arterial pumping following experimental myocardial infarction" (*Am. J. Cardiol.*, 1963: 11, 768). The eighth item, co-authored with S. Moore and D. G. Marpole, is "Shock Following Myocardial Infarction: A Clinical Survey of 140 Cases" (*C.M.A.J.*, 1965: 93).

Dr. Yvon Goulet; 1 May 1929, Montreal; Université de Montréal, M.D. 55; C.S.P.Q. Med. and Cardiol. 60; F.R.C.P.(C), F.A.C.C.

Dr. Yvon Goulet represents an early generation of students who could obtain a complete training in cardiology, either medical or surgical, in Montreal in either francophone or anglophone institutions. He completed his training in Internal Medicine at the Notre Dame Hospital and in cardiology at the Institute of Cardiology. Then he spent a year in Paris observing the work of Professor Soulié and his colleagues at l'Hôpital Lariboisière. Dr. Goulet was an early devoté of exercise in the prevention and treatment of cardiovascular disease. He organized a rehabilitation department at the Notre Dame Hospital.

With Drs. B. Leboeuf and R. Johnson, Dr. Goulet co-authored an article on "Pulmonary Oedema" (*Un. Méd. Can.*, 1958: 87, 1532-39). His bibliography includes reports of some unusual cases. The last item is, "Le Traitment des Troubles du Rhythme au Cours de l'Infarctus du Myocarde" (*Un. Méd. Can.*, 1967: 96, 818-22).

Dr. André Proulx, 4 November 1925, Montreal; Université de Montréal, B.A. (*summa cum laude*) 46, M.D. (*summa cum laude*) 51; C.P.S.Q. (Int. Med) 55; C.P.S.Q. (Cardiol.) 56; F.R.C.P.(C) 60; F.A.C.C. 64.

Ten years after Dr. Proulx completed his postgraduate education, he made an interesting comment. During the year that he spent in Paris his experience was restricted to making rounds with the great chiefs. He missed the opportunity of being responsible for clinical work. Apparently, in France at that time, there were very few opportunities for the equivalent of internships and residencies in departments of cardiology.

Dr. Proulx's postgraduate education began with two years internship in Internal Medicine at the Hôpital St. Luc in Montreal, followed by a year at l'Hôpital Boucicaut in Paris. His questionnaire comment about his experience in France is "Entrainement à Paris est plus difficile à cause de l'absence de pôste au responsabilités.

Travail consistant à observer et à suivre les grands patrons." (Training in Paris was more difficult because of the absence of positions of responsibility. The education consisted of observing and of following the big chiefs.)

After he entered practice, he continued to attend courses to maintain his ongoing education in electrophysiology, phonocardiography and cardiovascular physiology. Between 1952 and 1970, twenty-seven items accumulated in his bibliography. The titles of his publications are for the most part on pragmatic subjects relating to diagnosis and therapy.

In 1971, when Dr. Proulx updated his curriculum vitae, he held the post of Assistant Professeur en Médicine Interne at Université de Montréal, and chef des Service de Cardiologie and chef du service de Medicine at the Hôpital Sacré Coeur. Service on various important committees is listed in his curriculum vitae.

Dr. Proulx's bibliography grew to 27 items between 1952 and 1970. The first four deal with general medical topics. The fifth is a thesis for which he earned the title "Assistant-étranger en Cardiologie." The thesis contains a study of the literature plus what he observed in the activities of others at Hôpital Boucicaut. Its title is "Conformation électrique hemodynamique et anatomique dans l'Hypertrophie ventriculaire droite." The eleventh item is "S.G.O.T. in Myocardial Infarction," a paper he delivered at the meeting of the Canadian Cardiovascular Society in Quebec City in 1956. The 25th, co-authored with M. Doray is "Le Syndrome Post-Infarctus du Myocarde" (*Un. Med. Can.*, 1964: 93, No. 1).

Dr. Gaston Mercier, 9 April 1929, Matane, Quebec; St. Dunstan's, Charlottetown, B.Sc. 50; Laval, M.D. 55; C.S.P.Q. Cardiology 60.

Dr. Gaston Mercier's postgraduate education began with three years at Hôpital de l'Enfant Jésu followed by the Harvard University course in cardiology at the Massachusetts General Hospital (1958-59). He completed this phase of his career with a year at Hôpital Boucicaut in Paris. He returned to practise cardiology as the one cardiologist at l'Hôpital de l'Enfant Jésu, Quebec City.

His bibliography of six items includes the report of a case of congenital anomaly of the left coronary artery with myocardial infarction in an infant. This article is co-authored with Fernand Hould and Roland Leclerc (*Un. Méd. Can.*, 1963: 92). The sixth item, co-authored with George Patryis, is "Quebec Beer Drinker's Cardiomyopathy; Clinical Signs and Symptoms" (*C.M.A.J.* 1967: 97, 884-888).

Dr. Wilfred Howard Palmer, 3 April 1929, Montreal; McGill, B.Sc. 52, M.D., C.M. 56; F.R.C.P.(C); C.S.P.Q. Int. Med. and Cardiol.

Dr. Palmer's postgraduate education included internships at the Royal Victoria and Queen Mary Veterans hospitals and on the cardiorespiratory service jointly managed by the Montreal Children's and the Royal Victoria hospitals. Dr. Palmer has pursued an academic career. In 1968, he was Assistant Professor of Medicine at McGill and Assistant Physician at the Royal Victoria Hospital.

His bibliography grew to 12 items between 1958 and 1968, all co-authored with colleagues of the Royal Victoria Hospital. The fourth item, co-authored with Dr. M. McGregor, is "The Mechanism of Angina Pectoris" (*Proceedings of the 7th Hahnemann Symposium, 1962,* Grune and Stratton, N.Y., 1963).

Dr. Henry Frank Mizgala; 28 November 1932, Montreal; Loyola College, B.A. (*magna cum laude*) 53; McGill, M.D., C.M. 57; F.R.C.P.(C) 62; C.P.S.Q. (Cardiol.) 62; A.O.A., F.A.C.C., F.A.H.A.

After internship in Montreal during the years 1957-1960, Dr. Henry P. Mizgala was granted a Dazian Fellowship in Cardiology at Mount Sinai Hospital, New York. In this respect his training is unique for although this hospital had one of the best cardiology departments in the world and in 1957 Dr. Charles Friedberg, the author of the great textbook on *Diseases of the Heart,* was its chief, Dr. Mizgala is one of a very few Canadians who trained there. He spent the years 1960-62 there and returned to Montreal to develop his career.

In 1972, he was Associate Professor of Medicine at McGill University and Associate Cardiologist at the Montreal General Hospital. His bibliography grew to nine items between 1963 and 1970; all are co-authored and all deal with problems related to medical therapeutics of cardiovascular disease. He also presented six papers at medical meetings during these years. In 1971, he delivered a paper at the meeting of the Royal College of Physicians and Surgeons of Canada on "The Sick Sinus Syndrome: Clinical Manifestations and Pathology."

Dr. Reginald Antoine Nadeau, 18 December 1932, St. Léonard, N.B.; Loyola College 52; Université de Montréal, M.D. 57; F.R.C.P.(C), C.S.P.Q. (Cardiologie); F.A.C.C.

Dr. Nadeau began his postgraduate education with a year in the Department of Physiology of his alma mater and the following year served an internship at the Montreal Institute of Cardiology. There followed four years at the Henry Ford Hospital and a year (1963-1964) at the Nuffield Institute of Medical Research in Oxford, England. On returning to Montreal, he chose to continue his career in physiology. When he filled in the questionnaire in 1968, he was Associate Professor of Physiology at the Université de Montréal.

Between 1956 and 1968, his bibliography grew to 55 items. The first article is co-authored with J. Sternberg on "A Simple Method for the Determination of Protein-Bound Sugar" (*Can. J. Pub. Health,* 1956: 47, 44). The second item, co-authored with M. Savard and Y. Desrochers, is "Dextroversion du Coeur avec Transposition des Vaisseaux de la Base, sans autre Anomalié Associé" (*Un. Méd. Can.*, 1959: 88, 1435). Many of his articles are co-authored and deal with pharmacological studies.

Dr. Serge Renaud, 21 November 1927; Bordeaux, France B.A. 47; Université de Montréal Veterinary School, D.M.V. 57; Ph.D. 60.

When Dr. Renaud joined the staff of the Montreal Institute of Cardiology in 1963 as Chief of the Laboratory of Experimental Pathology, he had unique credentials which included the degree V.M.D. from the Veterinary School of the Université de Montréal (1959), Ph.D. (1960) from the same university, and the experience of working with Dr. Hans Selye in experimental medicine since 1957. By the year 1965, his bibliography listed 30 items, the first 24 on work done under Dr. Selye and the last six on arteriosclerosis and thrombosis, studies made at the Institute of Cardiology.

Dr. Benoit Tousignant, 7 September 1927, Ste-Thécle, Québec; Laval, B.A. 51; M.D. 57; C.P.S.Q. Cardiol. 62.

In his comments on the special questions, Dr. Tousignant relates that his chief, Dr. Adélard Tétrault, strongly advised him to seek training in cardiology so that the hospital in Trois Rivières would be assured of the services of a cardiologist when Tétrault retired. Accordingly, after two years of internship at the Hôtel-Dieu de Québec, he worked for two years (1963-1965) under Dr. Paul David at the Montreal Institute of Cardiology. In 1968, when he filled in the questionnaire, he was a member of the staff of the Hôpital St. Joseph de Trois Rivières. Concerning the influence of the Canadian Cardiovascular Society on his career, he wrote that by attending the annual meetings regularly, he enjoys the friendship of members from all parts of Canada and is stimulated in his activities in ongoing education.

Dr. John Herbert Burgess, 24 May 1933, Montreal; McGill, B.Sc. 54; M.D., C.M. 58; F.R.C.P.(C) 63; C.S.P.Q. Int. Med. 63; C.S.P.Q. Cardiol. 66; F.A.H.A.; F.A.C.C.; C.S.C.I.

In 1968 Dr. Burgess related the story of his postgraduate education, presenting a good picture of available opportunities during the decade 1958 to 1968.

> Interest in a career in Internal Medicine developed in second year of medical school and continued thereafter — interest in Cardiology developed about the same time. Interest in an academic career in Investigative Clinical Medicine especially cardiopulmonary research began as a junior intern and continued into the second year of residency training at the Montreal General Hospital. This interest was accelerated by an association with Dr. A. S. E. Reid and the cardiac clinic at the M.G.H. It was during this year that I tried to become acquainted with the reading of E.C.Gs and also took part in my first experiences with right heart catheterization.
>
> Half way through my second year at M.G.H. I decided to go away for two years of my pre-fellowship training in order to gain further experience in cardiopulmonary research and also clinical cardiology. It was at this time that I met with the only real problems in career planning — that is, the decision of where to go. After some discussion with various people in the field I decided against an appointment at the London Heart Hospital under the late Dr. Paul Wood in favour of two years with Professor W. Melville Arnott and associates in Birmingham, England. This later proved to be a very wise decision as it was here that I was able to get my first real taste of cardiopulmonary research on a ward that was oriented towards this. In England my major research interest was in the diffusing capacity of the lungs, but I also took part in the cardiac catheterization program. On leaving England to return to Montreal I had already decided to seek further training in this field in Dr. Comroe's laboratory if possible, on completion of my Canadian Fellowship.
>
> After two more years in general clinical medicine at M.G.H. I went to the Cardiovascular Research Institute in San Francisco. Here I continued my interest in cardiopulmonary research more on the haemodynamic side this time rather than pulmonary, and spent a major amount of time so far in a research project involving left heart catheterization. The present plan is to stay here

until the summer of 1966 before returning to the Department of Medicine, Division of Cardiology, at the Montreal General Hospital.

The major influence in determining Montreal as a place to live and work has been the long association with the M.G.H. through my father [Chief of Dermatology] and of course having been born and bred in Montreal. The practice of cardiology will probably be secondary to doing clinical investigation in this field on a geographic full time basis.

In 1971, when Dr. Burgess updated the questionnaire, he was Director of the Cardiorespiratory Laboratory at the Montreal General Hospital and Associate Professor of Medicine, McGill University. The first item of his bibliography is an article he co-authored with J. M. Bishop, "Pulmonary Diffusing Capacity and its Subdivisions in Polycythema Vera," (*J. Clin. Invest.*, 1963; 42, 997-1006). This article reflects the new departure in the organization of a research laboratory, the change from cardiovascular to cardiorespiratory for which Dr. Burgess had excellent training.

Dr. Paul-Emile Roy, 8 December 1929, Cap-Chat, Co. Gaspé N., Quebec; Laval, M.D. 58; C.S.P.Q. Anat. Path. 66.

Dr. Paul-Emile Roy, a pathologist who joined the team led by Yves Morin in the investigation of the Quebec beer-drinkers' cardiomyopathy, became intensely interested in matters cardiological. After internship at Hôtel-Dieu de Quebec, he studied pathology at the Mallory Institute in Boston. At the time that he filled in the questionnaire in 1972, he was Professeur Agrégé at Université Laval and Pathologist at the Hôpital Laval and the Institute of Cardiology.

The first item in his bibliography is "Xiphoid Mediastinoscopy for Permanent Myocardial Implantation of a Modified Electrode, Preliminary Report" (*J. Surg. Res.*, 1971; 11, 342-34). The seventh was co-authored with J. Dorais and P. J. Morin: "Les Foyers de Necrose Intracellulaire Focale dans le Muscle Cardiaque Humain" (accepted for publication in *Ann. Anat. Path.*, in 1972).

Dr. Martial G. Bourassa, 14 May 1931, St. Barnabé North; Laval, B.A. 54; M.D. 59; C.S.P.Q. Cardiol. 64; C.S.I.M.Q. 64; F.A.C.C.; F.A.H.A.; F.I.C.A.

Dr. Bourassa's postgraduate education began with two years of internship and residency at the Buffalo General Hospital (1959-1961), followed by a year of cardiology at the City of Hope Medical

Center in Los Angeles. In 1962, he joined the medical staff of the Montreal Institute of Cardiology. At the time when he filled in the questionnaire in 1972 his status at the Université de Montréal was Assistant Professeur de Clinique.

Dr. Bourassa's bibliography grew to 48 items between 1962 and 1972. The first item is co-authored with colleagues of the City of Hope Medical Center, G. M. Boiteau and B. J. Allenstein, "Haemodynamic Studies during Intermittent Left Bundle Branch Block" (*Am. J. Cardiol.*, 1962; 10, 792). All but two items are co-authored with both surgical and medical colleagues at the Montreal Institute of Cardiology, and deal with a wide variety of clinical subjects studied with the most modern methods. One of those two items concerns the description of an invention by Dr. Bourassa, "Preshaped Polyethylene Catheters for Percutaneous Haemodynamic and Angiographic Studies" (*Angiology,* 1971; 22).

Dr. Gaston Choquette, 13 March 1921, Montreal; Université de Montréal, B.A. 42, M.D. 50; C.P.S.Q. Cardiology 56; C.P.S.Q. Int. Med. 57.

Dr. Choquette composed an effective description of how he chose cardiology as his specialty and how he found opportunities for training.

> I chose to specialize in cardiology while I was in general practice. I spent my mornings at the Notre Dame Hospital at the cardiology and allergy clinics. After a few months of deliberation, I decided to train for the practice of cardiology. As soon as I made my decision I asked several of the doctors with whom I had worked in Montreal, for letters of recommendation so that I might apply for study in Boston, New York and then Philadelphia. In Philadelphia, I was immediately offered the opportunity to do research in endocrinology. During this period I obtained a position at the University of Pennsylvania to do research in cardiovascular physiology with Dr. Lysle Petersen. Following this I had the opportunity of working with Dr. Samuel Bellet in the Department of Cardiology at the Graduate Hospital of the University of Pennsylvania. Ultimately, I was offered the opportunity to complete my training in internal medicine there at this same hospital.
>
> As you may now realize, it was these offers at the opportune time which were decisive in determining the exact nature of my training. In 1957, when I came back from the U.S. I received my certification in cardiology, bought my electrocardiograph and entered the practice of cardiology.

In 1957, Dr. Choquette joined the staff of the Montreal Institute of Cardiologie. He has had a special interest in epidemiology of coronary heart disease and in rehabilitation after myocardial infarction. Dr. Choquette did not send his bibliography.

Dr. Reginald Johnson, 3 November 1918, Danville, Quebec; Université de Montréal, M.D. 47; C.S.P.Q. Int. Med. and Cardiol. 53; F.R.C.P.(C); F.A.C.C.; F.A.C.C.P.

Dr. Reginald Johnson filled the gap in the medical cardiology staff at Notre Dame Hospital of Montreal when Dr. Paul David resigned to undertake the creation of the Heart Institute in 1954. Dr. Johnson's comments on the special questions written in 1965 tell the story of his pioneering:

> My internship with Dr. Paul David at the Notre Dame Hospital was decisive in making my choice of cardiology and this happened during the first year of my senior internship in 1948.
>
> The main difficulty I had in arranging for post-graduate study was financial. I overcame this obstacle by making a loan at the bank and by receiving a scholarship of $1,000 per year for two years from the Provincial Government.
>
> I must add that by deciding on my specialty rather early I later had to do some special work to build up my experience in internal medicine. I achieved this by devoting six months to preparation for the examinations of the Royal College of Physicians in Internal Medicine. At the beginning of my career I had an appointment at St. Mary's Hospital and the City of St. Laurent Hospital. When Dr. Paul David resigned from the Notre Dame Hospital I gained the advantage of obtaining an appointment there. I first bought an electrocardiograph in 1952.

In 1971 when he updated his curriculum vitae he was chief of cardiology at the Notre Dame Hospital, and Professeur Agrégé at Université de Montréal. Dr. Johnson did not provide his bibliography.

Dr. Robert Potvin, 27 July 1930, Quebec; Laval, B.A. 48, M.D. 53, F.R.C.P.(C) 58; C.S.P.Q. Cardiol. & Int. Med. 59.

In his brief response to the special questions, Dr. Potvin summarized his postgraduate education.

I decided to specialize in Cardiology during my internship. I was very much interested in physiology and was attracted by its application to the practice of cardiology.

I believe that I was very much influenced in my training by Dr. Jean Fortier who had himself specialized in Cardiology in London, England. I worked under him as a senior intern and he helped me plan my trip to London. I was then fortunate enough to obtain a McLaughlin Scholarship which enabled me to spend a little over a year in London and a year at the Toronto General Hospital. After completing my training, I returned to St. François d'Assise Hospital to become assistant in the service of Medicine under Docteur Fortier. Shortly afterwards, I joined the staff of the "Institut de Cardiologie de l'Hôpital Laval" which had just been founded. I have been working there on a part-time basis ever since. I started practising in 1958 and bought my electrocardiograph then.

Ontario

Dr. Samuel Mirsky, 19 May 1899, Ottawa; McGill, B.Sc. 21; M.D., C.M. 24; R.C.P.(C) Cert. Int. Med.; F.A.C.P.

Dr. Mirsky had internships at the Mount Sinai Hospital in New York (1925) and the Sinai Hospital in Baltimore (1926-27). In 1965 he composed a succinct summary of the *status quo* of cardiology during his career as a pioneer internist in Ottawa.

> I have never considered myself a cardiologist, but do see myself as an internist with an interest in cardiology. When I left McGill in 1924, we had a fairly sound basic understanding of heart failure and the use of digitalis, but basically heart disease was known to be due to rheumatic fever, syphilis or congenital abnormality. Even though coronary thrombosis had been described by Herrick in 1912, it was never really discussed in our classroom or clinics. Angina pectoris was discussed as a peculiar vague illness sometimes causing death.
>
> Little wonder, therefore, when around the autopsy table at Mount Sinai Hospital in 1926, as Louis Gross was questioning the interns as to their diagnosis, I mentioned coronary thrombosis — he looked up at me and made one of his not unfamiliar

jibes — about how a fathead could be so bright as to think of coronary thrombosis.

In Baltimore, in 1927, there were a few very seriously interested men working in a little corner with the big Cambridge machine — but very few staff men were interested in their efforts. Our chiefs felt the machine was only helpful in arrhythmias and then they felt a good clinician could recognize the arrhythmias without the machine.

This was rather discouraging, and so I started practice in Ottawa in 1928 without any knowledge of the electrocardiograms. However, two internists in Ottawa about this time did get machines and needless to say, their misinterpretation on a few occasions did not help to instil faith or interest in the subject.

It was the recognition of the typical Pardee curve of myocardial infarction that gave a great stimulus to electrocardiography, and from then on, we began to ask for electrocardiograms on our patients [Pardee, 1920, 1928].

It was during the war, however, when I had the privilege of working with internists from all the medical schools in Canada that my interest and knowledge increased and in 1945 when I returned to Canada I bought an electrocardiograph.

I have to this day never mastered the fine points in interpreting the graphs, but I have developed a most intense admiration of the young men who come to us with such keen knowledge and wisdom and whose help I depend upon.

One of the men whose influence was very great on the profession in Ottawa was Elmer Plunkett. When I returned to Ottawa after the war, Dr. Plunkett was the Dean of Internal Medicine in Ottawa. He created an atmosphere among the internists that could be described as a fraternity dedicated to furthering knowledge of medical diseases. He was an excellent clinician, he read voraciously and remembered all he read. He shared his knowledge with us all. He was never too busy to discuss a problem, he was always willing to be of help.

His knowledge of cardiology spurred us on to learn more and this attitude of a scholarly fraternity prevails among Ottawa internists more so than in any other community in Canada. His premature death caused us much grief, but his memory lives on.

It was to Elmer I most frequently turned for an interpretation of an unusual cardiogram. After his death, it was the younger men, some of whom were inspired by the teachings of Dr. Harold Segall, whose assistance I obtained.

The advent of phonocardiography and cardiac catheterizations came to Ottawa in the last few years. Coronary angiography has as yet not been performed here.

Having served as Chief of Medicine for D.V.A. [Department of Veterans' Affairs] in the Ottawa District since 1951, having been Chief of Medicine at the Civic Hospital for four years, having been Treasurer of the Academy of Medicine of Ottawa for four years and President for one year, I have had an opportunity to learn not only about patients, but also about doctors. This I have found of great interest.

As I grew older I began to see the greater issues involved in medicine. I was the first President of our Rehabilitation Institute, and I am now engaged in trying to develop a Geriatric Study Centre for Ottawa.

Dr. Mirsky did not submit his bibliography.

Dr. Mitchell Kohan (17 October 1900-8 July 1965)

Dr. Kohan enjoyed the privileges of growing up in the small town of Midland, Ontario (population of about 7,000) situated near Georgian Bay. He entered a five-year course at the University of Toronto to study medicine in 1918 directly from high school. Consequently, he was only twenty-three years old when he graduated. His internship at the Buffalo General Hospital may have lasted at most two years. Thus, he began the practice of medicine at about the age of 25. He took the exams for the fellowship of the Royal College of Physicians of Canada and became a fellow at the age of 53. This phenomenon is an expression of his devotion to his own program of continual postgraduate education. He practised internal medicine with a special interest in cardiology. He gained the necessary expertise by persisting in reading, attending national and international meetings, and taking special courses in cardiology. He became Chief of the Department of Medicine of the New Mount Sinai Hospital and gave leadership to the successful effort which resulted in integration of the Mount Sinai Hospital with the University as a teaching unit. He was appointed Associate Professor of Medicine. A good measure of his influence as a teacher, especially on residents and interns, is gleaned from the fact that in 1963, the 'men in white' at the Mount Sinai Hospital presented him with their award for the best teacher of the year. At the time of his retirement from the active staff of the Hospital, he was presented with a portrait which now adorns a wall in the hospital auditorium.

He was a regular member of the audience at nearly all of the meetings of the Canadian Cardiovascular Society since 1948.

His career is of special interest because it exemplifies the scholarly physician who needed no special reward except that of achievement in his work to motivate his continuing education.

Dr. William Welmore Priddle, 1904, Eden, Ont.; University of Western Ontario, B.A. 1922; M.D. 26; F.A.C.P.; F.A.G.S.; Cert. Int. Med., R.C.P.

After internship and Assistant Residency at the Buffalo General Hospital, Dr. Priddle went to England and worked at St. Bartholomew's Hospital and at the National Heart Hospital.

When engaged in general practice in Almond, New York, (1928-29), he experimented with a low sodium regime in the treatment of hypertension and observed some favourable results. Later, when he settled in Toronto, he developed a special interest in Geriatrics and served as Consultant Cardiologist to the Geriatric Study Centre in Toronto.

His bibliography of thirteen items deals mainly with clinical observations in the treatment of hypertension and with problems related to geriatrics.

Dr. Hugh Addison Mitchell, 15 February 1898, Grand Valley, Ont., 10 Feb. 1968, Peterborough, Ont.; University of Manitoba, M.D. 27; F.R.C.P.(C).

The curriculum vitae of Dr. Hugh Addison Mitchell was composed by his widow in June 1968; he had died on 10 February 1968. After graduation M.D. from the University of Manitoba, in 1927, he interned at the Winnipeg General Hospital and then did general practice in Saskatchewan. He attended postgraduate courses in Toronto (1934) and in England (1936-37). He settled in Peterborough in 1937, acquired a string galvanometer in 1938, and practised as an internist with a special interest in cardiovascular disease. He was on the medical staff of the Peterborough Civic Hospital and the St. Joseph's Hospital. He was a charter member of the Canadian Cardiovascular Society.

Dr. Lewis Dewitt Wilcox, 1 August 1905, London, Ont.; University of Western Ontario, M.D. 1928; F.R.C.P.(C) 1937.

Dr. Wilcox began his postgraduate training with a rotating internship at the Brantford General Hospital, followed by an internship in Ophthalmology at the Royal Victoria Hospital, Montreal, and then in Medicine at Johns Hopkins and the Baltimore General Hospital. In 1965, Dr. Wilcox was Clinical Associate and Professor of Medicine at the University of Western Ontario and on the staff of the Victoria General Hospital.

My postgraduate training was all done in the field of general medicine and at no time did I ever practise Cardiology as anything more than an important part of medicine.

I was of course influenced by my contacts with Dr. Jonathan Meakins, W. De M. Scriver, W. F. Hamilton, G. R. Brow, H. B. Cushing and others during my Montreal experience. I spent a good bit of time with Dr. Maude Abbott when I was on the paediatric service there, and I continued to keep in touch with her after leaving Montreal.

In Baltimore I was influenced by Louis Hamman, T. R. Boggs, and especially W. S. Thayer, along with John King and William Reinhoff. While at Hopkins I strongly urged the ligation of a patent ductus, and I have an interesting letter written by John King twenty years later regretting that they had not followed my urging about this question on a patient I showed to Dr. Thayer in 1933. Dr. Reinhoff would have been the surgeon since he alone had done any chest work.

I began practice in London in the fall of 1934. Things were made to appear very congenial to me, so far as McGill and the Royal Victoria were concerned, but because of the smaller size of London and the presence of a medical school here I decided to try this area since it seemed to offer the advantages in practice and teaching which I was interested in at that time. My home town was Stratford and this meant proximity to the family base. Dr. E. R. Bartram bought his cardiograph here in 1935 and I well remember that I did not wish to be known as a heart specialist only, and it was not until 1950 that I acquired an electrocardiograph.

In the spring of 1935 Dr. Bartram and I had lines on two patients with patent ducti. At the same time we spoke with Dr. Henry Christian when he was speaking to the Tri-State Meeting in Detroit about the proposed operation. Dr. Christian felt that it was not a very good idea and he was very much afraid that an aneurysm would develop at the area where the ductus was tied. We had no chest surgeon in London until 1938 and of course Robert Gross preceded all by then.

A letter which the late Dr. Maude Abbott wrote to Dr. Wilcox on

March 25, 1935 is of considerable historical interest. The letter begins as follows:

> Dear Dr. Wilcox ... I was very glad to hear from you, and needless to say I am extremely interested in your case of patent ductus and your suggestion that the condition might be cured by ligation of this channel.

Dr. Abbott agreed that the operation should be feasible and effective, provided a good thoracic surgeon would do the work. She thought that the chief risk was an intercurrent subacute infection, involving the pulmonary artery. She referred to a case in which she had recommended resection of the ligamentum arteriosum in the case of a puppy when this had caused dysphagia. The comment appeared in *Blumer's Bedside Diagnosis,* Vol. II: 385.

This letter to Dr. Wilcox exemplifies the method in which she worked. The last paragraph of the letter reads as follows:

> On account of your interest in cardiac anomalies, I thought you would like to know more of the work of the Museums Association, so am sending you a copy of the new issue of our *Journal of Technical Methods,* which is just out. As you will see, we specialize not only on technical subjects, but also on cardiac anomalies and teratology, and we have a very full program and symposium in this field at our next meeting in April, of which I will send you a program as soon as it is issued. If you would like to join, I will send you an application form. The annual fee is $3.00 and includes the subscription to the Bulletin.

Regrettably, Dr. Wilcox does not list the Museums Association among his memberships.

An interesting item in Dr. Wilcox's bibliography is the presentation which he made at the 1964 Interamerican Congress of Cardiology in Montreal: "The Coronary Explanation to the Patient."

Dr. Walter Ford Connell, 24 August 1906, Kingston; Queen's University, M.D., C.M. 29; F.R.C.P.(C); F.R.C.P. (London); F.A.C.P.; F.A.C.C.; F.A.H.A.

Dr. Connell's postgraduate education included a fellowship in pathology at the Pathologisches Institut, Freiburg in Breisgau, and a period at Victoria University in Manchester (1931-32). During the next two years, he worked at the National Hospital for Nervous Diseases, Queen's Square and at the National Heart Hospital, London. In 1965, when he submitted his curriculum vitae, he was professor and head of the Department of Medicine at Queen's University, Chief of Medicine and Director of the Heart Department at the Kingston General Hospital.

Teaching and practising internal medicine as I do at Queen's, I cannot say that I ever made a conscious decision to specialize in Cardiology. In fact, during the 22 years that I have been Professor and Head of the Department of Medicine here, a goodly amount of my time has been spent in areas of internal medicine other than cardiology, and not an inconsiderable proportion of it in administration. Nevertheless, as my department has grown especially in the past 15 years, the time I have had left after carrying out my administrative duties has been increasingly spent in the specialty of cardiology — with a fairly even split between teaching, research and clinical work.

During my two years of internship at the Toronto General Hospital my interest in Cardiology was greatly stimulated by my contacts with Drs. John Oille and John Hepburn. I went abroad to study in 1931 and after obtaining my London Membership in April 1932 I spent some months at the Heart Hospital. I remember particularly and with gratitude my contacts with John Parkinson and Evan Bedford. I was back there for the summer of 1934 and that year, following conversations with William Evans, I purchased my first electrocardiograph, a Hellige ink-writer with which I struggled for a couple of years. Until its arrival at Queen's we had had access to a very early Cambridge model which was operated on request by Dr. Spencer Melvin, our Professor of Physiology. In 1935 I obtained a Westinghouse Orthodiascope and a few months later a Cambridge Hindle electrocardiograph with a heart sound recording attachment and set up an embryo Heart Department at the Kingston General Hospital. The following year I started the small Heart Clinic which still operates as one of the specialty clinics of the hospital.

Dr. George Carswell Ferguson, 8 October 1905, Pembroke, Ont.; University of Toronto, M.D. 1930, B.Sc. (Medicine) 1932; F.R.C.P.(C) 64; F.A.H.A.

Dr. Ferguson was present at the first meeting of the Canadian Cardiovascular Society in Winnipeg on 24 June 1947 and became a charter member. His comments on the special questions state that while he was serving as Medical Resident (1932-35) at the Toronto General Hospital, Dr. Oille and Dr. Hepburn initiated his special interest in the cardiovascular system. During the year 1931-32, he was a Fellow in physiology at University of Toronto. He became associated with a group practice clinic in Port Arthur and with both the Port Arthur General and the St. Joseph's Hospital as an internist with a special interest in cardiology. He served on the committee which led to the formation of the Ontario Heart Foundation and he organized its Lakehead Chapter. He was a member of the Medical Advisory Committee of the Ontario Heart Foundation.

Dr. Ferguson did not submit a bibliography.

Dr. John E. Plunkett (1901-1953)

Dr. John E. Plunkett was a Charter Member of the Society who died prematurely at the age of 52 on 11 January 1953 of acute coronary heart disease. He began his medical career as a student of pharmacy, graduating in the year 1922. Later, he studied medicine at Queen's University and obtained the degree M.D. in 1930. His postgraduate studies included three years at the Mayo Clinic and he began to practise medicine in Ottawa in 1935. He was appointed Assistant Professor of Clinical Medicine at Queen's University, teaching students who came to serve internships at the Ottawa Civic Hospital. In 1945 he became Honorary Secretary of the Royal College of Physicians and Surgeons of Canada. Among the societies to which he belonged were the Montreal Medical-Chirurgical Society, the Ontario Medical Association, and the American Heart Association.

Dr. Plunkett was greatly appreciated by his confrères in Ottawa as a teacher and as a consultant in internal medicine which included a special interest in cardiovascular diseases. He contributed much to maintaining a high standard in the practice of medicine in Ottawa.

Dr. Francis Staples Brien, 9 April 1908, Windsor, Ont.; University of Toronto, B.A. 30; M.B. 33; M.R.C.P. (London) 1937; F.R.C.P.(C) 46; R.A.C.P. 46; F.R.C.P. (London) 58; M.C.G.P. (HON).

Dr. Brien became a member of the Society at its inception. He was then already Professor and Head of the Department of Medicine at the University of Western Ontario. His interest in cardiology was inspired by his good fortune in having as teachers in Toronto John Oille, John Hepburn, and Harold Rykert. Thus, early in his career as a house physician it became obvious to him that "a study of hypertension, cardiovascular disease in general and of diabetes would be most rewarding." His bibliography of sixteen items between 1947 and 1964 reflects interest in a wide variety of subjects related to internal medicine. These include a study of "The Differential Diagnosis of Chest Pain" published in *Post-Graduate Medicine,* July 1957. In the same year he associated with N. M. Lefcoe and G. W. Manning in an article on "An Opening Snap Recorded in a Case of Tumor of the Left Atrium" (*N. Eng. J. Med.* 25 July 1957).

Dr. Carl Rutherford Burton, 23 October 1911, Toronto; University of Toronto, B.A. 33; M.D. 36; M.R.C.P. (London); F.A.C.P., F.A.C.C., F.A.H.A.

Dr. Carl Burton responded very promptly to the request of the archivist. In June 1965, he wrote the following reminiscences:

> After graduation from the University of Toronto in 1936 I became a junior rotating intern at the Toronto General Hospital. Unfortunately, after three months I was forced to bed by a neurological ailment. This was feared to be disseminated sclerosis at the time, but subsequently, fortunately, has proven to be an innocent disease. However, it kept me off duty for a year and resulted in sufficient physical weakness that I was unable to undertake any but the lightest of work in the hospital. I became a voluntary assistant on the Heart and Lung Ward under Dr. Oille, Dr. Hepburn and Dr. Rykert. As heart appealed to me more than chest disease I gradually concentrated on it to the exclusion of the latter. The dominant personalities of Dr. Oille and Dr. Hepburn probably accounted for this decision more than anything else. Dr. Oille was still in his hey-day as an excellent clinical teacher. His knowledge and clinical acumen were outstanding and were revered by such clever persons as Dr. John Hepburn.
>
> As the war came on, the staff of the ward gradually diminished and as Dr. Hepburn and I were ineligible for the armed forces we formed closer and closer association. Dr. Hepburn of course was well established in practice, and I opened an office adjacent to his in 1941, practising in a very limited way. This of course was in addition to our teaching and ward duties.
>
> At the end of the war Dr. John Oille retired and Dr. Hepburn became head of the ward. Dr. Rykert through illness had returned to us from the Army in the middle of the war and resumed his former prominent place on the cardiological staff.
>
> My appointment to the staff of both University and the General Hospital were temporary contingent upon my completing my training at the cessation of hostilities. I was able to sit the examination for fellowship of the Royal College of Physicians of Canada in 1945, and Prof. Graham sent me to England to study in August 1946. As the British Post-Graduate Medical

School in Hammersmith was the only school offering postgraduate courses at that time, I was fortunate indeed to have a letter of introduction to Prof. McMichael, who enrolled me as a student. I sat the London Membership in the Royal College of Physicians in January 1947, and became associated with the late Dr. Paul Wood temporarily while he was still at Hammersmith.

When I returned to Canada in the middle of 1947, Prof. Farquharson appointed me a clinical teacher in the Department of Medicine, and a junior attending physician at the Toronto General Hospital.

In 1948 the Section of Cardiology of the Ontario Medical Association was formed, and I was appointed to a committee on cardiology along with Dr. John Keith and others to look into the possibility of forming some organization to coordinate heart activities in the province. As a result of this, the Ontario Heart Foundation was established. It was the pioneer in the field and led to heart foundations across the country as well as the Canadian Heart Foundation.

I am not sure when the Canadian Cardiovascular Society, or as it was formerly called the Canadian Heart Association, was formed, but it must have been about this time and it of course was always a purely professional body requiring certain minimal qualifications to become associated with its membership. Dr. John Hepburn of course was one of the leaders in the formation of the Canadian Heart Association, and as I recall, I was also a charter member.

For some years after the formation of the Ontario Heart Foundation I used to attend their Board meetings in an ex-officio capacity and also sat on their research committee.

Dr. Burton's bibliography begins with an article on "The Value of Lead IVF in Cardiac Infarction" (*Am. Ht. J.* 1945). Among his later publications there is "Spatial Vector-cardiography in Proven Atrial Septal Defect" (*Br. Ht. J.*, 1962: 24, 163).

Dr. Ross Martin Lymburner, 8 May 1904, Warner, Caistor Township, Ont.; University of Toronto, M.D. 29; University of Minnesota, M.Sc. (Med); F.A.C.P.; C.R.C.P.(C); F.A.C.C.

After a year's internship at the Hamilton General Hospital, Dr. Lymburner had a Mayo Foundation Fellowship in Medicine (1930-1933). He then joined the staff of the Hamilton General Hospital and worked as an internist with a special interest in Cardiology. As part of his continuing education in cardiology, he attended the courses given by Dr. Paul D. White and also those by Dr. Samuel Levine in Boston, as well as some courses in Philadelphia. Dr. Lymburner pioneered cardiology in Hamilton. He did not submit his bibliography.

Dr. Alfred John Kerwin, 26 March 1909, Toronto; University of Toronto, M.D. 33; F.A.H.A.

Dr. Kerwin had all his postgraduate training in Toronto, namely internships in Medicine and Pathology (1933-37) at the Toronto General Hospital. He held the post of Attending Physician at Toronto Western Hospital since 1946 and reached the rank of Professor of Medicine at Toronto University when he submitted his curriculum vitae in 1968.

Dr. Kerwin came under the strong influence of the late Dr. Oille and the late Dr. Hepburn. Of his early years in training he wrote:

> I was of course inspired by the teachings of Doctors John Oille and John Hepburn, both as an undergraduate and as an intern. The particular focus in cardiology which attracted most attention was undoubtedly electrocardiography. I do not suppose I really decided to practise cardiology until late in the war. There was of course a hiatus of nearly thirteen years between graduation and starting practice, and at one time I fully intended to become a pathologist, but curiously enough in the mid and late 30s there seemed to be no call for pathologists except for the few positions in university centres. I therefore switched back to internal medicine at the suggestion of Doctor Duncan Graham and then went to Peru for three years as the silicosis consultant for one of the large mining companies.

In the 1980s it is of some historic interest that the first paper which Dr. Kerwin published was on "Persistent (Partial) Truncus Arteriosus Associated with Double Aortic Arch" (*Journal of Technical Methods and Bulletin of the International Association of Medical Museums,* 1936, XV, CXLII, CXLVII). Dr. Maude Abbott was the editor of this Journal at that time. She must have enjoyed very greatly including this article in her *Bulletin.* Dr. Kerwin is one of the few who have written about the effect of spinal deformity on cardiac function. He reported five cases (*Arch. Int. Med.,* April 1942). His bibliography contains a wide variety of items related to both congenital and acquired cardiovascular disease.

Dr. Irwin McAmmond Hilliard, 24 March 1911, Morrisburg, Ontario; Victoria College, Toronto, B.A. 33; University of Toronto, M.D. 36; F.R.C.P.(C); F.A.C.P.; F.A.C.C.

Dr. Hilliard began his postgraduate studies with internship at the Toronto General Hospital (1936-38). There followed six years in China as Physician-in-Chief of the Canadian Mission Hospital in Fuling Szechwan (1939-1945). He returned home to work as a research fellow in Cardiology at the Toronto General Hospital (1945-1947), after which he occupied a post at the Toronto Western Hospital. In 1954-62 he was Physician-in-Chief at the University Hospital in Saskatoon and Professor as Head of the Department of Medicine at the University of Saskatchewan. In 1962, he became Professor of Medicine at Toronto University and Physician-in-Chief at Toronto Western Hospital. He held those posts when, in 1965, he wrote of the early phase of his career:

> Two of the three really great undergraduate teachers our Clinic had were Cardiologists — Dr. John Oille and Dr. John Hepburn. In a way, they represented cardiology to undergraduates and their clear thinking and logical approach to problems and their warmhearted, sincere, though rather gruff relationship with patients, influenced many of us greatly.
>
> One other aspect of Medicine which at that time did not seem related to cardiology but which impressed me as an undergraduate was toxaemia pregnancy. The work that was being done in Toronto by Professor Harding stimulated my curiosity and made me wonder whether there might be some relationship between salt and water metabolism, toxaemia pregnancy and hypertension. When I came back from the East in 1945, I talked to Professor Graham about the chance of further study and doing some research. He asked me what I was interested in. I mentioned this undergraduate interest that had started so many years ago. He said they wanted someone in the department to work on this. I rather suspected that it would be in the field of kidney disease or renal physiology. Instead he sent me to Dr. Hepburn who had just received a letter from Dr. Paul White discussing the use of mercurial diuretics and the new theory of flooding the cardiac patient as Dr. Schemm was doing in Great Falls, Montana. During the two years I worked with Dr. Hepburn studying the effect of ammonium chloride and mercurial diuretics, high and low fluid intake in patients with congestive heart failure, I followed patients on Ward 1 at the Toronto General Hospital and

the Cardiac Clinic. The patients, the nurses and the staff all seemed a very happy and congenial family. It would have been very surprising if someone working as I did in that environment, hadn't developed this as his first love — Cardiology.

Dr. Hilliard attended the first meeting of our society in Winnipeg on 24 June 1947. He has served in a succession of offices, including the presidency for two years (1963-1964). As an inspiring teacher he has had a very significant effect on the evolution of cardiology in Canada. Dr. Hilliard did not provide his bibliography.

Dr. Elliot Maurice Heller, 15 October 1912, Sarnia, Ontario; University of Toronto, M.D. 37; M.Sc. (Med.); F.R.C.P. (Edinburgh); F.A.C.P.; F.A.C.C.; F.C.C.P.; R.C.P.(C) Cert. Int. Med.

Dr. Elliot Heller, a classmate of Dr. Greenwood and several other cardiology pioneers, had a very good postgraduate training, but unlike his classmates, none of his appointments were in Toronto. His comments on the special questions are quoted in full.

> I first began to consider specializing in Cardiology when I was in physiology class in medical school. We were given special hearing tests and my range was higher than anyone else in the group. The instructor suggested that I would be able to hear more on examining the heart than the average physician.
>
> During my first year at the Graduate School of the University of Pennsylvania in the internal medicine course, I discovered that I could pick up difficult murmurs and recognize the various heart sounds easier than my colleagues. Also, I have always been anxious to help the patient in the most significant manner and nothing could be more vital than heart disease. A final determining factor was that Dr. George C. Griffith, whom I felt to be the best Cardiologist I had ever been in contact with up until that time, wished to become my preceptor. Consequently my second year at the Graduate School was spent under his supervision.
>
> When I first decided to specialize in Internal Medicine, I had finished an internship at St. Mary's Hospital, St. Louis, in 1938. At that time there were certain [anti-Jewish] discriminations that made it difficult to obtain a residency in Internal Medicine in a teaching hospital [in Toronto] in spite of my very good qualifications. For that reason I went to the University of Pennsylvania Graduate School in Philadelphia and enjoyed the nine months course in Internal Medicine followed by the preceptorship under

George C. Griffith. It was easy for me after that to get my third year as resident at the Genessee Hospital, University of Rochester, New York, where I continued working towards my Master of Medical Science Degree in Cardiology. In 1942 I joined the R.C.A.M.C. and after serving in Canada, England, Holland and Germany, was granted a British Council Scholarship for further training at the University of Edinburgh under the auspices of Dr. Rae Gilchrist at the Royal Edinburgh Infirmary. Here I also took the Fellowship course and was successful in the membership examinations. I loved the Scots people and at one time thought I might settle there. I spent almost two years working under Dr. Gilchrist and his associate, Dr. Ian Hill, who is now Professor of Medicine at Dundee University. I was introduced to Sir John Parkinson and spent some time in London at the National Heart Hospital, etc., working under his auspices and through him met Dr. Frank Wilson, who invited me to spend some time with him at the University of Michigan Medical School in Ann Arbor. My association with Dr. Wilson was, as you might expect, memorable especially since at that time he knew more about unipolar leads than any man in the world. As a matter of fact, with my electrocardiograph bought early in 1948, I was probably the first in Toronto to routinely take unipolar 13-lead electrocardiograms. I chose Toronto because there was only one other physician specializing in heart disease — Dr. S. Carlen at the Mount Sinai Hospital. He had returned one year earlier and I felt that there was room for another well trained Cardiologist. Further events proved this judgment to be correct.

By 1971, Dr. Heller's bibliography had grown to thirty items. His early special interest in rehabilitation of patients with myocardial infarction is manifested in five papers he published during the years 1966 to 1971 on a standard exercise program for such patients.

Dr. George Adalbert Mayer, 7 June 1913, Budapest, Hungary; University of Budapest, M.D. 37; M.Sc. Queen's University (Med.), 56; Cert. Int. Med. Hungary 41; F.A.H.A.

Dr. Mayer, before emigrating from Hungary in 1951, had risen to the status of Assistant Professor of Medicine and Director of Clinical Research at the University of Kolozswar (1941-44). In Canada, he became associated with Queen's University, and in 1965, he was Assistant Research Associate when he resigned and organized his private laboratory for independent research.

Commenting on the special questions, he relates some interesting experiences during his undergraduate and internship years.

In Hungary where I was born and educated, cardiology was not a separate specialty. However, a good number of qualified internists restricted their practice to cardiology. My first encounter with cardiology was in 1933 or 34 when Professor Haynal asked my class to volunteer for experiments in the diuretic effect of a new mercurial diuretic, Novurit, which was apparently the precursor of the well known Salyrgan. Thereafter, Professor Boros in 1937 tried the first Digitalis Lanata product, the precursor of Cedilanid. I volunteered for both experiments and was fascinated by feeling the side effects of diuresis (we received quite high doses in the muscles): for two weeks after this experiment I could not play tennis because my muscles would not move properly. The high doses of digoxin produced vomiting for a couple of days and possible xanthopsia [yellow vision]. However, I am not sure today if this was not imagination since we were allowed to end the experiment when this symptom appeared. The big reward was when the Professor invited the volunteers to his office, shook our hands and addressed each of us by name. At that time the Professor was a demi-god and only assistant professors and high ranking staff members could speak to him. I think these two events aroused my interest in cardiology. After I came to Canada in 1951, the research post which I obtained at Queen's University gave me the unique opportunity to study and do full-time clinical research in atherosclerotic vascular disease.

My cardiology training was not planned in my native country. I saw and treated large numbers of patients and watched carefully what the more experienced staff members did. Since the University Hospital in Budapest was a closed hospital and the Professor could control the admitting material, we saw one year mostly decompensated valvular cases, or myocardial infarctions, etc.

I had and have now many obstacles which take the form of conservatism in the treatment of cardiac patients. I remember well that in 1937 the use of potassium in cardiac patients was prohibited as it was considered as quackery to prescribe a drug used by older country doctors, the effect of which was not then known. When one weekend I was alone on duty in a ward and had a desperately ill old lady, with intractable heart failure in spite of vigorous digitalis and diuretic therapy, a retired old physician who visited my ward daily suggested giving the patient some potassium chloride. He was so persuasive that I committed the 'crime' and gave potassium. She improved in 48 hours but I was almost 'fired' from the internship. We know today the value of potassium. I left my country, travelled to Canada and we are 25 years older, but today I am in the same spot with anticoagulant therapy. However, I am a little stronger today and will fight for what I consider right.

Dr. Mayer's bibliography begins with a paper entitled "Diet and Plasma Cholesterol Levels," 1954. Subsequently, he published principally on this subject as co-author with Drs. Beveridge, Connell, and occasionally Drs. Firstbrook, DeWolfe, Maximin, and Dorsey. The major part of his bibliography contains articles related to the management of anticoagulant therapy.

Dr. Donal Patrick Murnaghan, 2 November 1913, Ireland; M.B., B.Ch. 37; F.A.C.P., F.A.C.C., F.R.C.P.(C).

Dr. Murnaghan has been a familiar figure at meetings of the Canadian Cardiovascular Society and at reunions of Dr. Paul D. White's pupils. Very few of his many friends are likely to be aware of the kaleidoscopic pattern of his early career which began in Dublin, Ireland. The story of how eventually Dr. Paul White was instrumental in developing his career in cardiology is told by this talented raconteur.

Some kind of an answer now to your list of questions: While working in a medical outpatient department as a voluntary assistant in the second year after graduation I decided to do some extra study on some of our cardiac problems of interest to the attending physician. We had them come to his private office on a Saturday afternoon where I learned my first fluoroscopy and read a little of Dr. Paul White's first edition of *Heart Disease.* At that time I was pursuing a course of post-graduate anatomy, planning to do neurology.

I met Dr. Jason Mixter of Boston on a holiday in Dublin the following year and he expressed some interest in my plans and asked me to write him in case he could be of any assistance to me. At that time he was in charge of neurosurgery at the Massachusetts General Hospital.

I pursued my first postgraduate year abroad at the Department of Embryology, Carnegie Institution of Washington in

Baltimore, learning the vagaries of tissue culture and in particular neuronal cells. The war was going badly for the Allies in 1940 and I didn't see in my heart how spending another year in micro-neuro-anatomy could be any contribution to war service. I wrote my thoughts to Dr. Mixter and suggested I would turn my thoughts to clinical medicine and that I had an interest in the name of Dr. White from the tiny experience in Dublin. Imagine my delight when I had a letter back from Dr. White welcoming me to the department on the first of August, 1940, and suggesting that I take part in the postgraduate course starting at that time for the month of August. I would say during the month of August, 1940, my interest in Cardiology really got under way.

My scholarship from Eire in sterling only lasted another twelve months. With decreasing exchange during 1940 and early 1941 I knew what it was to have little to buy on my own at some stages. The kindness of many friends in Boston at this time will always be treasured. Due to Dr. White's kindness I continued my training in Boston. During the winter of 1942 I came to Canada to enlist in the Armed Forces because the Americans applied the draft to everyone shortly after Pearl Harbor and were about to grab me for a private's duty, hopefully in a hospital, they said, as an attendant, nursing assistant, or what have you.

My years in the R.C.A.F. provided an opportunity for cardiac consultation mainly on the Prairie. I decided upon further clinical training which was arranged at Toronto General Hospital through the kindness of the late Dr. Ray F. Farquharson — whose unfailing support shall always be a living memory — and the cooperation of the Professor of Medicine, Dr. Duncan Graham. There I came in close contact with John Hepburn and Harold Rykert and occasionally with Dr. John Oille. Their critical appraisal of cases, their vast fund of experience and constant prodding never let one forget the underlying scientific side of clinical cardiology. I began teaching with second year students, spent a lot of time at the hospital, and started clinical consultation in 1948. I decided to purchase a portable electrocardiograph and a fluoroscope early in 1949. This was the great mouth that ate up most of the income. From there it has been one period of enjoyment where any progress has been due to attention to clinical details taught by former experienced men and the application of scientific principles acquired from a variety of sources. As one progresses one realizes that the milk of human kindness is an important consideration in dealing with human nature.

Dr. Murnaghan's publications include an article on "Ganglion Cells in Tissue Culture," 1941, "Pulmonary Embolism," 1942, "Cardiovascular Examination of Air Crew," 1944, "The Optimistic Outlook in Rheumatic Heart Disease," 1965, and finally what Dr. Murnaghan describes as "Miscellaneous Talks."

Dr. Donald Bernard Moran, 27 October 1914, Warkworth, Ontario; University of Toronto, B.A. 36; M.D. 39; F.R.C.P.(C) 46; F.A.C.C. 70.

Dr. Moran began postgraduate training with internships and residency at St. Michael's Hospital, Toronto. There followed a year as Fellow-in-Medicine at the Toronto General Hospital. In 1971, when he submitted his curriculum vitae he was on the Active Staff in Cardiology at the Scarborough Centenary Hospital and Consultant in Medicine at St. Michael's Hospital.

Dr. Moran did not submit a bibliography.

Dr. James Edward Gibson, 10 November 1914, Kingston; Queen's University, B.A. 37; M.D., C.M. 40; F.A.C.P.; F.C.C.P.; F.A.G.S.; R.C.P.(C).

Dr. Gibson served a junior rotating internship at the Regina Grey Nuns Hospital in 1940. After the war, in 1946, he had a senior internship in Brownsville, New York, followed by an assistant residency at the Kingston General Hospital (1947-48).

In 1965, he was Assistant Professor of Medicine at Queen's University and on the staff of the Hôtel-Dieu, Kingston General and St. Mary's of the Lake Hospitals.

Dr. Gibson wrote that he became interested in cardiology as he witnessed his father using an electrocardiographic apparatus, in the early 1930s. Further inquiry revealed that Dr. William Gibson (1878-1942) had bought a Cambridge electrocardiograph in 1927, and pioneered cardiology in Kingston, practising as an internist and Associate Professor of Medicine at Queen's University and Chief of Medicine at the Hôtel-Dieu in Kingston. Dr. J. E. Gibson emulated his father and in addition developed a special interest in Geriatrics and in Rehabilitation.

Dr. Joseph Greenblatt, 21 February 1916, Russia; Queen's University, M.D., C.M. 40; F.R.C.P.(C) 49.

Dr. Greenblatt served internships and residencies in medicine at the Ottawa Civic, Kingston General, and Sunnybrook (Toronto) Hospitals until 1950 when he entered private practice. He acquired knowledge of clinical cardiology as part of internal medicine. In 1971, when he updated his curriculum vitae, he was Assistant Professor of Medicine at Ottawa University and Senior Physician at the Ottawa Civic Hospital.

He co-authored, with G. Cohen and I. Dardick, an article on "Post Myocardial Infarction Syndrome" (*C.M.A.J.* 1960: 82, 123). Dr. Greenblatt and his colleagues were among the earliest to recognize this syndrome which was first described by Dressler in 1959.

Dr. George W. Manning, 4 August 1911, Toronto; University of Toronto, B.A. 35; M.D. 40; M.A. 37; Ph.D. 47; F.R.C.P.(C) 48; F.A.C.P. 59; F.A.C.C.; Amer. Bd. Prevt. Med. 54; F.A.H.A.

After the second distribution of the questionnaire in 1968, Dr. Manning responded very generously. The letter which accompanied his curriculum vitae and bibliography tells a unique story.

> My interest in Medicine goes back to my high school days, and peculiarly enough to music, for it was a music teacher who first roused my interest in the profession of medical science. I entered the University of Toronto in 1931, registering in the Honour Sciences course. During my last years at high school and early years at University I managed to keep ahead of the game from my earnings as a teacher of piano music, which my former music teacher had encouraged me to do, so the first degree I held was one in music. In those years, when steak was 2 pounds for a quarter, a little money went a long way. However, by 1935 I had run completely out of funds, but also had completed my B.A. degree. Dr. Harry Gates, who was then professor of anatomy, felt he could get me a research position with Banting, and after a somewhat rigid and rigorous interview and oral examination I finally was appointed as a research assistant at the Banting Institute in the Department of Medical Research at a salary of $50.00 per month. Ed Hall had graduated that year, and I became his first graduate student. Ettinger was also at the Lab during this period, and fortunately within a month or two my salary was raised to $75.00 a month, where it remained for the next year. I spent two years at the Banting, published a few papers on experimental coronary occlusion, completed my M.A. degree while there, and then went back into Medicine in 1938, graduating finally in 1940, when the war was now upon us. I maintained a very close association with Banting's Department of Medical

Research, after I returned for the final three years in Medicine in 1937. Most of my spare time was spent in the Lab, all of my summers, Christmas holidays, etc., continuing our work on experimental coronary occlusion. My years with Banting and Hall were, indeed, very wonderful years, which I recall with pride and happiness, for they did represent the beginnings of my small career. Banting was truly a great man. He belonged to no clubs. Did not play golf, and as you know lived for research, which I am sure caused most of his domestic troubles. Banting had a tremendous imagination and seemed to be always coming up with ideas as to how this or that problem might be solved. He was most receptive to anyone who had an "idea." Shortly before I arrived at the Banting, Hall and Ettinger had attempted to produce chronic and continuous vagal stimulation in dogs in order to study its effect on the heart. They had been unable to come up with a technique to accomplish this. Fortunately, I was able to devise a rather simple technique from bicycle sprockets, speedometer cables, etc. which allowed us to stimulate the vagus for 15 seconds out of each minute continuously. The method is a bit of a Rube Goldberg setup, but was published in the *Journal of Laboratory and Clinical Medicine* shortly after the experiments were completed entitled "An Apparatus for Prolonged Stimulation Experiments in Unanaesthetized Animals." Another technique, for the continuous administration of acetyl choline, was also published in the *Journal of Laboratory and Clinical Medicine* entitled "The Continuous Intravenous Injection Apparatus for Unrestrained Animals." These experiments lasted up to three weeks and ran 24 hours a day. A number of dogs were run at the same time, and it was obvious that I would need considerable help in carrying out these experiments. Banting was intrigued with the technique, and volunteered to take the midnight shift from 12:00 to 8:00 in the morning, which he religiously carried out. I spent from 3:00 to 4:00 in the afternoon until the next morning with the experiments, and got some rest prior to the next day's shift. Some nights when the animals were under good control Banting had a little snooze on the couch in the Lab, and snored heartily for an hour or two. On other nights he might bring in a little drink for the two of us, swearing me to secrecy, for in those days the presence of alcohol in any university building at Toronto was an extremely serious offence, which if it ever became known, would certainly lead to "excommunication." On a number of mornings as the sun arose, Banting, sitting at the lab bench, with the windows looking to the West, made sketches of anything that might be within his view. These included the Conservatory of Music at the corner of College and University, Botany Building across a stretch of empty land that there was there at that time, the Police Commission on College Street, and the intersection of College, University, etc. Unfortunately, these sketches, which, indeed, were very good, for Banting, as you know, did have a good deal of artistic ability, were either thrown in the waste basket, at the time, or remained around for a few days only to be disposed of. I still have my day books describing in some detail these experiments, and which provide many an interesting story, however, the early morning sketches are not with them. This was the kind of a man Banting was — a researcher of international fame, who had been knighted by the King, and who insisted on assisting me, an undergraduate student at the time, with an experiment of really little importance, but which was an original idea. He was continually interested in new ideas, experiments that had never been done before, and this, of course, was the nature of his entire research life. Prior to the war years, and during his research in Aviation Medicine up until the time of his death, which would not have occurred had he not insisted on doing the job himself. Early in 1940, when the first decompression chamber was installed at the Banting Institute in his Laboratory (a big secret at the time) he was anxious and impatient to get on with high altitude research, for very little was known of this problem at that time. I can well remember undertaking a decompression run with him to compare British and German oxygen masks. We ascended at a moderate rate to an altitude equivalent of 40,000 feet, at which even with 100% oxygen we were both somewhat anoxic. Banting insisted on further altitude and we continued to decompress until we eventually reached an altitude equivalent of 45,000 feet. This was a record, and I am sure still is, considering the equipment we were using, however, Banting loved breaking records, and he was quite happy likely due to the euphoria of anoxia, however, I wasn't since I had developed some joint pain due to the bends and lost half of the vision in my left eye, and was feeling so faint that I felt I would be unconscious within seconds. Banting was all for continuing, however, the chamber operator could see that I had had it, and brought the chamber down. The descent was uneventful except for the fact that my vision did not return properly until after we compressed to ground level. Banting had been using the German mask, which was more efficient in oxygen delivery than the economizer type R.A.F. mask that I was using, and I am sure that Banting knew of this. When I explained to him that this was the reason I was having more difficulty than he, he looked at me with a sly grin, and said "No excuses, Manning. You are a sissy."

There are many more interesting tales during the years 1935 to 1941, however, I will not go into them, and would not have recounted even as much as I have about Banting, except that I remember you specifically asked me to include something about Banting in this letter to you. There is one other incident that you should know about, and perhaps do, which is related to cardiology, and which occurred during the Banting years, and this was a clinical diagnosis of myocardial infarction in the ape (based on history alone). Banting had introduced me to the curator of the Riverdale Zoological Gardens, and it was through this association that I had an opportunity to make this diagnosis, and do the post-mortem examination. This led to my first clinical publication in the *American Heart Journal,* entitled "Coronary Disease in the Ape."

And now to get on with the rest of it, as briefly as I can. From 1940 to 1945 I had the good fortune to be associated with Aviation Medical Research in Canada and England. I had a Research Unit in Regina until 1943, where a good deal of research in the fields of motion sickness, high altitude and cardiovascular problems as they applied to aircrew were carried out. The electrocardiographic studies, which are still going on were, of course, initiated in Toronto before I left for Regina. I returned to Toronto in 1943, and soon after proceeded to England, where I worked at Farnborough (R.A.F. Physiological Lab) for the next year. I did not get into much work actually at Farnborough but fortunately was seconded to the Medical Research Council, and carried out some interesting work on anoxic collapse with Barcroft and Edholm in Belfast. On return to Canada in 1945, at the request of Ottawa, since they were not happy with me being loaned to the R.A.F. and M.R.C., however, their objections were put off long enough to allow us to complete the work in Belfast and publish the results. On return to Canada I was posted to Ottawa, given the job of historian, sent to the second floor of a barrack block in Rockcliffe. This banishment and removal from research resulted in my complete refusal to cooperate. I returned to Toronto at my own expense, stated flatly to Ken Ferguson, who was then in charge of the I.A.M. in Toronto, that I would not accept. After a week I was informed that unless I returned to Ottawa the charge would not only be A.W.O.L., but likely desertion. I had, however, returned to some reasonable thinking by this time, and on my arrival in Ottawa found that the episode had been very worthwhile, for the situation was very greatly improved, and I actually did a good deal of collecting from the various Medical Units throughout the R.C.A.F. in connection with the part the R.C.A.F. Medical Branch had played throughout the War.

Following discharge from the Service, I spent a year at the Toronto General Hospital as a Senior in Medicine, and was fortunate enough to receive a Nuffield Scholarship to take me back to England in the Fall of 1946. This left me with three months during the summer of 1946, during which myself and a chap named Caldwell, a surgeon, carried out a very satisfactory series of experiments on coronary occlusion, again in my old Lab. at the Banting Institute. Dr. Best was very friendly, and cooperative, and provided me with facilities (since it was the summer holiday), and animals to carry out a series of experiments, which was published shortly after in the *British Heart Journal.*

I proceeded to London, England early in September, 1946 on one of the first Nuffield Travelling Scholarships. I am sure that Professor Duncan Graham had been influential in obtaining this scholarship for me. He also made the arrangements for me to work with Parkinson during the year in London.

The year 1946-47 at the London Hospital Cardiac Dept. was of tremendous interest and stimulation. Parkinson and Evans were at their peak. This was perhaps one of the last years of pure classical clinical cardiology, for we were on the brink of 'Laboratory Cardiology.' Fluoroscopy and electrocardiography, although well established tools of the cardiologist, were all we had. Phonocardiography usually confirmed our clinical findings and this was really just beginning as a frequently used procedure. It seems to me that the diagnosis of acquired or congenital heart disease was just as accurate then as it is today with all our complex haemodynamic equipment. We had to rely, as you know, entirely on the clinical findings. The management of the patient depended on the signs and symptoms and not on 'the degree of haemodynamic disturbance' (since we didn't know this). If the patient needed help, he got it, today he gets it whether he needs it or not — modern 'prophylaxis' — for example, the 'prophylactic' Vineberg procedure!

Parkinson like Banting was truly a great man, dedicated to his work and a man who commanded and demanded a great respect for cardiology. Parkinson and Evans, in addition to being great teachers, provided me with solid clinical cardiology which added to my basic science years with Banting and Hall and was the background that has led to my continued interest in cardiovascular research, teaching and practice.

Following this year in England, I returned to Canada, completed my Ph.D. in Physiology (experimental coronary occlusion) in 1947, and my F.R.C.P.(C) in 1948. I came directly to London, Ontario from London, England in 1947 and have been here since.

Since the war years I have continued with the R.C.A.F. ECG Program, and this work is still going on. Except for my year in England, I have carried on with these programs continuously since 1940. You know the rest of the story. I worked with you in the early days of the Canadian Heart Association and was a member of the Committee on Cardiology of the O.M.A. in 1949. I was also one of the original members of the Medical Committee of the Ontario Heart Foundation and having been associated with heart affairs of Ontario during the transition and incorporation of the Ontario Heart Foundation in 1952. I remained on that Committee a bit too long, however, in those days there was no mechanism for terminating committee membership and appointing new ones. This came into being, and rightly so some years ago so that each committee member serves for a period of 2 or 3 years only. However, that original committee did serve for a very long time, and perhaps looking back on it, there may have been some design and justification for all of the members of the committee held grants in aid from the Ontario Heart Foundation. We must remember that the Ontario Heart Foundation was established for the support of clinical research. We were criticized in the early days for being too clinically orientated, however, this group you must remember had no support from basic science for clinical research, whereas basic science had enjoyed support for some period. Naturally some criticism developed strictly from the basic science side, however, the situation has now balanced out very satisfactorily with a proper balance between basic science and clinical research, I think to everyone's satisfaction. As you know I have been associated with our Canadian Heart Foundation and encouraging financial support of clinical cardiovascular research since the days we had nothing at all.

Canada has gone a long way in the past 10 to 12 years. This was clearly apparent at the recent meeting held in Geneva in September 1969 of the International Cardiology Foundation. This was a planning meeting to prepare for the setting up of an international cardiology federation to replace the Foundation and to take effect next September in London at the Congress. During this meeting the various nations were asked to give a brief review of their activities and fund-raising efforts and results. Canada, I was proud to see, led the world in activity (i.e. Foundations, Research and Fellowship support, etc.) and in fund-raising for heart research. On a per capita basis, Canada equalled the great U.S.A. in fund-raising.

To conclude, I hope this letter will give you something of which you requested, however, there are of course very many gaps; if I were to go on reminiscing I might write a whole book which would be of little or no interest to anyone. May I tell you again that one of the very first articles I referred to in connection with my early cardiovascular research was one by Anrep and Segall which I read with great interest and used in the preparation of both my M.A. and Ph.D. theses. Perhaps one of the first references I ever quoted. Finally, may I say that the greatest encouragement to my continuing with a medical career, particularly in my younger days, came from my parents, both of whom have passed away during the past year and whom I miss very much. I trust that I have finally completed my assignment from you.

In the 1970s, Dr. Manning's list of publications exceeded 100. In his letter, he mentions the various fields of interest in which he worked. He has covered every phase of cardiovascular research. A wide variety of methods culled from physics and chemistry, applied with great mechanical skill have been used by George Manning. His statistical study "The Normal Electrocardiogram and Its Variations in 20,000 Cases" (*Circulation,* July 1960) is an example of his ability to organize a clinical investigation. He had 31 co-authors. They represent the many men who have come under his stimulating influence.

Dr. W. Stanley Hartroft, 5 August 1916, Calgary; University of Alberta, B.Sc. in Med. (Anatomy and Histology) 41; M.D. 41; Ph.D. University of Toronto, 49; LL.D. University of Alberta, 61; F.A.I.N. 61; F.R.C.P.(C) 63; F.A.A.C. 68; F.R.S.C. 69.

Dr. Hartroft earned his Ph.D. with work carried on in the Department of Pathology and Bacteriology at the University of Toronto. His academic career has taken him to various institutions including the Banting and Best Department of Medical Research, the Washington University School of Medicine, and the Hospital for Sick Children in Toronto. No member of the Canadian Cardiovascular Society is associated with as many other societies as he is. He belongs to 42 scientific organizations. He has served on 14 advisory committees of scientific bodies. Between 1943 and 1967 his bibliography grew to 191 items. They include studies of pulmonic histology and pathology; renal embryology, histology and pathology; experimental and clinical diabetes; experimental and clinical hepatic cirrhosis; experimental hypertension; experimental and clinical arteriosclerosis.

In 1961 he left Washington University School of Medicine where he had occupied the post of Mallinckrodt Professor and Chairman of the Department of Pathology for seven years. He returned to Toronto where he became Director of the Research Institute of the Hospital for Sick Children and Professor of Physiology at the University of Toronto. He has received many honours including the Claude Bernard Medal and numerous visiting professorships, and he is an honorary member of four societies in North and South America. He is one of a small number of basic scientists among the members of our society.

Dr. Robert Laidlaw MacMillan, 23 May 1917, Toronto; University of Toronto, B.A. 1938, M.D. 1941; John Oille Scholarship in Cardiol.; M.R.C.P.; F.R.C.P.(C); F.A.C.P.; F.A.C.C.; F.A.H.A.

Immediately after graduation Dr. MacMillan served a rotating internship at the Toronto General and then enlisted in the Royal Canadian Navy. On returning to civilian life in 1946 he had a Fellowship in Pathology followed by a senior internship in Medicine at the Toronto General Hospital. When he submitted the questionnaire in 1965 he was Associate in Medicine at Toronto University and Physician at the Toronto General Hospital.

In 1965 when Dr. MacMillan submitted the completed questionnaire and very brief comments on the special questions, he was the first John Oille Scholar at the University of Toronto. This scholarship bears some similarity to the Markle Scholarship. The scholar has it for five years and engages in teaching, research, and patient care. He is expected to have special interests in cardiology and cardiorespiratory diseases. Dr. MacMillan considers himself an internist who has been concerned with the use of anticoagulants, and thus became involved particularly in cardiovascular disease problems. Together with Dr. Kenneth W. G. Brown he organized the first coronary care unit in Canada and their report about such a unit was the first in world literature. He did not submit a bibliography; reference to his report appears in the chapter on pacemakers, monitoring, and coronary care units.

Dr. Alexander Dunbar McKelvey (1920-1972)

From an obituary resolution of the Council of the Faculty of Medicine of Toronto University that was composed by W. F. Greenwood we learn that Dr. McKelvey graduated with the degree M.D. at Toronto University in 1943. After a year of internship at the Toronto General Hospital, he served in the Royal Canadian Army Medical Corps until the end of the war. He resumed postgraduate education in 1946 in Toronto and Vancouver.

In 1949, he became a National Research Council Fellow in Cardiology, at the Toronto General Hospital. He was a most valued member of the group which dealt with the techniques of cardiac catheterization. He limited his practice of cardiology, and was a popular teacher of undergraduates and graduates from 1951 to the time of his premature demise.

Dr. John T. M. Fraser, 25 February 1919, Halifax; Queen's University, M.D., C.M. 43; F.R.C.P.(C); F.A.C.P.; F.A.C.C.P.; F.A.C.C.

Dr. Fraser served internship in medicine and pathology at the Ottawa Civic Hospital. In private practice, he became associated with A. M. McNabb, who had pioneered electrocardiography in Ottawa since about 1930. Dr. McNabb initiated Dr. Fraser's interest in cardiology. In 1965, Dr. Fraser had retired from his posts at the Ottawa Civic Hospital and Ottawa University.

Dr. James Alexander Little, 8 December 1922, Detroit; University of Toronto, M.D. 46; M.A. (Biochemistry) 50; F.R.C.P.(C) 52; F.A.H.A.

Dr. Little's postgraduate training and the posts he has occupied were those of a man dedicated to research. In 1963, he became Director of the Clinical Investigation Unit at St. Michael's Hospital and in 1969 he attained the rank of Professor in the Medical Faculty of Toronto University.

His bibliography lists 30 items published between 1951 and 1965, concerned mainly with biochemistry related to the study of atherosclerosis.

Among his brief comments on the special questions, there is:

> Although I am not a cardiologist in the strict sense of the word, I am interested in cardiovascular disease, particularly atherosclerosis. I became interested in this aspect of cardiology during my postgraduate training, because atherosclerosis is the single, largest cause of mortality in our population.

Dr. Kenneth William Gordon Brown, 11 June 1923, Toronto; University of Toronto M.D. 46; B.Sc. (Med.); F.R.C.P.(C); F.A.C.P.; F.A.C.C.; F.A.H.A.

Dr. Kenneth Brown had all his postgraduate training in Toronto, through internships and residencies at the Toronto General and Sunnybrook hospitals.

When he prepared his curriculum vitae in 1968, he was Attending Physician at the Toronto General Hospital and Assistant Professor of Medicine at the University of Toronto. His response to the special questions reveals that he and his colleagues were the first to organize a coronary care unit.

> For as long as I can remember, I always felt an urge to become a physician and, in particular, to specialize in heart disease. I think this probably is due to the fact that my father was a pharmacist and, for this reason, we had many physician friends in our home from the time I was an infant. I can remember the prevalence of heart disease in the discussions that went back and forth around our home whenever these friends came to visit.
>
> I think that the obstacles of obtaining special training were removed by Professor Duncan Graham and the late Dr. Ray Farquharson and the difficulties encountered to going into practice were largely removed through the kindness of the late Dr. John Hepburn, the late Dr. Harold Rykert and my great friend, Dr. Ross Jamieson.
>
> Early on in my career as a practising cardiologist, I attached a good deal of pride in my membership in the Canadian Heart Association and in attending their meetings and in the association with the revered and respected senior cardiologists also in attendance.

I think that the greatest thrill of my career has been my good fortune to be closely associated with Dr. R. L. MacMillan and the fact that, jointly, he and I set up the first coronary care unit anywhere in the world. When we opened up our coronary unit at the Toronto General Hospital and admitted the first patient on March 13th, 1962, we did not know what to expect from this approach, but it appears now that this type of care has made some definite improvement in the mortality figures for this dread disease. The second coronary unit to open up was that of Hughes Day in Kansas City and he began operating on May 28th, 1962.

Dr. Brown's bibliography begins as co-author of an article on cardiac failure in 1949 and by 1968 it grew to 28 items, all on subjects related to the cardiovascular system. The first article on the subject of coronary care units is "Coronary Unit, an Intensive Care Centre for Acute Myocardial Infarction," Brown, MacMillan, Forbath, Meligrana and Scott (*Lancet,* 17 August 1963).

Dr. Goodman Cohen, 28 August 1922, Reserve Mines, Nova Scotia; Mount Allison University, B.A. 43; McGill, M.D., C.M. 47; F.R.C.P.(C) 53; F.A.C.P. 64.

Dr. Cohen's postgraduate studies began with a rotating internship at the Montreal Jewish General Hospital (1947-48) followed by senior internships (1948-49) and assistant residency (1949-50) in Internal Medicine at the Bronx Hospital, New York. There followed two years in the Department of Cardiology at the Massachusetts General Hospital (1950-52) and a year at Johns Hopkins Hospital as Research Fellow in Environmental Medicine. He chose to settle in Ottawa. He became Chief of Cardiology and Director of the Pulmonary Function Laboratory of the Ottawa Civic Hospital. In 1965, he was Assistant Professor at the Ottawa University School of Medicine.

Following are some excerpts from the letter to the archivist which accompanied his curriculum vitae in 1965.

I am providing a curriculum vitae and I think it is reasonably detailed and should furnish the necessary information for the form. In thinking about your questions (a) and (b) I have had to do some reflecting and this takes me back a number of years to my time in McGill. I was trying to decide whether your instruction in my third or fourth year, that is 1946 or 1947, on the virtues of cardiac auscultation preceded or was contemporary with my purchase of *Diseases of the Heart* by Thomas Lewis. I still have that book of course and my name on the fly leaf is dated January 9, 1947. I am a little uncertain on priorities but I think I was exposed to your teaching first, perhaps in 1946 in my third year. Naturally at this time it is difficult to transplant oneself back a number of years and be sure of just what his plans were. At best they must have been very tentative ones since the internship was still to come with its varying influences. But I am certain that the germ of cardiology was planted by you at the bedside with the stethoscope and the note pad, and reinforced perhaps simultaneously by Lewis's book which I read in my fourth year from cover to cover. I am leafing through it at this moment and perhaps I was influenced as much by the beautiful firm style of the writing which carried such a tremendous amount of information with such economy of words, as by the scientific information drawn therefrom. I distinctly recall to this day and can look back in my mind's eye to an afternoon in the McGill Library poring over perhaps your original description of the method of recording heart sounds and murmurs and marvelling at what could be gleaned by the relatively crude method of listening through a couple of pieces of tubing. I have just drawn down from the shelf a book on *Auscultation of the Heart* by Ravin to search the bibliography for the actual date and reference. I find that in chapter 3 he devotes the whole of several pages to your method and acknowledges that he uses it with minor modifications throughout the book. I see that the original article to which I devoted myself that afternoon was written in the *American Heart Journal* in 1933. So without belabouring the point further I can say that the early seeds were planted at the bedside by you and Lewis' *Diseases of the Heart* followed shortly thereafter. I can truthfully say that I recall no other important influences.

My interest in respiratory disease and respiratory physiology which you will see in the curriculum vitae forms a prominent part of my work. It came about while I was at the Massachusetts General Hospital in 1951 and 1952 where one of the Fellows was a Fulbright Scholar from Italy, Dr. P. Curti. Curti could not speak a word of English and was basically unintelligible to most of us for a full three months. However, the tremendous range of his physiologic knowledge of the heart and lungs quickly made its influence felt and somehow and for what reason I am not sure he was determined to make a respiratory physiologist out of me. Together we pored over some of the outstanding publications from Cournand's laboratory in New York dealing with such things as "ideal alveolar air," diffusion, ventilation-profusion relationships, and succeeded in applying this to a study on mitral stenosis, referred to in my bibliography. It was an exciting time and I have maintained my interest in respiratory physiology to this date. I subsequently went on to Johns Hopkins, invited there by Riley, originator of much of the theory referred to above, to complete the work on mitral stenosis.

In 1965 Dr. Cohen's bibliography consisted of six items published between 1953 and 1960. The first is co-authored with Dr. Curti — "Respiratory and Circulatory Studies in patients with mitral stenosis" (*Circulation,* December 1953). The sixth article is "The Place of Function Tests in Chronic Respiratory Disease" (*The Medical Services Journal of Canada,* December 1960).

Dr. John Edward Fay, 3 September 1925, London, England; King's College and Charing Cross Hospital Med. Sch., University of London, M.B., B.S. with Honours Distinction in Med. 49; F.R.C.P.(C) Med. 58; F.A.C.C..

Dr. Fay's postgraduate education began with internship at Charing Cross Hospital (1949), followed by an appointment as Demonstrator in Physiology at his alma mater (1950). During the next four years, he served as a medical officer in the Royal Navy. He returned to physiology as an Assistant in the Charing Cross Hospital Medical School in 1955. The following year, he served as Assistant Resident in Medicine at the St. Raphael Hospital in New Haven, Connecticut. Specialist training began with Fellowship in Cardiology at the University of Saskatchewan (1950-57) followed by an assistant residency in medicine at the University Hospital in Saskatoon. He then received a National Research Council of Canada Research Fellowship to work at Queen's University (1958-59). He concluded formal postgraduate education with a Fellowship in Cardiology at the Sick Children's Hospital, Toronto (1959-60).

In 1971, when Dr. Fay updated his curriculum vitae, he was Associate Professor of Medicine at Queen's University and a member of the Attending Staff of the Kingston General Hospital and the Hotel Dieu.

Dr. Fay comments:

I first began to consider the study of cardiology while I was working as a resident in the United States, following my service in the Royal Navy. I had been offered various fellowships at Yale in subspecialties and then having applied to some Canadian schools for further residency training, I received a most warm and enthusiastic letter from Dr. Irwin Hilliard who was then Professor of Medicine in Saskatoon. As a result of this, I accepted a fellowship in cardiology and worked for a year with Dr. Louis Horlick. I have never regretted for one moment my decision to go to Saskatchewan and from that time on decided to devote my time to cardiology.

Dr. Irwin Hilliard and Dr. Louis Horlick were most helpful during my time in Saskatoon and as a result of their recommendation, I came to Queen's University to work for a year in the Department of Physiology with Dr. Don Hatcher. During this year, I was offered a post in Queen's University in the Department of Medicine to have a special interest in Paediatric Cardiology.

Dr. Fay's bibliography of twelve articles, all co-authored, published between 1963 and 1967 deal with a variety of subjects related to clinical cardiology.

Dr. Teruo Izukawa, 15 December 1930, Vancouver; University of Toronto, M.D. 50, A.O.A., F.A.H.A., F.R.C.P.(C).

During internship in 1956, Dr. Izukawa read Paul Wood's book, *Diseases of the Heart and Circulation.* This inspired him to seek training for a career in cardiology. Thus, he went to England in 1958, and remained there seven years during which he worked with Professor John Goodwin and Paul Wood in London, and Hugh Fleming in Cambridge. Then he spent three years (1965-1968) with Dr. Rowe at Johns Hopkins. He returned to Toronto and joined the Department of Cardiology at the Sick Children's Hospital. In 1972, when he composed his curriculum vitae he was Assistant Professor of Paediatrics at Toronto University.

His bibliography of 14 items published between 1962 and 1971 are all related to the cardiopulmonary system and are all co-authored.

Dr. Evan M. B. Patrick, 24 December 1927, Liverpool, England; University of Liverpool, M.B., B.Ch. 51; M.R.C.P. London 65; L.M.C.C. 66; F.R.C.P.(C), F.A.H.A.

Dr. Patrick served internships and registrarships in Internal Medicine and in Cardiology in Liverpool and its neighbourhood until 1966, when he emigrated to Canada and settled in Port Arthur for about two years until in 1968 he moved to Ottawa. In 1971, he was Lecturer in Medicine at Ottawa University and visiting consultant at the Winchester and District Memorial Hospital.

Dr. Patrick's comments about his postgraduate education and quest for a place in which to settle are of special interest.

> In 1961-62 I was working in Whiston Hospital, assisting in the setting up of an Intensive Care Unit (the first in Liverpool region). At the same time as this I was also assisting in the Cardiothoracic Clinic with a visiting cardiothoracic surgeon, which occurred about once every week or two. Between both of these, my interest in cardiology was stimulated. In 1963 the opportunity to join the Regional Cardiothoracic Unit in Liverpool arose and I obtained the post because of my experience in Intensive Care. My prime duty initially was to assist in the monitoring of the patients following by-pass surgery. Prior to 1961 I had been a general internist, with no very special interest in any particular field.
>
> After serving in the Royal Navy for four years, the major obstacle on returning was to find a suitable post in internal medicine at all. Other obstacles were the fact that training was largely "learning by doing," in the National Service, except in a very few favoured posts in special areas. Obviously this approach takes rather longer than the more formal training program in vogue on this side of the Atlantic. There is, however, a possible advantage of wider practical experience. (For example, during part of my career, while doing acute medicine at Whiston Hospital, I also 'ran' a geriatric block of 100 beds for my Chief. This took probably one to two hours a day of my time and considerably more of the interns' time, but gave me some experience in administration and management of waiting lists, as well as in rehabilitation of geriatric patients.)
>
> The lack of formal training was largely off-set by part-time courses from the University of Liverpool and meetings at the Liverpool Medical Institution (these were weekly events), and informal discussions with the consultant physicians. Once on the Cardiac Unit, however, training was rather more formal in that there was a weekly Unit meeting and several Journal Clubs, as well as the informal sessions with the consulting cardiologists.
>
> I had planned to emigrate many years ago due to frustration with the National Health Service (slow promotion, etc.) The opening in Port Arthur arrived at an appropriate time and provided me with a foothold in the New World. From here I have been able to get my Canadian qualifications. My practice so far, however, is only about 40% cardiological.

Dr. Walter Zingg, 29 March 1924, Kloten, Switzerland; University of Zurich, M.D. 51; University of Manitoba, M.Sc. Med. 52; F.R.C.S.(C) 58.

Dr. Walter Zingg, early in his career, decided to be an "experimental surgeon." Cardiovascular studies have always played an important part in his work. In his remarks about the special questions he wrote in 1965:

> A career in experimental surgery is still considered to be somewhat unusual.... It should be pointed out that my work with pump oxygenators although strictly speaking not research at all, led to some early clinical application which has helped me greatly in establishing myself in surgical research.

In the course of his training and in the development of his career he travelled extensively, changing jobs more frequently than is usual in North America. As an undergraduate student he served internship at the Hôpital du Samaritain in Vevey, Switzerland in 1946. During his senior undergraduate year, he had an internship at the Bethesda Hospital in Cincinnati, Ohio (1950-51). He experienced a residency in Pathology in 1949-50 at the University of Zurich. The year after the internship in Cincinnati he worked in the Department of Physiology of the University of Manitoba (1951-52). He then returned for training in surgery in Switzerland at the Winterthur General Hospital (1952-53). He returned to Manitoba in 1954 to "do" a residency in Medicine at the Winnipeg Municipal Hospital. The following year he devoted to surgery at Deer Lodge Veterans Hospital as Chief Surgical Resident (1955-56). He held an appointment as Lecturer in Physiology and also in the Department of Surgery of the University of Manitoba (1957-61), when he was promoted to Assistant Professor. He became Associate Professor in 1964. During these seven years he was in charge of the Surgical Research Laboratory. Among his appointments during his sojourn in Winnipeg he was in charge of extra-corporeal circulation at the Winnipeg Children's Hospital from 1959-1964. He moved to Toronto in 1964.

When he prepared his curriculum vitae for the archives in 1965, he was Assistant Professor of Surgery at the University of Toronto and both Associate Scientist and Associate Surgeon at the Hospital for Sick Children. This post provided him with ample opportunity to exercise his skills and special interest in the physiology of the cardiovascular system.

The first item in his bibliography appeared in 1950. It concerned a study of the duration of effectiveness of a preparation of heparin in animal experimentation (*Experimenta*, 1950: 6, 299). The forty-first item, the last in the list prepared in 1965, *Investigations on a Plastic Bonding Agent in Vascular Surgery*, was co-authored with M. Khododadeh, H. N. Ross, and C. C. Ferguson. The remaining thirty-nine range very widely in general surgery and experimental physiology.

Dr. John Robert Evans, 1 October 1929, Erindale, Onario; University of Toronto, M.D. 52; D. Phil. Oxon. 55; F.R.C.P.(C) 58; F.R.C.P.(C).

Dr. John Evans' postgraduate education began with a year at the Toronto General Hospital, then as a Rhodes Scholar in 1953-55 at Oxford. In 1955-56 he studied at the National Heart Hospital in London with Dr. Paul Wood. Between 1956 and 1960 he served residencies at the Toronto General, the Sunnybrook, and the Sick Children's hospitals. His postgraduate studies concluded with a Fellowship in Research at the Harvard Medical School. He returned to Toronto in 1961 to appointments on the staff of the Toronto General Hospital and the University. In 1965, when he prepared his curriculum vitae, he was Professor of Medicine and Dean of the Faculty of Medicine at McMaster University.

In his brief comments on the special questions, Dr. Evans states that he was "strongly influenced by the exciting approach of Dr. Paul Wood at the National Heart Hospital."

Between 1955 and 1965, his bibliography grew to 26 items. The eleventh item is related to the cardiovascular system, titled "Spontaneous Closure of Ventricular Septal Defects," co-authored with R. D. Rowe and John D. Keith *(Circulation,* 1960: 13, 1044). Of the remaining 15, all but two are on some aspect of myocardial metabolism, the 14th is on "Murmurs of the Patent Ductus Arteriosus in Normal Newborn Swine," co-authored with R. D. Rowe, H. G. Downie, and H. C. Roswell (*Circ. Res.*, 1963: 12, 85). The 25th is on "Coarctation of the Aorta," co-authored with R. J. Baird and C. L. Labrosse (*Arch. Surg.*, 1964: 89, 466).

Dr. Kyohei Joe Kako, 29 May 1928, Tokyo, Japan; Tokyo Jikei University, M.D. 1953.

Dr. Kako, born in Tokyo, was educated in his native city, graduating M.D. at Tokyo Jikei University in 1953. His interest in basic science was triggered by one of his teachers in Tokyo and further enhanced when he worked with Dr. Richard Bing at Wayne State University (1959-61).

He has continued his research on cardiac metabolism. When he composed his curriculum vitae in 1972 he was Associate Professor of Physiology in Ottawa University.

Dr. James Fraser Mustard, 16 October 1927, Toronto; University of Toronto, M.D. 53, Cambridge University, Ph.D. 56; F.R.C.P. 65; F.A.H.A.

Dr. James Mustard's postgraduate studies, mainly in Pathology, began with a year at the Toronto General Hospital, followed by two years at Cambridge University where he received the degree Ph.D. and finally two years (1956-58) at Sunnybrook Hospital.

In 1971, when he updated his curriculum vitae, he was Professor and Chairman of the Department of Pathology at McMaster University and visiting Professor of Pathology at the University of Toronto.

His researches on thrombosis are world-renowned. In 1967, he was honoured with the Gairdner Foundation International Award.

Dr. Walter Govan Waddell, 3 April 1928, Ottawa, Ontario; Queens University, M.D., C.M. 53; F.R.C.S.(C); F.A.C.S.

After internships at the Ottawa Civic Hospital (1953-54) and the Kingston General Hospital (1954-55), Dr. Waddell worked as a Fellow in Cardiovascular Surgery Research at the University of Toronto (1955-1957) then as assistant resident in Surgery at the Hospital for Sick Children, Toronto.

During the years from July 1958 to July 1960 (with the exception of 6 months, July 1959 to January 1960) he served as chief resident in Surgery at the Sunnybrook Hospital. He finally began his career in his native city, Ottawa, as chief resident in Surgery at the Ottawa Civic Hospital during the year 1960-61. In 1972, his academic status was Professor of Surgery, University of Ottawa and he was on the Active Staff of the Ottawa General and the Courtesy Staff of the Ottawa Civic Hospital. He also held the appointments of Consultant in Vascular Surgery at the Ottawa Grace Hospital and the National Defence Medical Centre.

Dr. Waddell made no comments about the special questions but did include his bibliography of ten items. The first two represent work done in 1955-57 on hypothermia and are co-authored with W. G. Bigelow and H. B. Fairley. There are several items related to vascular surgery; one is concerned with "Canine Myocardial Thresholds and Tissue Responses to Chronic Pacing" co-authored with Dr. O. Z. Roy and H. A. Heggtveit (*Med. & Biol. Eng.*, 1969: 7, 501-506). One is entitled "Jejunal Intussuseption: A Complication of Small Bowel Bypass for Intractable Obesity," and is co-authored with M. R. Tanga and J. L. Willinton. As a general surgeon with a special interest in vascular surgery, Dr. Waddell should more properly be placed among his fellows in Chapter Eleven.

Dr. Bernard Sean Langford Kidd, 7 July 1931, Belfast, Northern Ireland; The Queen's University, M.B., B. Ch., B.A.O. 54; M.D. with commendation by thesis 57; M.R.C.P. (Edin.) Cardiol. 60; F.A.C.C.; F.A.H.A.

As good luck would have it for all concerned, Dr. Kidd accepted Dr. John Keith's invitation to work at the Hospital for Sick Children in Toronto where he has remained since he came to Canada. The course which led him to enter the field of cardiology is well described in his comments.

> As a student, my ambition was to become a specialist in Internal Medicine. However, at this time, I was interested in Cardiology and attended clinics with the cardiologist in our teaching hospital. During my intern year, I arranged to acquire a broad education in this area, i.e., neurology, general medicine, endocrinology, renal physiology, etc. At the conclusion of this year, I felt that I should secure the two higher qualifications (M.D. and Membership) necessary for consultant practice in Britain as soon as possible, and to this end entered the Physiology Department in Belfast with the aim of writing a thesis for my M.D. This Department was a very active research centre in Circulatory Physiology, and I was a member of the unit for two years, and being engaged in research, obtained my M.D. in 1957.
>
> On re-entering the clinical fold, I was invited by the Cardiologist to become a Registrar in his unit, and I suppose it was at this point that the decision was made that this would be my main field of interest. For the next three years, I assisted my chief in the care of adults and children with acquired and congenital heart disease at the Royal Victoria Hospital, Belfast and at the Royal Belfast Hospital for Sick Children. I obtained membership of the Royal College of Physicians of Edinburgh with Cardiology as a special subject, in 1960. In this year, I was offered and accepted a post in the Department of Medicine of the University of Edinburgh, where Professor K. W. Donald was setting up a unit for research and investigation of problems in the cardiopulmonary area. In addition to work in the laboratory, I had teaching duties in the university and clinical care of patients in the Royal Infirmary, Edinburgh.

While working in this unit, I was invited by Dr. John Keith of the Hospital for Sick Children, Toronto, to consider whether I might possibly emigrate to Toronto to become the member of his unit with a responsibility for the cardiac catheterization laboratory, which invitation I accepted. Since 1961, I have worked in the Department of Cardiology at the Hospital for Sick Children, Toronto, and am currently Assistant Physician and Physiologist in the Unit, Research Associate in the Research Institute and Clinical Teacher in the Department of Paediatrics, University of Toronto.

Between 1956 and 1971 Dr. Kidd co-authored more than forty publications. They deal with a wide range of subjects related to physiology and pathology of the cardiovascular system. Since 1961 his co-authors have frequently been men and women who received their training as fellows of the Department of Cardiology at the Hospital for Sick Children. Dr. Kidd has contributed richly to the education of cardiologists in Canada and in all parts of the world.

Dr. H. Alexander Heggtveit, 3 March 1933, Montreal; University of Ottawa, M.D. 1957; F.C.A.P. 62; Cert. Royal Coll. of Path. 67; F.A.C.C.; F.C.C.P.; F.I.C.A.

Dr. Heggtveit's postgraduate education prepared him for a career as pathologist. In addition to two years at the Ottawa General Hospital (1957-59), he had three years at King's County Hospital, Brooklyn, New York.

In 1972, when he responded to the questionnaire, his principal appointments were Professor of Pathology at the University of Ottawa and Pathologist at the Ottawa General Hospital.

He wrote, commenting on the special questions:

My interest in cardiovascular diseases was engendered during the latter years of my residency training in pathology when I studied and subsequently published several series of cases of rheumatic and luetic aortitis. An additional year of training in electron microscopy was devoted to a study of the effects of experimental magnesium deficiency on the myocardium. For the past ten years I have been involved in the academic practice of pathology at the University of Ottawa and Ottawa General Hospital and during that time have become exclusively involved in the sub-specialty of cardiovascular pathology in all of my research, teaching, and service activities. Major areas of interest include human and experimental cardiomyopathies and ultrastructural pathology of the myocardium.

Dr. Heggtveit's bibliography begins with senior authorship in an article on "Panaortitis," (*Am. J. Path.*, 1942: 151, 1963). His bibliography grew to sixty-eight items which reflect the comments he has made about the evolution of his interests.

One of his affiliations places him in the forefront of current investigation of the cardiovascular system. He is a member of the executive of the International Study Group for Research in Cardiac Metabolism.

Dr. Geoffrey Frank Trobridge, 8 October 1926, Birmingham, England; University of Birmingham, M.B., B.Ch. 48; M.D. 58; M.R.C.P.(E) 57; F.R.C.P.(E) 70.

Dr. Trobridge's experience in England included Registrar in the Chest Clinic at Leeds (1953-54) and Registrar and Senior Medical Officer at Hawkmoor Chest Hospital, Devon, 1955-1965. His comments on the special questions describe his unique experience before coming to Sudbury where he established a cardiopulmonary laboratory in 1966, the first in that region of Canada. When he submitted his curriculum vitae in 1972 he held the following posts: University Research Associate in the Department of Biology, Laurentian University; Consultant at the Sudbury Memorial, the Sudbury General, the Sudbury St. Joseph's, the Copper Cliff, Espanola, Little Current, Elliot Lake and South Porcupine Hospitals. Among the services he pioneered is ambulatory electrocardiographic monitoring with the early models of the Holter apparatus. He wrote as follows about his entry into the field of cardiology:

> I specialized in respiratory diseases starting in 1953. From working in close association with Thoracic Surgery, I was encouraged to work in the field of pulmonary physiology from 1955 onwards and by 1966 it was quite apparent that in this type of work, cardiac catheterization was necessary. As soon as I studied this, the demand for my services in this field was such that I became extremely interested in this.
>
> From 1957 to 1965 I continued this work in cardiopulmonary physiology in England. In 1966 I came to Canada to set up a Cardio Pulmonary Physiology Department in Sudbury and this was preceded by further training for three months at the Toronto General Hospital.

My formal training in England was in chest clinics and chest hospitals. My subsequent transition into Cardiology resulted from the work in cardio-pulmonary physiology. There were considerable obstacles to acceptance of anyone specializing in the field of cardio-pulmonary physiology even in a Thoracic Surgical Unit. As a result of my rather unusual development in this specialty I did not buy my first electrocardiograph until 1967.

Membership in the Canadian Cardiovascular Society inevitably appeared rather late in the development of my career but has proved a most valuable meeting ground with specialists all over Canada.

Dr. Trobridge did not provide a bibliography.

Manitoba

Dr. Hubert Daniel Kitchen, 31 January 1895, Brandon — 4 November 1966, Winnipeg; University of Manitoba, Med. Coll. M.D. 21; C.R.C.P. 45; F.A.C.P. 48.

Dr. Kitchen is mentioned by Dr. Robert Beamish as one of the senior men of the Manitoba Clinic who had a special interest in cardiology. He was present at the first meeting of the Canadian Cardiovascular Society, 24 June 1947 in Winnipeg.

The following obituary appeared in the *Canadian Medical Association Journal,* 21 January 1967, Volume 30, and is quoted in full:

> Dr. Hubert Daniel Kitchen, 71, died at Deer Lodge Hospital, Winnipeg, on November 6, 1966. Born in Brandon, he received his early education at Souris, Manitoba. During the First World War, he served with the 11th Field Ambulance C.E.F. and received the Military Medal.
>
> He graduated from Manitoba Medical College in 1921, winning the Gold Medal for the highest aggregate during the course and the Rockefeller Scholarship for three years. This period was spent at the Mayo Clinic and he became a member of the Clinic in 1924. He was medical director for the Arctic and Central Divisions of the Hudson's Bay Company at Winnipeg. In 1945, he was certified in internal medicine by the Royal College of Physicians of Canada, and in 1948, he became a Fellow of the American College of Physicians.
>
> A founder of the Manitoba Clinic in 1946, he served with that clinic until his retirement in 1963. He was Associate Professor of

Medicine at the University of Manitoba and for 29 years he served on the staff of the Winnipeg General Hospital.

He was President of the Manitoba Medical Association in 1941 and President of the Manitoba Club in 1958. He was made an Honorary Member of the Canadian Medical Association in 1966. Other interests were curling, golfing and fishing.

His widow, a son, a daughter and two grandchildren survive him.

Dr. Benjamin H. Lyons, 1 December 1908, Rosthern, Saskatchewan; Alberta Med. Sch., M.D. 1931; L.M.C.C: F.R.C.P.(C): F.A.C.P.

As a medical student, Dr. Lyons harboured the ambition to become an internist. How he achieved this eventually, he tells in his brief comments on the special questions:

> While a medical student, I found I was interested in Medicine. After graduation, I had an appointment with Dr. Louis Katz at Michael Reese Hospital, but this was 1931 — for economic reasons, I had to go out into rural practice in Birch Mills, Saskatchewan, population 500. I retained hope of eventually doing postgraduate work in Medicine. I bought an E.C.G. at about 1936. In 1945, I disposed of the practice, put the family in a car and drove down to Philadelphia to Internal Medicine Post Graduate School and Hospital.
>
> Having lived all my life in Western Canada, Winnipeg was a natural choice to practise in, especially as I had family and friends here.

Dr. Lyons did not provide a bibliography.

Dr. Francis Alexander Lavens Mathewson, 1 February 1905, New Westminster, B.C.; University of Manitoba Med. Coll., M.D. 31; B.Sc. (Med.) 33; Amer. Bd. Preventive Med., Aviation Med.; Cert. in Int. Med., Roy. Coll. Phys. 46; F.A.C.P. 42; Fellow, Aerospace Med. Assoc. 47; F.A.H.A, F.A.C.C.

Dr. Mathewson devoted the first year after graduation to internship at the Winnipeg General Hospital and the second year to residency at the Vancouver General Hospital. For the year 1933-34, he had a Gordon Bell Research Fellowship.

In 1971, when his curriculum vitae was updated, he had retired from the Directorship of the Department of Electrocardiography at the Winnipeg General Hospital, which he held from 1954 to 1967. He was a member of the Honorary Attending staff of the Winnipeg

General Hospital and Associate Professor of Medicine, University of Manitoba. His curriculum vitae lists many affiliations with scientific societies and posts of responsibility, including that of Medical Director of the Great West Life Assurance Company.

Dr. Mathewson's contribution to the creation of the Canadian Heart Association in 1947, and his effective work as a councillor and president are alluded to in the chapter on Societies and Foundations. His bibliography of 18 items, published during the years 1935 to 1965, reflects his keen interest in electrocardiography. The articles he has written about the long term follow-up of the pilots he began to study during World War II represent a major accomplishment very much appreciated throughout the world, especially by those interested in aviation medicine.

Dr. Mathewson supplied a detailed curriculum vitae and bibliography. He did not comment on the special questions.

Dr. Laurie Coke, 12 June 1913 Winnipeg; University of Manitoba, M.D. *cum laude* 36; F.C.C.P.; F.A.C.P. Cert. R.C.P.(C), F.A.H.A.; C.H.A.; F.A.C.P.; F.A.C.C.P.

Dr. Coke began postgraduate training with three years of internships and residencies in Winnipeg, then a year at the London Hospital, England and three months at the Massachusetts General Hospital, Boston. In 1971, when he updated his curriculum vitae he was Associate Professor of Medicine at the University of Manitoba, on the active staff of the St. Boniface Hospital, cardiologist at Deer Lodge Hospital, and consultant at the Grace Hospital.

In brief comments about the special questions, Dr. Coke relates that he became interested in cardiology in the first year of his internship. He notes that in 1946 the Professor of Medicine at the University of Manitoba did not recognize the existence or the necessity of cardiology as a specialty. With respect to the Canadian Cardiovascular Society, Dr. Coke states it "will establish our specialty." Dr. Coke's publications include several on the relation between nutrition and the cardiovascular system. This observation arose out of his sustained interest in the study of 391 veterans of the Japanese prison camps in Hong Kong who suffered from dietary deficiency from December 1941 to August 1945. In 1961, he published a twelve-year follow-up of these men (*Medical Services Journal,* May 1961). The twenty-year follow-up study was to be published in 1972.

Dr. Paul Kinley Tisdale, 6 July 1913, Bradwardine, Manitoba; University of Manitoba, B.Sc. 33; M.D. 38; F.A.C.P.; C.R.C.P.

Dr. Tisdale's first experience in postgraduate training was as junior intern at the Winnipeg General Hospital (1937-38). He spent the following year as an intern in the Winnipeg Children's Hospital. He served in the Royal Canadian Army Medical Corps from 1939 to 1945. After the war, he spent a year at Deer Lodge Hospital. He then entered practice. He attended courses for continuing medical education organized by the American College of Physicians and also by the University at Minnesota. Dr. Tisdale did not provide a bibliography.

Dr. Tisdale's stationery has these words under his name — "Internal and Occupational Medicine," — a unique specialty title which immediately initiates thoughts related to rehabilitation of cardiacs. The men who have given major attention to this field are very few. Dr. Tisdale's comments in 1965 on the special questions are of considerable interest.

> Your request for supplementary remarks dealing with the special questions is unusual and certainly provokes thoughtful and nostalgic reflections on these aspects of one's career. Concerning how and when my specialization in cardiology was born, my interest in cardiology was certainly first stimulated in undergraduate years by Professor W. H. K. Moorehouse, my professor of physiology, and by the late Drs. John McEachern and Hubert Kitchen, my clinical instructors in cardiology. I declined Dr. McEachern's suggestion to me at the time of graduation that I embark then on a career in cardiology. This decision in 1938 was made on the basis that I wished to acquire a broader base for cardiology or whatever specialty I might eventually practise. The Second World War intervened and though one did encounter more than one's share of cardiological problems, the scarcity of ECG photographic paper was the major handicap in electrocardiographic investigation even of our diphtheritic patients.
>
> My qualification in internal medicine immediately followed the Second World War but without any special emphasis on cardiology. It might be truly said that subsequently in my practice of internal medicine, as I developed my consulting practice, I found an increasing preponderance of cardiovascular patients, particularly among those referred to me. This trend continued until 1965 when I restricted my practice to referred patients only,

patients with cardiac and/or general cardiovascular problems have constituted over 75% of the patients referred to me.

I never experienced a formal course of training in cardiology as this phenomenon of our educational postgraduate activities has really only come into its own since I completed my qualification in internal medicine, and at a time when I could ill afford the time or money to drop out of practice for several years to undertake such a formal course. My training therefore has been self-organized through attendance at short courses of one or two weeks duration occasionally and fairly regular attendance at professional association meetings superimposed on regular perusal of the usual periodicals.

In my younger days formal training in cardiology per se was not available in Canada and not too readily available in the U.S.A. The advent of World War II interrupted my plans for postgraduate study in Britain. I did not really choose a place to practice cardiology but rather the place in which I chose to practice seemed to 'force cardiology upon me.'

I purchased my first electrocardiograph machine, a Cambridge string galvanometer photographic unit in about 1947 I think.

My career was fairly well developed before the Canadian Cardiovascular Society had become a significant force in clinical cardiology in Canada or at least on the Prairies. I have found the two Annual Meetings of our Society, which I have so far attended, have been fascinating and extremely stimulating. I think the mingling of investigators, full time educators and those of us involved in the clinical practice of cardiology, is one of the major roles which our Society has to play in promoting the highest standards of medical care, education and investigation in Canada. I look forward to experiencing a major degree of stimulation from our Society in the remainder of my practising life.

The combination of opportunity and interest — the opportunity to see many patients with cardiovascular problems and the interest which this experience stimulates — was of course the channel through which most of our generation arrived at an exclusive or predominant preoccupation with cardiology and cardiovascular diseases. This pathway is obviously no longer suitable for those who have not had the opportunity of growing up with the development of modern cardiology and particularly those who wish to devote a major part of their time to investigation and/or educational work. They must compress into three or four short years the knowledge that has developed and grown over thirty and more years.

Dr. Leon Michaels, 1 March 1925, London, England; University of London, St. Mary's M.B., B.S. 46; M.D.; Ph.D.; M.R.C.P. London; F.R.C.P.(C).

In 1965, Dr. Michaels submitted his curriculum vitae together with a letter about how he chose cardiology and obtained special training in England.

> The decision to become a cardiologist was based partly on an emotional attraction to the glamour of the advances linked with catheterizing techniques as they were being developed in the late 1940s. I was also influenced by chance making me a resident to a cardiologist whom I found extremely stimulating. This was before leaving Great Britain.
>
> The special training was carried out at Guy's Hospital. Some of the obstacles were:
>
> 1. Lack of any formal training program. I just had to pick up Catheterizing and Investigative techniques.
> 2. The fact that many techniques were reserved for surgeons. I had no experience of angiography, for example, and the investigative and clinical sides were largely divorced.
> 3. The training was based on the then-existing English system of having paediatric cardiology down to about the age of four united with adult cardiology. As a result of their separation here, I am not practising an appreciable part of that branch of cardiology in which I have trained.

Before settling in Winnipeg he spent a year (1957-58) at the Mayo Clinic. Items 14 and 16 of his bibliography are co-authored with colleagues of the Mayo Clinic. Number 14 is "Detection of the Retrograde Passage of Indicator from Aorta to Left Ventricle in Days" *(The Physiologist,* 1960: 3, 10). Number 16 is "Detection and Measurement of Experimentally Produced Aortic Regurgitation by Means of Indicator-Dilution Recorded from the Left Ventricle" (*Cir. Res.*, 1963: 12, 169). Number 19, for which he is sole author, is "Cancer: Incidents and Mortality in Patients Having Anti-Coagulant Therapy" (*Lancet,* 1964: 2, 832).

In 1965 Dr. Michaels was Lecturer in Medicine at the University of Manitoba and on the staff of the Winnipeg General Hospital and the Manitoba Clinic.

Dr. Peter Gaskell, 24 June 1917, England; University of Western Ontario; M.D. 50; University of London, Ph.D. 55; A.O.A.

Dr. Gaskell wrote the following about his training and his subsequent career.

> Began medical education as veteran in veterans' class at the University of Western Ontario in 1945. Graduated in 1950 and during 1950-51, while interning at Victoria Hospital, London, was influenced by Professor A. C. Burton, Department of Biophysics of the Medical College and induced to enter an academic career. Began research career in his department in July 1951. (I had come to know Dr. Burton during war years when I was a Technical Assistant Medical in RCAF and worked in the unit in Toronto in which he was carrying out research as a civilian). From his department, I went to work under Professor Henry Barcroft of the Sherrington School of Physiology, Saint Thomas's Hospital, London, England in 1952, where I obtained my Ph.D. on the basis of research concerned with the peripheral circulation in the limbs. In 1955, I was appointed Assistant Professor in the Department of Physiology, University of Manitoba, and am still in this Department as Professor of Physiology since 1970.
>
> The research under Professor Barcroft was arranged through Professor Burton. During the period July 1951 to July 1955, I was supported by the Life Insurance Medical Research Fund for the last year — all arranged through the University of Western Ontario.

Dr. Gaskell's bibliography contains articles mainly related to peripheral circulation. Among the items of clinical importance is one by Dr. Gaskell and Dr. Krisman on "An Auscultatory Technique for Measuring the Digital Blood Pressure" (*Can. J. Biochem. & Physiol.*, 1958: 36, 883).

Dr. Violet Marie Storrie, 3 January 1923, Winnipeg; University of Manitoba, M.D. 1950; Cert. Int. Med. R.C.P. 54; F.A.C.P. 1960.

Before graduation, Dr. Storrie had a rotating internship (1949-50) as part of the final undergraduate year, followed by an assistant residency in Pathology and Medicine. The following year she was assistant resident in Medicine. All these appointments were at the Winnipeg General Hospital. She spent the next two years in Boston at the New England Centre, 1953-54, as assistant resident in Medicine and 1954-55 as Fellow in Medicine. She then returned to

Winnipeg to develop her career. In 1971, she held the following posts: Assistant Physician on the Honorary Attending Staff of the Winnipeg General Hospital; she is on the Courtesy Staff of the Winnipeg Municipal Hospital and the Manitoba Rehabilitation Centre; she is Lecturer in Medicine at the University of Manitoba. Her curriculum vitae lists active membership in many organizations.

Dr. Storrie has a firm opinion, namely, that she definitely has had no problems related to discovering her identity. While doing postgraduate work in Boston, 'they' tempted her to remain and make her career there. But she believed firmly that Canadians "who go away to train should return to Canada." Her comments on the special questions are quoted in full:

> I believe that my interest in cardiology resulted from working with and being inspired by Dr. R. E. Beamish of Winnipeg. I had decided to specialize in Internal Medicine, and during part of my resident training in Winnipeg, I was closely associated with Dr. Beamish. I assisted Dr. Beamish in clinical practice at the Manitoba Clinic for one year before continuing postgraduate studies in Boston, Massachusetts.
>
> My training in Boston included some time in the Cardiology Department, but I spent time in various departments of Medicine, and very nearly remained in Boston when I was invited to work permanently with Dr. Ted Astwood in Endocrinology. However, I felt that Canadians who go away to train should return to Canada. I had known all along that I would be welcomed in practice at the Manitoba Clinic, and knew that Dr. Beamish was planning expansion of our Cardiology Department. I returned to start practice here in 1956, and of course, our Department already had several electrocardiograph machines. As you see, my work in the field of cardiology has been largely clinical and not academic. As I am a lady physician, I find that cardiovascular work is particularly well suited to women.

Dr. Storrie's bibliography includes several articles in the field of endocrinology between 1953-56, then the subjects become related to cardiology, notably, "Impending Infarction and the Management of Anticoagulant Therapy."

Dr. Gordon R. Cumming, 2 March 1929, Winnipeg; University of Manitoba, M.D. 53; B.Sc. (Med.) 53; F.R.C.P.(C) 1958; C.A.S.S., F.A.H.A., F.A.C.C.

Dr. Cumming's postgraduate training began with internship at the Winnipeg General Hospital followed by assistant residency at Deer

Lodge Hospital. There followed a teaching fellowship at the University of Toronto, chief residency at the Winnipeg General Hospital, and a Fellowship in the Cardiovascular Division of the Cleveland Clinic.

In 1968, he held the following posts: Assistant Physician at the Winnipeg General Hospital, Director of Cardiology at the Winnipeg General Hospital, Director of Cardiology at the Winnipeg Children's Hospital, Associate Professor of Medicine and Paediatrics, University of Manitoba.

Dr. Cumming did not submit a bibliography.

Dr. Reubin Kaufman, 5 June 1930, Winnipeg; University of Manitoba, M.D. 53; L.M.C.C. 53; C.R.C.P.(C).

After two years of residencies, one at the St. Boniface and one at Deer Lodge Hospital, he entered general practice for a year (1955-56). Because he developed a great interest in cardiac arrhythmias, he proceeded to obtain training in cardiology at the Cedars of Lebanon Hospital in Los Angeles, where after one year as Resident in Medicine he was a Fellow in Cardiology for two years (1958-60).

In 1972, he was on the Active Staff of St. Boniface and the Victoria General Hospitals and clinical instructor, University of Manitoba.

Dr. Kaufman did not provide a bibliography.

Dr. Stefan Andrew Carter, 25 March 1928, Warsaw, Poland; University of Manitoba, B.Sc. (Med.) 54; M.D. 1954; M.Sc. 1956; C.S.C.I.; F.A.H.A.; F.A.C.A. 69.

Dr. Carter started postgraduate training with internship in Medicine at the Winnipeg General Hospital (1954-55), then he spent a year working with Professor M. Nickerson in Pharmacology at the University of Manitoba. Having become interested in peripheral vascular disease, he next studied with Dr. Irving S. Wright at Cornell University (1956-57), followed by a year at the Mayo Clinic with Dr. E. H. Wood. On returning to Winnipeg he was appointed Director of the Medical Peripheral Vascular Clinic at the St. Boniface Hospital. He still held the post in 1971 when he updated his curriculum vitae. At the University, he was then Chairman of the Cardiovascular Subject Committee, Co-ordinator of Didactic Teaching, 2nd year Medicine and Associate Professor of Medicine. He commented on the special questions as follows:

> My specialty is not Cardiology, but rather Angiology and Cardiovascular Investigation. I am interested and involved in clini-

cal care and diagnosis of patients with peripheral arterial disease and research in the same areas.

My activities include testing of patients with arterial disease by measurements of skin temperatures and local systolic pressures, investigation and improvement of methods for studying arterial disease, long term anticoagulant therapy, teaching cardiovascular physiology, and clinical angiology.

I began to consider work in this field during my first postgraduate year spent doing internal medicine and research in experimental shock. Various stages of my postgraduate training were spent and arranged with the essential help of Professor J. Doupe, late Chairman of the Department of Physiology, University of Manitoba.

Between 1955 and 1971, Dr. Carter published twenty-eight papers. The first item in his bibliography set the course of his future work, "The Pathogenesis of Atherosclerosis," 1955. A year later his second paper reported work carried out with Dr. Beamish on the use of Danilone as an anticoagulant. Later he published many papers on occlusive disease of peripheral arteries of the lower extremities.

Dr. Robert Gerald Handford, 1 July 1929, Winnipeg; University of Manitoba, B.A. 1950; M.D. 1955; Cert. R.C.P.(C); F.A.C.P.

Dr. Handford had all his postgraduate education in Winnipeg, at the Deer Lodge and the Winnipeg General Hospitals. He was Resident Fellow in the Renal Vascular Department of Deer Lodge Hospital in 1957-58. When he submitted his curriculum vitae in 1972, he was Assistant Professor of Medicine at the University of Manitoba, on the Attending Staff of the Winnipeg General Hospital and Medical Director of the Monarch Life Assurance Company.

Dr. Handford made no comments on the special questions and did not provide a bibliography.

Dr. Robert Arthur Corne, 5 June 1936, Winnipeg; University of Manitoba, B.Sc. (Med.) 59, M.D. 59; University of Minnesota, M.S. 64; University of Manitoba Med. Coll. Dept. of Med. 67; F.R.C.P.(C) 66; Dip. Amer. Bd. Int. Med., F.A.C.C.P.; F.A.H.A.; F.A.C.C.

Dr. Corne's postgraduate training took place chiefly at the Mayo Clinic (1960-64). In the last year of this period, he worked in the Department of Cardiology of the Mayo Clinic and the University of Minnesota and earned the degree M.S. He returned to Winnipeg to occupy posts at the University and at the St. Boniface Hospital. In

1971, he was Assistant Professor of Medicine, Assistant Physician at the Winnipeg General Hospital and in that year became Assistant Medical Director of the Great West Life Assurance Company.

Dr. Corne made no comments on the special questions. Between 1960 and 1965, he published six papers. The first item is a thesis on a haematological subject for which he earned the degree B.Sc. (Med.) at the University of Manitoba. Three articles deal with the electrical axis of the electrocardiogram.

Dr. Robert James Hoeschen, 16 September 1935, Winnipeg; University of Manitoba, M.D. 59; M.Sc. 62; C.S.C.I.

Dr. Hoeschen started postgraduate training as a junior intern at the Winnipeg General Hospital (1959-60), followed a year as Resident Fellow in Cardiology and one year as assistant resident in Medicine at the same hospital. During the next two years he worked at the Royal Victoria Hospital in Montreal, one as Research Fellow in Cardiology and one as senior assistant resident in Medicine. During the next two years (1964-66), he studied at the Graduate School of Public Health, University of Pittsburgh, with a special interest in Nutrition.

In 1968, he was Assistant Professor of Medicine, University of Manitoba, Tutor in Biochemistry, and Assistant Physician at the Winnipeg General Hospital. Between 1962 and 1971 he published five articles, mainly concerning the pharmacology of nitroglycerine, digoxin, and persantin.

Dr. Bryan William Kirk, 12 February 1937, Winnipeg; University of Manitoba, M.D. (Hons) 60; F.R.C.P.; F.A.C.P.

Immediately after graduation, Dr. Kirk served internship and residencies at the Winnipeg General Hospital, then he devoted a year to pharmacology after which he was resident in Medicine at the Montreal General Hospital, and lastly, he served as resident on the Services of Respiratory System, University of Manitoba.

In 1972, he was Director of the Cardiovascular Department of the Winnipeg General Hospital, Consultant at the Winnipeg Children's and the St. Boniface Hospitals, and the P.A. Stewart Centre. His status at the University of Manitoba was Assistant Professor.

Between 1958 and 1972 his bibliography grew to 16 items which reflect broad interests; the first two are on a sociological subject, statistical studies of the academic progress of Manitoba High School students beyond grade XI. The third is on "Sensory Deprivation"

(*Man. Med. Stud. J.*, 1960). Beginning in 1965 the articles are related to cardio-respiratory physiology and pharmacology.

Dr. Robert Earl Beamish, 9 September 1916, Shoal Lake, Manitoba; McMaster University, B.A. 37; University of Manitoba, M.D. 42; B.Sc. (Med.) 44; L.C.M.C. 48; M.R.C.P. (London) 48; M.R.C.P. (Edinburgh) 49; F.R.C.P.(C) 50; F.A.C.P. 51; F.A.C.C. 57; F.R.C.P. (Edinburgh) 61; F.I.C.A. 62; F.C.C.P. 62; F.A.H.A. 63.

Dr. Beamish was among those who attended the first meeting of the Society on June 24, 1947. He had resumed civilian status in 1946 and joined the group which became the Manitoba Clinic. The two senior physicians of this clinic, the late Dr. John M. McEachern and Dr. H. D. Kitchen, were both specially interested in cardiology, and were also present at that meeting. Dr. Beamish was at the very beginning of his career when the Society was born. He has been intensely interested and very helpful in advancing the work of the Archives Committee. Although he sent the questionnaire and the comments on the special questions about a year after he had received the request, he compensated for the delay by the excellence of the material. The letter he wrote in 1966 that accompanied the curriculum vitae is quoted in full.

> Dear Harold:
> It is with dismay that I note that your request for biographical information is dated June 9th, 1965. I regret that I was unable to give this its proper attention until now — while I am on vacation. No doubt this has some significance in a historical sense — the doctor of today is besieged by so many demands that even the best intentioned cannot meet them all. Although many members of society can look forward to increased leisure in the coming years, it does not appear that this will apply to physicians for a good while yet.
>
> Attached is the form which you supplied, and also a copy of my curriculum vitae as well as a bibliography. The following is an attempt to answer your specific questions.
>
> Following discharge from the Army (May 1946), I entered practice with the MacCharles Surgical Clinic, which had plans for developing into a larger Clinic — and became the Manitoba Clinic in December 1946. The two senior physicians were the late Doctor John M. McEachern (an old friend of yours) and Doctor H. D. Kitchen. Both of these had extensive cardiac practices. Thus, I at once came in contact with a large variety of cardiac diseases. However, I did not plan to become a cardiolo-

gist until I was stimulated in this direction during a year spent at the National Heart Hospital in London, England. By the time I returned to Winnipeg (November 1948) I was quite secure in the intention to become a cardiologist. At first, practice was general internal medicine but as rapidly as possible it was restricted to cardiology.

After Doctor McEachern's death, I restricted entirely to cardiac patients and a few years later, further restricted to consultative work.

My first major interest in a segment of cardiology was acquired through the influence of the late Doctor J. D. Adamson who was Professor of Medicine at the University of Manitoba from 1943 to 1952. In 1941, while I was his junior intern, he suggested that I might investigate the use of thiocyanates in the treatment of hypertension. This was pursued through my senior internship and residency and resulted in my first publication "The Treatment of Essential Hypertension with Sodium Thiocyanate" (*C.M.A.J.*, 1945, 53, 236). After returning from England, I established an out-patient clinic for hypertension at the Winnipeg General Hospital and this was carried on for some years. Studies on the mode of action of thiocyanates were carried out and led to papers on thyroid function and adrenal function in hypertension treated with thiocyanate. About this time, new and better drugs developed and our interest in this subject waned. It is with some satisfaction that one notes the contributions to hypertension now made by Doctor Sheldon G. Sheps (Mayo Clinic) who first became interested in hypertension in my little clinic.

When I returned from postgraduate work, senior members of the department of medicine discouraged specialization in the now well-recognized sub-departments of medicine. It was said that one's first objective was to become a good general physician and in this area there was no encouragement (in fact opposition) to pursuing a sub-specialty. By 1952, it was clear that I was not going to realize my desire to have a sub-department of cardiology in the hospital and University setting, and I began to develop a department of cardiology in the private practice clinic (Manitoba Clinic) where I still work. This endeavour prospered and we soon had four physicians and a cardiac surgeon and later a vascular surgeon associated in this unit.

The reason I returned to Winnipeg was that I had a private practice to come back to, and an appointment in the hospital and in the University and it seemed like a good place to start. However, I was soon invited to Vancouver by the late Doctor G. F. Strong and spent three days with him, seriously considering a move to join him. I am not sure just why I did not go — probably mainly inertia.

Having joined practising cardiologists, electrocardiographs were already in daily use when I commenced practice.

Membership in the Canadian Cardiovascular Society was of great benefit to me from the beginning. Coming back to Winnipeg (where cardiology was not appreciated as a specialty) from the stimulating environment provided by the small group around the late Doctor Paul Wood in London, I had a great need to meet other young men interested in cardiology. The annual meetings of the Society thus became very important to me. Continued participation in the activities of the Society has been one of the most pleasant and rewarding experiences in my professional life.

One of the most interesting developments in my experience has been the evolution of the concept of "impending myocardial infarction." While with Doctor Paul Wood, I became interested in his early attempts to postpone or forestall myocardial infarctions in patients with what he called acute coronary insufficiency. His concept was that such patients had coronary thrombosis without infarction, and that anticoagulants might prevent the process going on to actual infarction. In the early years after returning to Canada, this concept was considerably extended so that we finally arrived at three categories of 'impending infarction.' It is interesting to note that the third edition of Friedberg's classic *Diseases of the Heart* now describes these categories following our (with Dr. V. M. Storrie) original description of them. This work led to presentations in this province, Edmonton, Regina, Montreal, North Dakota, Chicago, St. Louis, Atlantic City, and to participation in international conferences on anticoagulants, Toronto 1961, and Miami, 1964.

Like yourself, I have been most interested in the welfare of the Heart Foundations. I was one of the founding members of the Manitoba Heart Foundation and served as the first secretary-treasurer (1957-59), then as vice-president (1957-61) and now, chairman of the scientific committee. As honorary secretary-treasurer of the Canadian Cardiovascular Society, I have been a member of the Board of the Canadian Heart Foundation since 1963.

It was most interesting to serve as a member of the council, College of Physicians and Surgeons of Manitoba, for eight years beginning in 1954. This culminated in presidency of the College whereupon I transferred my activities to the Manitoba Medical Association, serving on the Executive Committee and now as an officer. These are strenuous but interesting days in the political and economic aspect of our profession.

Dr. Beamish's bibliography begins with an article on "The Treatment of Essential Hypertension with Sodium Thiocyanate." This article was written with Dr. J. D. Adamson and published in the *Canadian Medical Association Journal* of 1945. After 1948 most of his publications are concerned with various aspects of clinical cardiology. An interesting exception is on "The Diagnostic Use of Curare in Myasthenia Gravis," 1951. He devoted much attention to anticoagulant therapy and his article on "Impending Myocardial Infarction — Recognition and Management" (*Circulation,* 1960: 21, 1107) was abstracted in several journals which gave it world-wide circulation. He had served on the Editorial Board of the *Manitoba Medical Review* and in 1968 edited a special number on coronary heart disease.

Dr. Beamish responded to the request for information about the introduction of cardiac catheterization Winnipeg with the following:

> Since our conversation, I have talked with Dr. John A. Hildes who, unfortunately, is ill with an intracranial tumour. He was able to recall the first catheterization quite well. Early in 1949, Dr. Hildes and I performed the first cardiac catheterization in Winnipeg at the old Winnipeg General Hospital (now Health Sciences Centre-General). I had returned from the National Heart Hospital — London in November 1948 and had been a member of Dr. Paul Wood's first catheterization team. Dr. Hildes had been at the Hammersmith Hospital where he had done catheterizations, mainly in respect to the liver as he was primarily interested in gastroenterology at that time. At any rate, we combined our talents to perform several cardiac catheterizations, but we turned it over to Dr. John Armstrong some months later. John then performed this procedure in succeeding years. Later, Dr. Gordon Cumming established a unit at the Children's Hospital in Winnipeg.
>
> Many years later, Dr. Paul Wood visited Winnipeg and told me that when he wrote the first edition of his book (1950) the only catheterization cases he could use were those which I had written up. Knowing Paul Wood, you will realize that this was high praise indeed!

In response to the request for updating his curriculum vitae in 1971, Dr. Beamish submitted a twelve-page document, a model for a C.V. He had resigned from the Manitoba Clinic in 1970 and had become Medical Director of the Great West Life Assurance Company. He had served as president of the Canadian Cardiovascular Society in 1968-70. His bibliography had grown to 56 items between 1945 and 1972; 17 items have appeared since 1965. These reflect his continued special interest in various aspects of coronary artery disease and also his expertise in medical administration. Item 4 is his report, as moderator of the committee to study standardized accounting systems within clinics *(Quart. Bull. Can. Assoc. Med. Clin.*, 1968; 2, 1). Item 42 is on "Epidemiology of Coronary Heart Disease" (*Man. Med. Rev.*, 1948; 48, 366) and item 56 is "Prophylaxis in Vascular Disease" (*Modern Med. of Canada*, 1972; 27, 343-345).

Saskatchewan

Dr. Harold Sugarman, 22 September 1906, Poland; University of Saskatchewan, 26-30; University of Manitoba, M.D. 33; F.A.C.P.

Dr. Sugarman, in commenting on the special questions, states that he does not confine practice to cardiology, but has always had special interests in it. He began his career as an apprentice to Dr. David Baltzan in 1934, and this association has continued ever since. He maintained a regular program of continuing postgraduate education by attending courses and national and international meetings. His bibliography reflects the interests of an internist rather than a cardiologist.

In 1965, Dr. Sugarman was Assistant Clinical Professor of Medicine at the University of Saskatchewan, and on the Active Staff of St. Paul's and the University Hospitals, as well as Consultant in Medicine at the City Hospital.

Alberta

Dr. John William Scott, 5 February 1894, Ireland; McGill, M.D. 21; F.R.C.P.(C); LL.D. (Hon) University of Alberta, 70, F.A.C.P.

Dr. John Scott joined the group that in June 1947 organized the Canadian Cardiovascular Society. He was invited to become a member of the first council because he was Professor of Medicine and we knew of no one who was then actively engaged in cardiology in Edmonton. His bibliography reflects wide interests and some degree of special interest in endocrinology. His recollections about Dr. Hurlburt and Professor Downs (see their minibiographies) are interesting contributions to our present task.

Dr. John Creasey Hopkyns, 15 July 1915, Felixstowe, England; University of Oxford, M.A. Physiology 37; University of Oxford and London, England B.M., B.Ch. 40; M.R.C.P. (London) 1948; Cert. Int. Med. R.C.P. & S.(C) 53; F.A.C.P.; F.A.G.S.

Dr. Hopkyns did not comment on the special questions, nor submit his bibliography. In 1971, he was Clinical Lecturer in Medicine, University of Alberta, and on the Active Staff of the Misericordia Hospital in Edmonton.

Dr. Frank H. MacInnis, 25 January 1914, Souris, P.E.I.; Queen's University, M.D., C.M. 41; Cert. Int. Med. R.C.P.(C) 53; F.A.C.P. 58.

Dr. MacInnis began postgraduate education with internship at the Regina General Hospital (1941-42), followed by work at the Toronto Western Hospital in 1944 and the Deaconess Hospital, Great Falls, Montana in 1951-52. He joined a 12-doctor group clinic in Camrose, Alberta and although he practised general internal medicine, most of his work is related to cardiology.

His bibliography of six items published between 1946 and 1959, includes one which represents a breakthrough in electrocardiographic technique. He was associated with Dr. Norman Holter in the invention of tele-electrocardiography and wrote an article on "The Clinical Application of Radioelectrocardiography" (*C.M.A.J.*, 1954; 70, 574-576). This work led to the development of the Holter Dynamic Electrocardiograph manufactured by the Avionics Co. The fifth item reveals a healthy critical attitude, "Sympathectomy for Hypertension. An Analysis of a Failure" (*Alberta Med. Bull.*, November 1953).

Dr. David Lloyd George Howard, 18 January 1922, Harris, Saskatchewan; University of Saskatchewan, B.A. 45; University of Toronto, M.D. 48; Minnesota State Boards 53; Spec. in Int. Med., Alberta 55; F.R.C.P.(C) 55; F.A.C.P. 66.

Dr. Howard's postgraduate studies included cardiology as part of internal medicine with special studies in pathology and arthritis.

When he updated his curriculum vitae in 1971, his principal appointments were Chief of Staff and Director of the Division of

Rheumatic Disease, Calgary General Hospital, and Part-Time Associate Professor of Medicine, University of Calgary.

Dr. Howard's bibliography reflects the internist rather than the cardiologist. A significant item in the latter field is "Long Term Management of the Patient with Coronary Heart Disease," an address delivered at the Annual Meeting of the Canadian Medical Association, Alberta Division, in 1965.

Dr. George Sigurd Balfour, 17 January 1920, Edmonton; University of Alberta, M.D. 43; F.R.C.P.(C) 50; F.A.C.P. 60; F.A.C.C. 70.

During the years 1946-1949, Dr. Balfour engaged in postgraduate studies at the Montreal General Hospital and the following year in 1950 studied at the Trudeau Sanitarium in Saranac Lake. He chose to join the Campbell Clinic in Lethbridge, Alberta, as the only internist in the group.

In 1965, his curriculum vitae was accompanied by a letter in which he comments on the special questions.

> The only special training I had in cardiology was working under yourself and Dr. Birchard at the Montreal General Hospital. I came to this clinic primarily to cover the field of Internal Medicine. Since 1950 when I came here, we have always had an electrocardiograph. I was instrumental in bringing in a second internist soon after I arrived and he and I share the work. From the law of averages, we find that most of our work is cardiology but neither of us limits ourself to this entirely.
>
> I do not consider myself a cardiologist but rather a hanger-on. However, I rationalize that somewhere along the line the remarkable strides in cardiology must be offered to as broadly based a population as possible and perhaps this is a useful function which people like myself may serve.

Dr. Balfour published a paper on "Inheritance of Diabetes Mellitus" (*C.M.A.J.*, 1959: 80, 891-83); and co-authored with Drs. Fraser and Logan, a report of "Aneurysm of the Right Coronary Artery" (*Am. J. Cardiol.*, 1960: 61, 830-833).

Dr. Richard Edward Rossall, 26 January 1926, Lytham St. Annes, England; University of Leeds, Eng. B.Sc. 47; M.B., B.Ch. 50; M.R.C.P. London 52; M.D. Leeds 58; Cert. Int. Med. 58; F.R.C.P.(C); F.A.C.C. 65; F.I.C.C. 66; F.A.C.P. 69; F.A.H.A.

Dr. Rossall exemplifies the well-trained specialist who has had his undergraduate and postgraduate education in Great Britain, and later settled in Canada. He brought both technical and cultural influences to mesh with the Canadian scene.

Immediately after graduation, Dr. Rossall had an internship in medicine and in surgery in Leeds; he spent 1950-51 at the postgraduate medical shool, Hammersmith, London, and at the Brompton Hospital. In 1952-54, he served in the British Military Forces in England and Germany. During 1954-57, he worked in the Leeds General Infirmary in the Department of Medicine and in Radiology. He emigrated to Canada in 1957.

In 1971, Dr. Rossall was Professor of Medicine, on the Active Staff of the University of Alberta Hospital, and Director of Graduate Training in the Department of Medicine. He was also consultant cardiologist in four hospitals in Edmonton and vicinity.

Dr. Rossall supplied his bibliography for the years 1956 to 1967. His bibliography contains fourteen items, one of which concerns the use of radioactive isotopes in diagnosis and treatment of thyrotoxicosis, another is on "Radioactive Tracer Investigations of Absorption of Serum Albumin on Glass Surfaces," printed in *Radio Isotopes in Scientific Research,* Volume 2, Proceedings of the First UNESCO International Conference in Paris, 1957. The remaining twelve items deal with subjects related to congenital and acquired cardiovascular diseases.

Dr. Clinton Bruce Hatfield, 18 July 1926, Calgary; University of Alberta, B.Sc. 48, M.Sc. 51, M.D. 53; M.R.C.P. (London) 58; F.R.C.P.(C) 59; Dip. A.B.I.M. 62; F.A.C.P. 62.

Following graduation, Dr. Hatfield had a year of internship in the University of Alberta Hospital, then two years (1954-56) as Fellow in Medicine, followed by a year as chief resident in Medicine at the University of Minnesota Hospital.

In 1958, he was a Volunteer Research Assistant at Hammersmith Hospital in London. He returned to his native Calgary and joined the Active Staff of the Foothills Hospital. He also served several other hospitals: Sarcee Auxiliary, Glenmore Auxiliary, Cross Bow Auxiliary, and the Calgary General. These hospitals were his affiliations in 1965.

Dr. Hatfield made no comments on the special questions. His bibliography of four articles published between 1954 and 1959 all deal with subjects related to endocrinology.

Dr. David Walter Irving, 28 July 1932, Calgary; University of Alberta, M.D. 57; C.R.C.P.(C); L.M.C.C.; F.A.C.C.; F.A.C.P.; F.A.C.C.P.; F.A.H.A.; F.A.C.C.

Dr. Irving continued his postgraduate training from 1957 to 1964. His posts included internship and residencies at the University of Alberta Hospital, a Research Fellowship in Cardiology at the Cedars of Lebanon Hospital in Los Angeles (1959-61), a research fellowship at the London Postgraduate Medical School (1961-62), and a Teaching Fellowship at the University of Alberta, 1962-63, followed by a year as senior resident at the Alberta University Hospital.

In 1968, he was Instructor in Medicine at the University of Alberta, a member of the Active Staff of the Alexandra Hospital, and a member of the Baker Clinic Group.

His brief comments on the special questions indicate that he decided to specialize in cardiology during the second year of the residency program. Dr. Irving's bibliography grew to 18 items during the years 1960 to 1966. One of the first is a book, co-authored with Dr. Elliot Corday, *Disturbances of Heart Rate, Rhythm, and Conduction,* W. B. Saunders Co., 1961. All but three items are co-authored. The eighteenth item is authored solo: "Beta Blocking Drugs in Angina" (*Man. Med. Rev.*, Nov. 1966).

British Columbia

Dr. Lawrence E. Rampa, Director of Medical Services at the Vancouver General Hospital, was extremely helpful in our search for the earliest signals of the arrival of cardiology in British Columbia. Mr. Barron's list of purchasers of electrocardiographs, obtained from the Cambridge Instrument Company, revealed that Dr. Newton Drier of Vancouver had bought a Cambridge electrocardiograph before 1915, presumably in 1914. In December of 1915, the minutes of a medical board meeting record that it was proposed that the Vancouver General Hospital purchase Dr. Drier's electrocadiograph. This proposal was not approved. In December of the following year, the minutes of the board record that Mrs. B. T. Rogers presented the hospital with the gift of a Cambridge electrocardiograph. In fact, Dr. Gillies, who was nominally in charge of the Heart Station at the Vancouver General Hospital from 1916 until his retirement in 1947, had much to do with this donation and "It was installed on Ward F at a cost of $150.00."

The minutes of the medical board staff meeting in May 1918 had this note concerning the apparatus: "It would have to be disposed of if not used more."

Dr. Gillies was born in 1875, graduated M.D. at McGill 1898, and began to practise medicine in Vancouver in 1906. His principal contributions to cardiology are that he succeeded in bringing an electrocardiograph to the Vancouver General Hospital as early as 1916 and that he allowed Dr. George F. "Fritz" Strong to exercise his talents in building the Department of Cardiology without any restraints. Dr. Gillies died in 1948.

Dr. Ezra Newton Drier, 1871-27 June 1941.

Mr. Brian Berubé of the Canadian Medical Association assisted in finding information about Dr. Drier. Following is the obituary which appeared in the *Vancouver Medical Association Bulletin* of August 1941.

> Dr. Drier was born at Woodstock, N.B., seventy years ago. He graduated at McGill in 1899, practised a year at Kelowna, B.C., then in Vancouver till 1915. In 1906 he took a six months' postgraduate course at Harvard and spent 1909 studying abroad, in Vienna, London and Edinburgh, where he obtained his F.R.C.S.
>
> He joined the R.C.A.M.C. [Royal Canadian Army Medical Corps] in 1915 and went overseas, when he was attached to the Cambridge Hospital, but resigned after a year on account of ill health. Following a sea voyage he started a practice in New Zealand and continued there for 16 years.
>
> Then came two years travelling with his wife and daughter, visiting Australia, India, Ceylon, Japan and Europe, where he visited every state except Russia.
>
> He finally settled in Vancouver in 1931, where he led a retired life.
>
> In 1913 he studied the electrocardiograph in London under Lewis, and brought to Vancouver the first electrocardiograph, which he placed in St. Paul's Hospital.
>
> It was a pleasure to talk with him in his retirement, and he had a fund of information, both on professional and lay subjects, and his description of the customs and manners, the ways of living, the various grades of sanitation in various countries was very interesting.
>
> Not many of the old-timers are left here but those who remain have a vivid memory of his personality. To the younger members

of the profession here he was only a name. We extend our sympathy to his wife and daughter in their loss.

It would appear that his sojourn with Thomas Lewis was not of the kind which results in the publication of some observations, as was the case with Paul White and Jonathan Meakins who worked with Lewis in 1913. Apparently, Dr. Drier did not maintain an active interest in electrocardiography.

Dr. Philip Alexander Clyde Cousland, 15 October 1898, Edinburgh, Scotland; Edinburgh University Med. Sch., 1919-20; University of Toronto, M.D. 24; L.M.C.C. 24; M.C.P.S. (Ontario) 24; Cert. R.C.P.(C) 44; F.A.H.A.

Dr. Cousland had postgraduate training at the Royal Infirmary, Edinburgh and Westminster Hospital, London in 1926, at the London Hospital in 1936-37, and the Toronto General Hospital in 1947.

He became the Chief of Cardiology at the Royal Jubilee Hospital in Victoria, B.C. in 1952. However, he had been practising internal medicine with a special interest in cardiology in Victoria since 1934. Because of illness he retired in 1957. Of his medical school experience he wrote as follows in 1965:

> I think that I arrived at the decision to specialize in cardiology in my last year in Medical School, when Dr. John Oille was one of my teachers. This became so much so that when I spent a year in London, I made sure I got into the London Hospital where I could get instruction from Sir John Parkinson in the Bernard Barron Cardiac Institute. I had always practised in Victoria, so I came back confining myself to Internal Medicine until I felt that the city was large enough to have a cardiologist. I felt the time was ripe in 1947; I bought an electrocardiograph, X-ray, etc.

Presumably, people in Victoria consulted cardiologists in Vancouver until Dr. Cousland became rather officially the cardiologist for the community. Dr. Cousland represents one of the earliest pioneers who gained his inspiration during his student experience in Canada. He obtained some training in Toronto and also abroad in London, and then returned to practise in Victoria, B.C.

In 1965 Dr. Cousland was on the Active Staff of the Royal Jubilee Hospital. He had served as Chief of Cardiology in this hospital from 1952 to 1957. He did not submit his bibliography.

Dr. Charles Lock Hunt, 10 August 1903, Salisbury, S. Rhodesia; University of London and St. Bartholomew Hosp., M.R.C.S. (England) and M.R.C.P. (London) 25; L.M.C.C.; Cert. Int. Med. C.R.C.P.(C).

Dr. Hunt lists the following as subjects he studied in the course of postgraduate education: obstetrics, radiology, electrotherapeutics, tropical medicine, cardiology, and rehabilitation medicine; he names the following institutions in which he worked: St. Bartholomew's Hospital, London; a hospital in Bangalore, India, the Vancouver General Hospital, and Lions Gate Hospital in North Vancouver.

When he submitted his curriculum vitae in 1968, he was Director of the Division of Venereal Disease Control in the Provincial Department of Health, British Columbia.

Dr. Hunt's principal contribution to cardiology stems from his special interest in rehabilitation medicine. He was one of the few who prescribed early ambulation, early in the history of our knowledge related to the treatment of myocardial infarction. He urged the use of graduated exercises in cases of coronary heart disease and stressed, in his teaching, the dangers of excessive bed rest in heart disease. In his special comments about his career he wrote in 1968: "Iatrogenic cardiac cripples have always appeared to abound and have been a difficult problem to overcome in patients and employers alike."

Dr. Bernard B. Moscovitch, 6 March 1910, Lethbridge, Alta.; University of Alberta, M.D. 34; F.R.C.P.(C).

Dr. Moscovitch did pursue some postgraduate education during the years 1935-37 and 1945-46 but in preparing his curriculum vitae he did not mention any other details. In 1968, when he submitted the questionnaire, he was a member of the Attending Staff of the Vancouver General Hospital and Clinical Assistant Professor at the University of British Columbia. Dr. Moscovitch did not provided a bibliography.

Dr. Donald Spencer Munroe, 19 October 1911, Welwyn, Sask.; University of Saskatchewan, B.Sc. 32; University of Manitoba, M.D. 36; M.R.C.P. (London); F.A.C.P.; F.R.C.P. (London); F.R.C.P.(C).

Dr. George F. (Fritz) Strong attracted young professionals to the cardiology service of the Vancouver General Hospital which developed, as might be expected, into a modern progressive unit.

Among the early associates there were Donald S. Munroe and Hugh Stansfield, who played leading roles in the organization of the British Columbia Heart Association and, a little later, the B.C. Heart Foundation.

After obtaining a B.Sc. degree at the University of Saskatchewan in 1932, Munroe studied medicine at the University of Manitoba, graduating in 1936. During the next two years after graduation, Dr. Munroe served internship at the Vancouver General Hospital. In 1938, he entered private practice as Fritz Strong's assistant. In 1937, Munroe and Strong published a paper on "Gumma of the Heart" (*C.M.A.J.*, 1937: 36, 513) and in 1940, two papers, namely "Paroxysmal Ventricular Tachycardia" (*Am. Ht. J.*, 1940: 19, 486) and "Cardiac Hypertrophy—Forty-Two Hearts Weighing 750 grams or more" (*Ann.I.Med.*, 1940: 13, 2253).

During the academic year of 1939-40, Munroe was Research Assistant to Dr. William H. Kerr, Professor of Medicine at the University of California in San Francisco; Dr. Kerr, an early pupil of Paul Dudley White, had a special interest in cardiology. Munroe then returned to resume his association with Fritz Strong in Vancouver.

In 1941 he joined the Royal Canadian Air Force and served overseas until the end of the war. While in England he passed the examinations for membership in the Royal College of Physicians, London. After war service he returned to Vancouver and resumed his career in solo practice as an internist with special interest in cardiology. In 1971, when he updated his curriculum vitae, he was Senior Physician at the Vancouver General Hospital, Consultant in Medicine at the Grace Hospital, Medical Director of Fidelity Life Assurance Co., and Associate Professor of Medicine at the University of British Columbia. His partial bibliography of 14 items published between 1937 and 1964, reflects the internist as well as the cardiologist. In 1960 he delivered the Osler Lecture of the Vancouver Medical Association on "The Practitioner of Medicine."

Dr. Maurice D. Young, 20 September 1912, North Vancouver; London Hospital Med. Sch., M.R.C.S. and L.R.C.P. 36; University of Cambridge, M.B., B.Ch. 38, M.A. (Cantab); M.R.C.P. (Lon.); F.R.C.P.(C); Cert. Paediatrics, F.A.H.A.; F.A.C.P. (Cardiol.).

Following is the list of appointments Dr. Young held after graduation in 1938: House Phys., Receiving Room Office, Jr. Resident Anaesthetist — London Hosp.; House Phys. Children's Dept., Sr.

House Phys. & Surgeon — London H.; Res. Med. Officer, Private Wards — London Hosp. 37-40; First Asst. Children's Out-Patient Dept., London Hosp. 40-44; Res. Med. Officer, Warleywoods E.M.S. Hosp. 40-44; Physician-in-Charge, Paediatric Unit, Warleywoods E.M.S. Hosp. 41-44; Surgeon Lieut. RNVR 44-46; Sr. Rot. Int. Children's Mem. Hosp. Montreal 46-47; Resident-in-Charge, Med. Out-Patient Children's Mem. Hosp. Montreal 47; Fellow in Paediatrics Johns Hopkins Univ. and Asst. Phys. Cardiac Clinic, Harriet Lane Home, Johns Hopkins Hosp. 48-49.

When Dr. Young submitted his curriculum vitae in 1965, he was Associate Professor of Paediatrics at the University of British Columbia, Senior on Attending Staff of Vancouver General Hospital, consultant at the Lions Gate Hospital, and on the visiting staff of the Children's Hospital and St. Paul's Hospital.

Dr. Young's comments on the special questions reveal that he pioneered paediatric cardiology in Vancouver.

> My decision to undertake further training in Cardiology as related to paediatrics resulted from purely fortuitous circumstance. While [I was] acting as senior rotating intern at the Children's Memorial Hospital, Montreal, Dr. Graham Ross casually mentioned that Dr. Helen B. Taussig was looking for an assistant physician. Taking this as a hint, I applied and was duly appointed as a Fellow in Paediatrics of Johns Hopkins University and Assistant Physician to the Cardiac Clinic of the Harriet Lane Home. It was therefore not until after I had obtained my certification in Paediatrics that my special interest in Cardiology arose.
>
> After an absence of 19 years I returned to Vancouver and started to practise paediatrics in 1949 with the hope of obtaining requests for consultations in paediatric cardiology. In 1953 an offer was received from Dr. Taussig to return to Johns Hopkins Hospital on a permanent basis and this led to an offer from the Professor of Paediatrics at the University of British Columbia to become the second full-time member of the Department of paediatrics at U.B.C. Accordingly, an appointment as Assistant Professor of Paediatrics was accepted and commenced in July 1953. Although this appointment was nominally full-time, consultations were permitted and within a year these were limited to paediatric cardiology.

Dr. Young's bibliography includes a chapter on "Disease of the Cardiovascular System" in *Pediatrics,* edited by Patterson and McCreary, Chap. 10, 180-208, J. P. Lippincott, 1956. He has written on a wide variety of topics related to cardiovascular disease in children. In 1960 he co-authored an article on "Comparison of Arterial and Arterialized Bloods in Normal Newborn Infants and Older Children with Congenital Heart Lesions" (*J. Ped.*, May 1960, 56, 630-634).

Dr. Victor O. Hertzman, 9 November 1918, Toronto; University of Toronto, M.D. 42; F.R.C.P.(C) 49; F.A.C.P. 60; F.A.H.A.

Dr. Hertzman provided a minimum of information in his curriculum vitae and did not make any comments on the special questions, nor did he provide his bibliography. His postgraduate education consisted of a year at Michael Reese Hospital in Chicago, 1942-43; a year at the Sunny Acres Hospital, Cleveland, 1946-47; and three years at the Vancouver General Hospital, 1947-50.

In 1972, when he submitted his curriculum vitae, he was Instructor in Medicine at the University of British Columbia, a member of the Attending Staff and of the Cardiology Department at the Vancouver General Hospital, and on the Attending Staff of the Wellan Chest Centre.

Dr. Hertzman has played a dynamic role in the development of cardiology in Vancouver. He belongs to the group of pioneers who founded the British Columbia Heart Foundation. He is one of the few men in Canada who has worked in the field of ballistocardiography. He organized the cardiac rehabilitation service and is a leading authority on this subject in Canada.

Dr. Hugh Stansfield, 19 February 1916, Ottawa; University of Alberta, B.Sc. 37; M.Sc. 39; M.D. 42; Dip. Int. Med. McGill; F.A.C.C.; L.M.C.C. 42; C.R.C.P.(C) 49.

Dr. Stansfield enjoyed the advantage of close association with the late Dr. George F. ("Fritz") Strong. He played a leading role in organizing the Vancouver Heart Association and the British Columbia Heart Foundation. These organizations constitute very significant contributions to the development of cardiology in Canada. His comments on the special questions take the form of a brief autobiographical sketch written in 1968 which is reproduced below, in full.

> I have always been interested in things medical, perhaps because of a grandfather and three uncles in the field. I have also been very interested in biochemistry, probably as a union of my father's profession as a chemist with my uncles' profession of

medicine. I became particularly interested in biochemistry when my father read me some of the essays of J. B. S. Haldane's *Possible Worlds,* when I was a boy.

To bring these ambitions to reality, I took Honours Chemistry, followed by an M.Sc. in Physiology and an M.D. I spent one summer holiday working with Doctor J. B. Collip in Montreal. When I graduated I went to Montreal to work with Collip and was assigned to a war research project on blood transfusions with Orville Denstedt. I later went up to the Royal Victoria Hospital as an Assistant Resident in Medicine prior to joining the Army in April 1943.

Following basic training I was assigned to the Research Directorate and specifically to a group under Doctor Hebbel Hoff and J. S. L. Brown investigating psychosomatic heart disease. With this group I developed my first real interest in cardiology. I became very interested in the electrophysiology of the electrocardiogram as Doctor Hoff and his group were working it out. I also became familiar with the works of Sir Thomas Lewis who had worked on Effort Syndrome during the First World War. One of the young Canadians who was fortunate enough to work with him at that time was my uncle, the late Doctor R. S. Stevens of Ottawa. I spent many happy leaves from Montreal in Ottawa and had opportunities to discuss these problems with Doctor Stevens.

At the time of the invasion I was sent overseas and served in eight different Canadian General Hospitals. In most of these I found myself trying to get the electrocardiograph machine, which was usually out of order, back into operating condition again, and to take and attempt to read electrocardiograms. It is of interest that at this time I made one diagnosis of death by potassium intoxication based on some very unusual electrocardiograms which I felt fitted with Hoff's animal work on potassium. This diagnosis was made three or four months prior to the first published paper on potassium intoxication in humans with E.C.G. confirmation. Colonel J. A. Dauphinee intended to publish this case, but has never done so.

At the end of the War, I returned to Montreal to work with Hebbel Hoff and to take the Diploma course in Medicine at McGill. It was at that time that I took part in the early organization meetings of the Montreal Cardiac Society and the original plans leading to the formation of the Canadian Cardiovascular Society.

In 1949, I came out to Vancouver to work with the late Doctor G. F. Strong, and was appointed to the Heart Station Staff at the Vancouver General Hospital. I felt that the seminars in the Vancouver General Heart Station could easily form a basis for a Vancouver Heart Association. This was ultimately organized and I had the honour to be elected as the First President. Soon after the organization of the Vancouver Heart Association, we were becoming increasingly aware of the need for a lay medical organization to help with fund raising for cardiovascular research. At this time Ontario was the only province with a Provincial Heart Foundation, and the time seemed ripe for this movement to spread. I therefore set up a committee to discuss this possibility which included Doctor Victor Hertzman, Doctor Bruce Shallard, Doctor James Foulks and Doctor Sidney Friedmann and me. We met at my home on several occasions and then sent in an application to the Provincial Government to have the B.C. Heart Foundation registered under the Societies Act. The $25.00 fee was provided by a $5.00 levy from each of us. By a happy coincidence the B.C. Heart Foundation was officially registered on the same day that the meeting of the Canadian Cardiovascular Society in Toronto adopted the resolution to ask Paul Martin's assistance in forming a National Heart Foundation [June 1955].

The five original doctors then each promised to get four or five lay members to form the first Board of Directors for the Foundation. We felt very strongly that a lay medical organization should have a lay president and this principle has been followed until I broke it in the year 1966-67. As you know, the late Gordon Caine was our first Provincial President and so, with Doctor Strong, he appeared on the founding charter of the Canadian Heart Foundation the following year. As you know, I attended Paul Martin's meeting to explore the possibility of a National Heart Foundation and as a B.C. representative attended its actual founding at St. Helen's Island the following summer [June 1956]. For about eight years I was the Chairman of the Medical Advisory Committee for the B.C. Heart Foundation and in 1967, I spent one year as President of the B.C. Heart Foundation. I have been on the Board of the Canadian Heart Foundation for some years, because of the B.C. connection, and following Doctor Strong's death, when John Keith moved up to President, I was elected Secretary of the Canadian Heart Foundation. I was on the Council of the Canadian Cardiovascular Society at the time the plans were going forward for starting the Canadian Heart Foundation.

In private practice, as you know, I started with the late Doctor G. F. Strong in 1949. On October 1, 1952, I opened my own office and acquired my own first electrocardiograph. For the past two years I have also had Sanborn Heart-Sound Equipment. I have integrated this with its electrocardiograph, into a single unit which contains an electrocardiograph, heart sound equipment, oscilloscope and tape recorder. I am trying to build up material to use in teaching heart sounds to medical students. For some years my only special equipment in this field was a small pad of your heart sound diagrams. As you can well imagine, I have in the first few months been teaching myself more than I have taught my students.

I am interested in electronics and carpentry. This has produced stereo equipment for me at home and it has also produced the table and the oscilloscope for my heart sound equipment in the office.

In 1968, Dr. Stansfield was Clinical Associate Professor of Medicine at the University of British Columbia, Senior in Medicine at the Vancouver General Hospital, Consultant in Medicine at the Grace Hospital, and Medical Officer of the Fidelity Life Insurance Company. His curriculum vitae lists the many important executive offices he held and was holding in organizations related to cardiology. He did not submit his bibliography.

Dr. Max Benjamin Walters, 3 April 1921, Canada; University of Manitoba, M.D. 44; F.R.C.P.(C); F.A.C.P.; F.A.C.C.; F.A.H.A.

Dr. Walters served an internship during his final undergraduate year. During the next four years he worked in the group medicine Winnipeg Clinic. In 1949 he studied cardiology at the Massachusetts General Hospital, followed by a residency in Medicine at the new England Center Hospital in 1949-50, and a Fellowship in Cardiology at Mount Sinai Hospital, New York, 1950-51. When he submitted the questionnaire in 1965 he was Clinical Instructor at the University of British Columbia, member of the Heart Station at the Vancouver General Hospital, and head of the Department of Cardiology at the Shaughnessy Military Hospital.

Dr. Walters responded to the special questions and also to a request for comments on the late Dr. George F. Strong.

My decision to specialize in cardiology occurred early in my postgraduate training. After my term as a general intern, I decided to go into Internal Medicine, and after working for a year with Dr. C. R. Gilmour in Winnipeg, I became interested in electrocardiography and thyrotoxic heart disease. I pursued this interest and published an article with Dr. Gilmour on this condition. This stimulated my further interest in cardiovascular disease and led me to seek more training in this sphere.

In deciding to obtain special training in cardiology, I felt that I would like to complete most of my requirements for the Fellowship in Internal Medicine in Winnipeg and seek further training in Boston and New York. Accordingly, I went to the Massachusetts General Hospital as a postgraduate student in cardiology. At this institution I got a lot of stimulation, did a lot of reading, and decided without question that I would make cardiology my main and entire future interest. At the end of six months I felt that I was not receiving sufficient training in physiologic investigation and in direct patient handling in the position that I had at the Massachusetts General Hospital. Accordingly, I spent a year as resident in medicine at the New England Center Hospital and from there went to the Mount Sinai Hospital in New York where I was Fellow in Cardiology with Dr. A. M. Master. This was a very hard-working, fruitful year in which I received further training in all aspects of physiologic investigation in cardiology, had the opportunity to do a little clinical investigation, and worked actively on the ward with patients. The decision to come to Vancouver was based upon the fact that my wife and myself wished to return to Canada. The climate in the United States at the time we were there was not very healthy in our eyes because it was the time of McCarthyism and violent emotions. Both in Boston and in New York I received tempting offers to stay, but our feeling was that we would be happier in Canada. We chose Vancouver because it was a new and growing city, a medical school had recently been established, and there appeared to be a need for specialists in this area. My electrocardiograph was purchased in 1951 which was the year that I began to practice in Vancouver.

I cannot truthfully say that membership in the Canadian Cardiovascular Society played a significant role in the development of my career in cardiology. Our local Vancouver Heart Association was perhaps more important in that it led to an opportunity to organize the Cardiac Symposium which we have been holding yearly for the past seven years in which we have the opportunity of inviting two or three outstanding people in the field of cardiology to conduct a two-day symposium on some aspect of heart disease. I feel that in the future, the Canadian Cardiovascular Society might play a more important role in establishing a sub-specialty in cardiology and providing stimulation through its scientific sessions.

Finally, re the request for information that I might be able to mention regarding Dr.Strong, I might say that I consider that Dr. Strong was an extremely forceful person who had the interest of the development of cardiology in the city of Vancouver closest to his heart. When I came to Vancouver, I knew nobody and the first person that I met was Fritz Strong. I found him extremely forthright, direct, and honest. He was extremely interested in my previous training, my possible ability, and what sort of contribution I might make to progress in cardiovascular disease in Vancouver. He gave me every opportunity to prove myself, he accepted me into the Heart Station and allowed me to participate in the activities of this group, and he encouraged me to carry out any investigation or other work which might be of benefit to the group as a whole. Among other things, it was his attitude and approach to me on my first contact with him that finally decided that I would come to Vancouver. In this respect, I have always had the greatest admiration for the late Dr. Strong.

The first article in Dr. Walters' bibliography reflects his early special interest in cardiology. Together with Dr. C. R. Gilmour he wrote "Thyrotoxic Heart Disease" (*C.M.A.J.*, Oct. 1949: 61, 396-400). During his association with Dr. A. M. Master in New York, he was involved in the investigation of hypertension. He co-authored "New and Old Definitions of Normal Blood Pressure: Clinical Significance of Newly Established Limits" (*Bull. N.Y. Acad. Med.*, 1951: 27, 452-465). In 1952, a book titled *Normal Blood Pressure and Hypertension — New Definitions* was written by A. M. Master, C. I. Garfield, and M. B. Walters, and published by Lea & Febiger, 1952. Subsequently, he has published articles on a wide variety of subjects of clinical importance. A good example is "Mitral Regurgitation Simulating Aortic Stenosis" (*C.M.A.J.*, 1965: 93, 413).

Dr. Dorrance Bowers, 8 May 1925, Exeter, Ont.; University of Toronto, M.D. 49; M.S. (Med.) University of Minnesota, 56; F.R.C.P.(C) 56; Cert. Amer. B. Int. Med. 59; C.V. Dis. 66; F.A.C.C. 69.

Dr. Bowers began postgraduate training with a junior internship at the Vancouver General Hospital, followed by a senior internship at the Shaughnessy Hospital (1952-1953). Next, he became a Fellow of the Mayo Foundation and worked in Rochester, Minnesota from 1953 to 1956. He joined the Knox Clinic at Kelowna, B.C. as an internist with special interest in cardiology. In 1965 he wrote that he planned to take a postgraduate course in cardiology at the National Heart Hospital in London, England beginning in April, 1966 and on returning to Kelowna, he was to restrict his interest to cardiology. Dr. Peretz, in his letter of 1 November 1983, refers to the fact that in the later 1970s Dr. Bowers and Dr. Denton Corrigall, together with Dr. Brossuek, set up a cardiac catheterization laboratory in Kelowna. In 1971 when he updated his curriculum vitae he held the post of Internist at the Kelowna General Hospital.

His partial bibliography, 1952 to 1963, contains 20 items on a wide variety of subjects which reflect his scholarly interests. Beginning in 1959 he wrote a very important series of articles on Marfan's Syndrome based on a thorough study of the S. Family. He identified 33 cases of this condition in six generations of the family. The article which summarizes his study of this family is "Marfan's Syndrome: The S. Family" (*C.M.A.J.*, 1963: 89, 337-340). An interesting contribution he has made appears in an article entitled "Williams' Prior Description of Marfan's Syndrome" (*Am. J. Ophth.*, 1960: 50, No. 1). He quotes two paragraphs of a paper by Elanah Williams, an ophthalmologist of Cincinnati, published in 1876. The main features of Marfan's Syndrome are described in two patients, a brother and sister.

Dr. Chava Eve Rotem, 15 January 1928, Berlin, Germany; University of Geneva, M.B. 47; M.R.C.P. (Edinburgh) 58; M.R.C.P. (London) 58; E.C.F.M.G. (Edin.) 63; L.M.C.C. (Edin.) 67; F.R.C.P.(C) 68.

In responding to the special questions, Dr. Rotem summarized her postgraduate training.

> I started off in my training with the idea of becoming a thoracic surgeon. At that time, in 1954-55, the tendency was to do chest surgery, including pulmonary and the rather limited cardiac surgery done at that time. I enjoyed doing that very much, but for various personal reasons I found it too hard to consider complet-

ing training in chest surgery. I, therefore, decided to shift my interest to the medical aspect of diseases of the chest, again including initially both respiratory and cardiac ailments. Eventually, around about 1958, when cardiac catheterization became a somewhat more common diagnostic procedure, I became more and more attracted to the specialty of cardiology, and started training in cardiac catheterization under Dr. David Verelat, Sheffield, England. At that time I was a registrar (Resident III) at the Groby Road Hospital, Leicester.

The initial training I had in cardiology was somewhat haphazard and more a traineeship than planned training as we tend to do it now for our residents. I learned by watching my superiors and being actually responsible for patients on the cardiology ward. Similarly, interpretation of E.C.G.S was also initially learned just by watching the Chief Cardiologist interpreting E.C.G.S and comparing the one he had interpreted with new ones. As far as training in cardiac catheterization is concerned, my training was a little bit more organized since it developed practically in step with what was known at the time, namely, I started off by doing right heart catheterization from the arm; later learning to do brachial artery or femoral artery punctures with a needle only; then doing left atrial pressures through the bronchoscope; later via transthoracic method; and still later direct puncture of the left ventricle through the anterior chest wall. By 1960 I was doing the occasional trans-septal cardiac catheterization using the Ross technique. By that time I was senior registrar at the same hospital and becoming more and more involved in cardiology, doing both adult and paediatric cardiology.

In 1963 I decided that I had enough purely clinical and apprenticeship type of experience in cardiology and I applied for a research fellowship in cardiology at Stanford, Palo Alto, where I stayed for one year, learning new techniques, particularly the Brockenborough technique and various experimental techniques.

In 1965 I came to Canada and was employed initially at St. Paul's Hospital and later at Shaughnessy as a consultant cardiologist.

In 1972 when Dr. Rotem submitted her curriculum vitae she was Clinical Lecturer at the University of British Columbia, Consultant in Cardiology at Shaughnessy Hospital, Visiting Consultant at Vancouver General Hospital, and on the Attending Staff of St. Vincent's Hospital in Vancouver.

Dr. Rotem is married and has two children.

Dr. Rotem's first publication, co-authored with H. N. Hultgren, was on "Congenital Corrected Transposition of the Great Vessels" (*Am. Ht. J.*, 1965: 305-318), representing work she did in Stanford University before coming to British Columbia. By 1972 the bibliography had grown to twelve items, the last on "Carotid Sinus Nerve Stimulator — A Three Year Follow-Up Study" (*Br.Ht.J.*, 1972). The remaining ten items deal with subjects related to diagnosis and treatment. Several items are noteworthy as important contributions to the literature of unwanted side-effects, such as "Air Embolism of the Pulmonary Artery During Insertion of Transveneous Endocardial Pacemaker," co-authored with J. H. Greig and M. Walters (*J. Thorac. & Cardiovasc. Surg.*, 1967: 58, 562-565), and "Complications of Central Venous Pressure Catheters," co-authored with M. B. Walters and H. A. D. Stanger (*J.A.M.A.*, 1972: 1455-57).

Dr. Peter John Banks, 12 June 192, Gidea Park, Essex; University of London, M.B., B.S. 46; M.R.C.S. (Eng.) 46; L.R.C.P. (Eng.) 46; M.R.C.P. (Eng.) 52; M.D. (London) 52; L.M.C.C. (St. Bartholomew) 54; F.R.C.P.(C) 54; F.A.C.P.

Dr. Banks came to Canada at the age of 31, a well-trained physician. His postgraduate training included internship and residencies in medicine and paediatrics at St. Bartholomew's Hospital as well as a year in Physiology, and a year in Pharmacology and Applied Therapeutics at the University of London. He came to Canada in 1953; of this he wrote in 1965:

> I arrived in Canada on Christmas Day of 1953. The reason I left England was because their Health Services are appallingly organized and there are too many people in too small an Island with a progressive deterioration of their standards of living because the control of the country has slid too far to the left. I came to Victoria because I was offered a job teaching the interns and as a Registrar in St. Bartholomew's Hospital 7,000 miles away, I thought the University was in Victoria. I was most disappointed for about two weeks then I opened my eyes and realized that there could be few more beautiful places in the world in which to work, which opinion I now would change to, that there are no more beautiful places in the world to work.

In 1968-70 Dr. Banks was Chief of Staff of St. Joseph's Hospital and on Visiting Staff of the Royal Jubilee Hospital Victoria.

Dr. Banks took active part in the development of medical services in British Columbia and in Canada as a whole, as evidenced by the following committees on which he served and offices he has held.

C.M.A. Appointments

Economic Committee — 1959-62
Executive — 1966-68
Deputy Speaker — 1969, 1970, 1971
Member, Canadian Delegation to Study Australian Health Services — 1961
Chairman, National Committee on Relative Value Fee Schedule
Chairman, Committee on the Ideal Medical Insurance Plan
Member, National Committee on Intern Training
Member, Committee on C.M.A. Reorganization — 1968
Member, Furnishing Fund Committee, C.M.A. House

Government Appointments

Medical Advisor to the Board of B.C.Government Employees Medical Service
Director, B.C. Medical Plan, 1965-69
Member, Medical Services Commission, 1967-70
Member of Advisory Committee to Minister, 1965 onwards
Member, Appeal Board, Motor-Vehicle Licencing
Medical Referee, Canada Pension Plan

University — Government Appointments

Member, Committee of Open Heart Surgery in British Columbia, 1962, 1965
Chairman, Committee on Open Heart Surgery, 1971
Member, Committee on Provision of Coronary Care Units for British Columbia
Member, Committee on Provision of Chronic Renal Dialysis Units for British Columbia

Dr. Bank's bibliography contains a few articles which reflect his skills as an internist and several related to administration of organized medical services.

Dr. Shirley Glenda Hazell, 12 May 1934 England; University of British Columbia, B.A. University of Toronto, M.D. 60; F.A.C.C.

Dr. Hazell began postgraduate training with a rotating internship at the Toronto East General Hospital (1960-61). The following year she was senior intern in medicine at the Shaughnessy Military

Hospital (1961-62). During the next two years she was Resident in Paediatrics at the Vancouver General Hospital, and devoted the year 1964-65 as Resident in Paediatric Pathology at the Children's Hospital Medical Center, Boston. She returned to Vancouver and in 1965-66 she was a Teaching Fellow at the Vancouver General Hospital. She completed her course of training with a Fellowship in Paediatric Cardiology at the Mayo Clinic, 1966-68.

When she submitted her curriculum vitae in 1972 she was Clinical Instructor in Paediatrics at the University of British Columbia, on the Active Staff at the Vancouver General Hospital, on Associate Staff at the Children's Hospital, and on Medical Staff of the Grace Hospital.

Dr. Hazell made interesting comments related to the special questions.

> As a student I worked for my board and room at Women's College Hospital where I met Dr. Joan Vale and began to be interested in electrocardiography. My interest was further stimulated when working in internal medicine at Shaughnessy where I really decided to do cardiology, but felt that I was attracted more to congenital defects — I also felt that I would prefer to work with younger patients — hence paediatric cardiology.
>
> Dr. Maurice Young suggested that I must first concentrate on paediatrics — which was sometimes difficult as I preferred to read cardiology books! Dr. Dennis Vince suggested further paediatric cardiology training at the Mayo Clinic, after I had spent a good amount of time in my paediatric residency years working with him on the wards in O.P.D. [outpatient department] and in the Cardiac Catheterization Laboratory. After an exciting 18 months in Rochester I felt that I had barely skimmed the surface of paediatric cardiology, but returned home in January 1968 to begin practice. I began in Vancouver, since my parents and friends were here — since this was a good and growing centre for paediatric cardiology — and because of our beautiful mountains! My first and only ECG machine was bought immediately on starting practice and paid for itself within the first year.
>
> I have not been a member of the Canadian Cardiovascular Society for very long — but as in the American College of Cardiology — it is valuable to keep in touch with friends from other centres, to compare notes, ideas, procedures and to keep up in a way that one cannot do just from reading journals.

Dr. Hazell did not provide her bibliography.

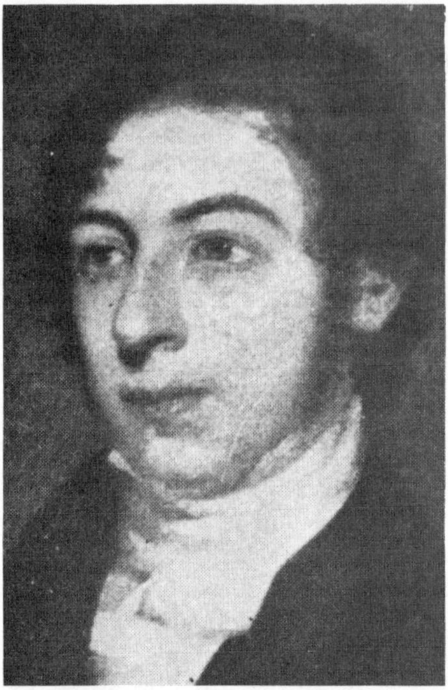

Andrew Fernando Holmes, 1797-1860. One of the four physicians who founded the Montreal Medical Institute in 1823, which became the McGill Faculty of Medicine in 1829; Holines was its first Dean.

Robert Palmer Howard, 1823-1889. Osler's revered teacher at McGill.

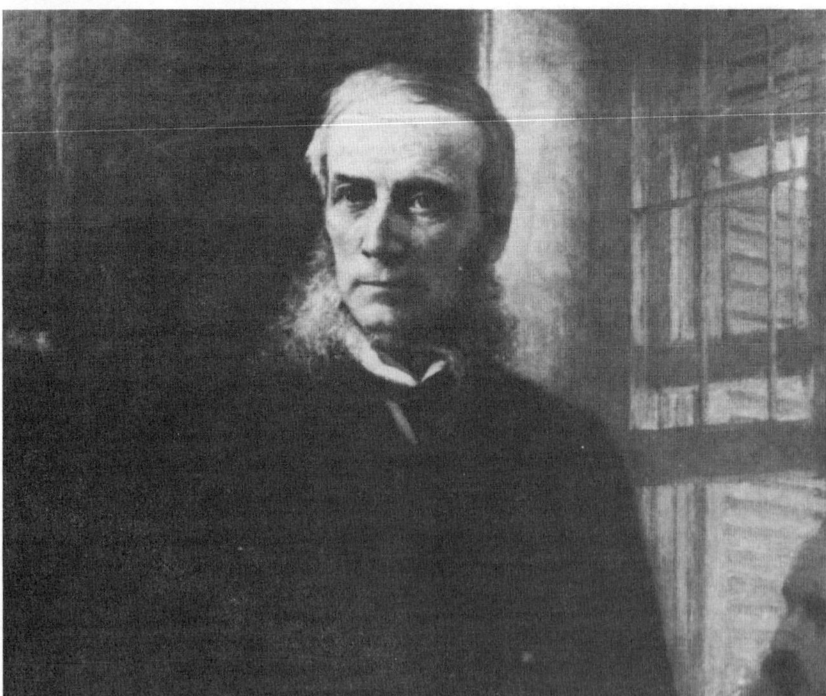

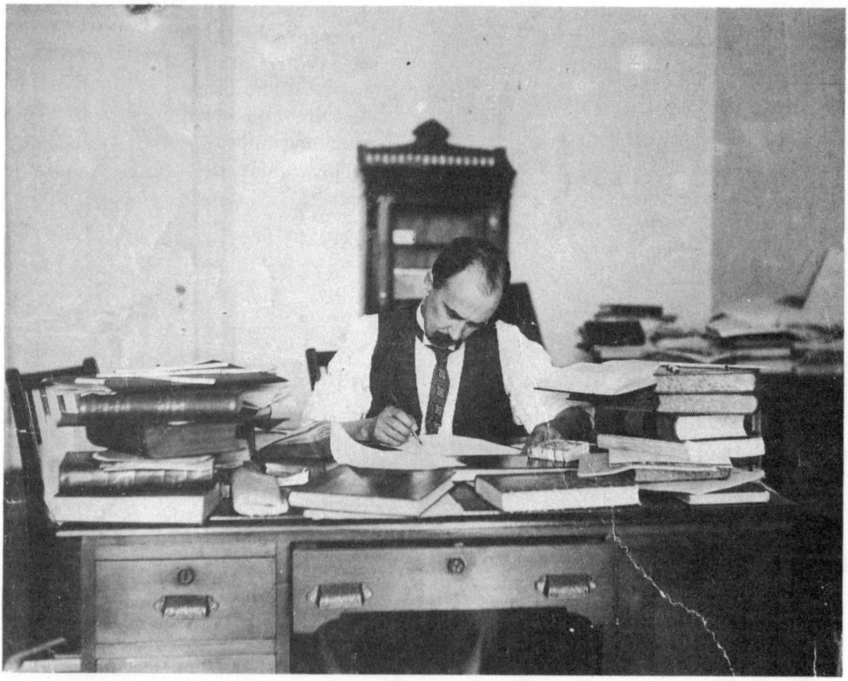

William Osler,
1849-1919. Legendary
physician, teacher and
bibliophile.

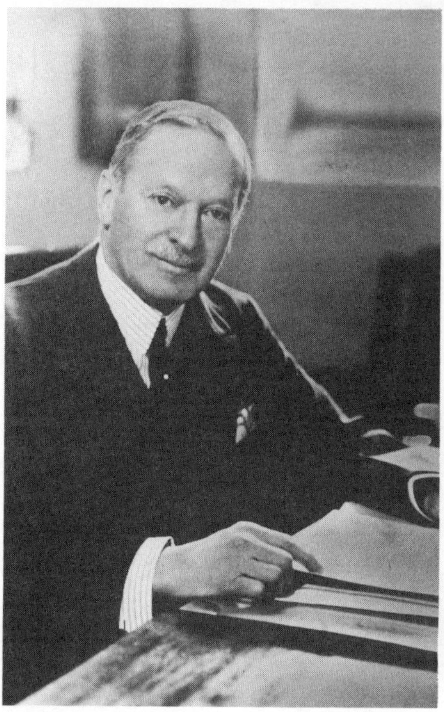

Charles Ferdinand
Martin, 1868-1953. First
full-time Dean of the
McGill Medical Faculty.
He contributed very
greatly to its vigorous
growth in quality and
in size.

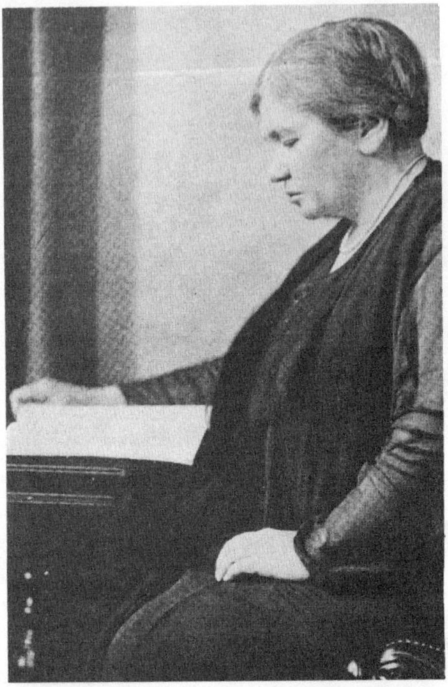

Maude Elizabeth Seymour Abbott, 1869-1940. Curator of the McGill Medical Museum, and world renowned authority on Congenital Heart Disease.

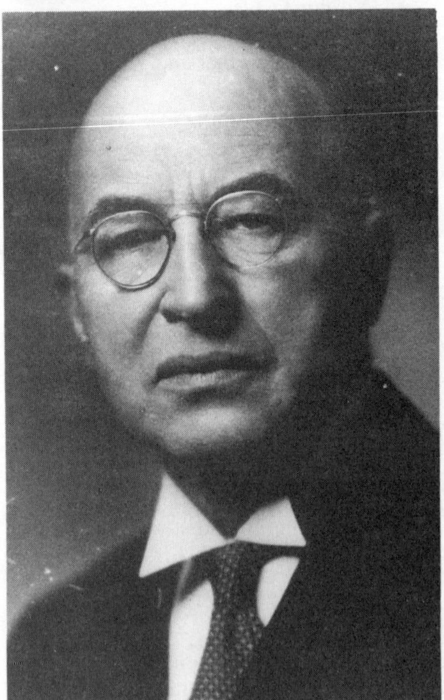

Julian Loudon, 1881-1959. One of the earliest pioneers of electrocardiography in Canada. He published the first article on the subject in a Canadian journal.

Thomas Forrest Cotton, 1884-1965. First Canadian to train for cardiology with Thomas Lewis.

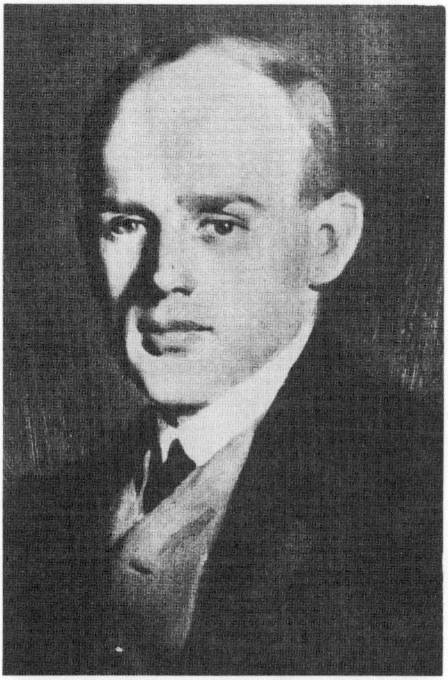

John Campbelll Meakins, 1882-1959. Second Canadian to train for cardiology with Thomas Lewis.

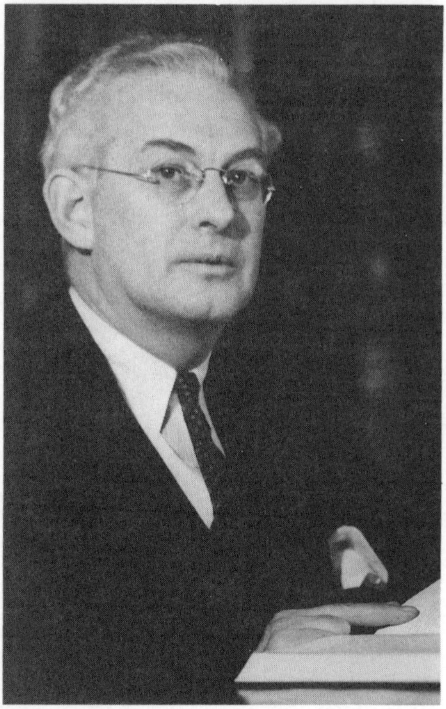

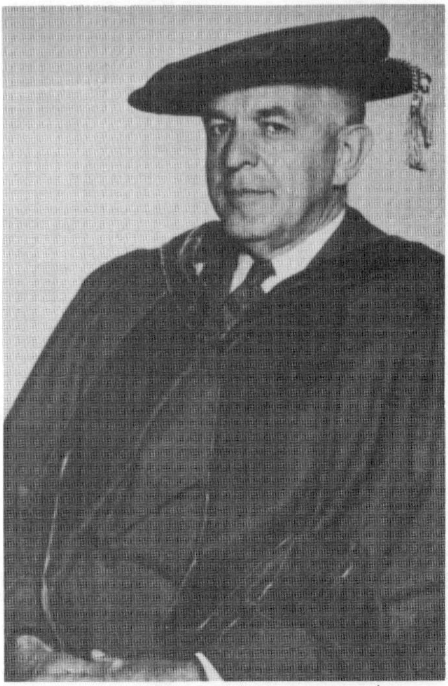

Cecil Clifford Birchard, 1886-1951. Succeeded Cotton in electrocardiography at the Montreal General Hospital. First president of the Canadian Cardiovascular Society.

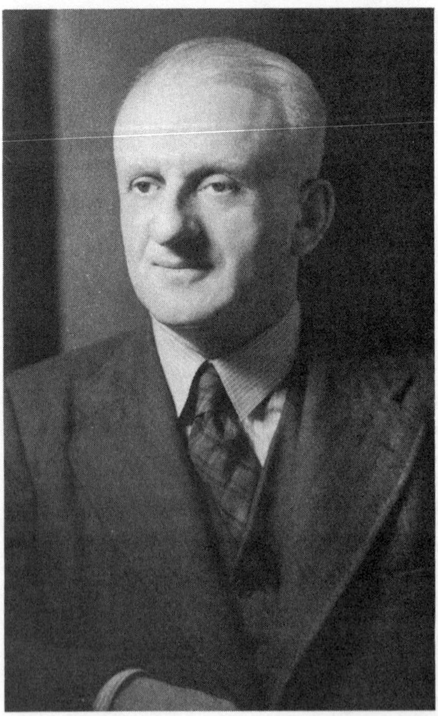

George Frederick Strong, 1897-1957. Founding president of the Canadian Heart Foundation.

Please note that the captions for these two illustrations have been transposed.

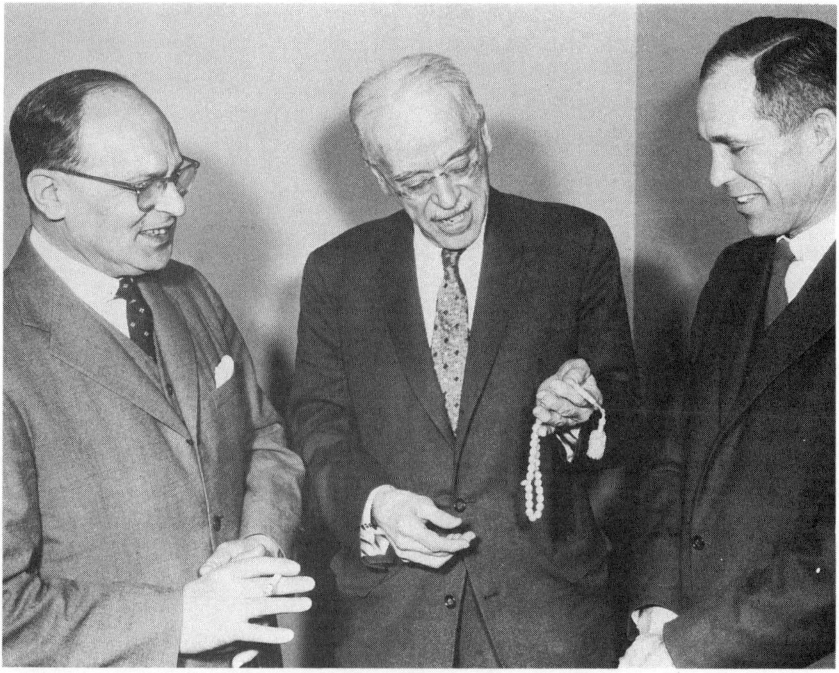

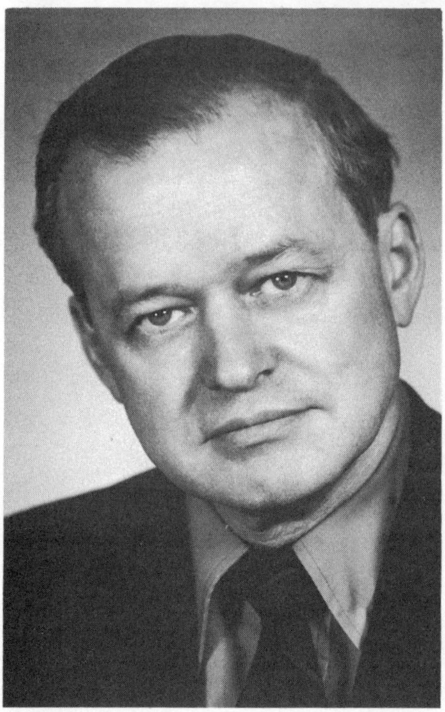

Photographed in February 1958, in the Toronto CBC radio station when Paul Dudley White (1887-1973) was interviewed about the opening of the first annual Canadian Heart Fund campaign; Harold Segall (left) and John Keith accompanied him. Dr. White is showing some prayer beads he acquired in Lebanon. Keith was president of the Heart Foundation and Segall, chairman of the Medical Advisory Committee.

John Buchanan Armstrong, M.D. Executive Secretary of the Canadian Heart Foundation, 1956-1972.

CHAPTER TEN

Cardiovascular Roentgenology

Wilhelm Conrad Roentgen (1845-1923), Professor of Physics at Wurzburg University, performed the first, critical experiment on Friday, 8 November 1895. During the next few weeks he explored and determined that he found a "new kind of rays which he named 'X-rays,'" X being the mathematical symbol for unknown. These rays passed through a variety of substances with different degrees of intensity and were blocked by lead and platinum, but not by aluminum. His first paper was promptly published in the *Proceedings of the Wurzburg Physical Medical Society* for 28 December 1895 (Roentgen 1895) and on 23 January 1896 he addressed the Society on "A New Kind of Rays." The first English translation appeared in *The Lancet* on 23 January, 1896. About three weeks later on 14 February, another English translation appeared in *Science,* the first in the Americas. Within the first year, 1044 scientific papers and 49 books were published dealing entirely with Roentgen rays (Sarton, 1936).

> But stranger still are the revelations of looking through the living flesh of the body by aid of the fluoroscope. First are seen the vertebrae, the greater bones, the ribs, and then to the astonished gaze, in dark outline but moving, may be seen the beating of the heart, the rise and fall of the ribs in respiration, and the movements and rhythmic displacement of organs. I have seen these organs plainly outlined and noted changes in their density due to disease.

These sentiments were expressed by Dr. William J. Morton (1845-1920) in New York City on 27 April 1896 (Brecher, 1969), four months after the appearance of Wilhelm Conrad Roentgen's first publication on what he named X-rays. It is of some special interest that this Morton was the son of William T. G. Morton (1819-1868) who introduced ether anaesthesia at the Massachusetts General Hospital in Boston on 16 October 1846.

In Boston, Francis Henry Williams (1852-1936) pioneered clinical roentgenology. After graduating from the Massachusetts Institute of Technology in 1873, he enjoyed the educational advantage of a trip around the world and then joined the Harvard class of 1877 in medicine (Willius and Keys, 1941). He was a member of the staff of the Boston City Hospital in 1896 when, learning of Roentgen's discovery, he assembled the necessary apparatus with the assistance of friends in the physics department of the Massachusetts Institute of Technology. At first he had to bring the patients to the M.I.T. laboratory; eventually the hospital trustees granted him some space in the basement of the hospital where he worked until 1915. His first publication (1896) was entitled "A Method for More Fully Determining the Outline of the Heart by Means of the Fluoroscope Together with other Uses of this Instrument in Medicine." Five years later, there appeared the first edition of his book, *Roentgen Rays in Medicine and Surgery* (Williams, 1901). In this volume of 658 pages he presented the work done to improve the efficiency of the apparatus and methodology, and clinical applications to diagnosis and therapy related to all systems of the body. The book contains 391 illustrations. From the very beginning Williams chose to protect his body from the rays. He has been quoted as saying "I thought that having such power of penetrating matters as X-rays had, must have effect upon the system and therefore I protected myself" (Brown, 1936).

According to Henri Vaquez, his teacher Pierre Carl E. Potain (1825-1901) (Willius and Keys, 1941) established one of the first X-ray laboratories in Paris (Vaquez, 1921). He had a special interest in the cardiovascular system, an interest which may have stemmed from his having been a pupil of J. B. Bouillaud (1796-1881) who had had Laennec as his teacher. Potain was to cardiology in the francophone world what Sir James Mackenzie was to the English-speaking world, although their special interests were somewhat different. Mackenzie focused attention on the myocardium, Potain on the function of the heart valves. Mackenzie found arterial pressure measurement of doubtful significance. Potain welcomed the new methods of measurement and, keeping in character at the age of 71, he was the first to apply X-rays to the study of the heart. His pupil Vaquez continued the tradition. In 1913, Bordet and Vaquez coauthored a book on *Radiology of the Heart and Aorta* (Vaquez and Bordet, 1913). Among the earliest books on radiology, G. Rosenfeldt's *Diagnosis in Internal Medicine* (1897) gave much attention to the heart and great vessels. The first German monograph on this subject, analogous to the book by Vaquez and Bordet, was written by Hans Dietlen in 1918 and published in 1923 (Dietlen, 1923). The author ascribed the delay to difficulties in acquiring the illustrations he had collected. The earliest book in English, *Clinical Roentgenol-*

ogy of the Cardiovascular System (1937), was written by Hugo Roesler, of the Vienna Herzstation. Soon after Roesler emigrated and settled in Philadelphia, a second edition appeared in 1943 (Roesler, 1937; 1943)

I have not found any clue to a radiologist in Canada who specialized in this field as Vaquez, Bordet, Dietlen, and Roesler did. However, in common with physicians and physicists elsewhere in the world, X-rays were used for medical diagnoses in Montreal a few weeks after Roentgen's discovery was announced. On 7 February 1896, at a meeting of the Montreal Medico-Chirurgical Society, Dr. J. Cox, Professor of Physics at McGill, demonstrated an X-ray picture of a man's leg to locate a bullet lodged in the patient's leg. The X-ray procedure aided Dr. R. C. Kirkpatrick, a surgeon at the Montreal General Hospital, in performing the operation to remove the bullet. Dr. J. P. Lipinski has written an informative article concerning four Canadian pioneers in the X-ray procedure (Lipinski, 1983). Dr. Gilbert Girdwood (1832-1917), Professor of Chemistry at McGill, who constructed a primitive apparatus in 1896, used the device on patients at Montreal General and the Royal Victoria Hospitals. He acquired new apparatus as improvements became available, and in 1901 was appointed the Director of the Medical Electrical Department (Lewis, 1969: 155), a post he held for ten years. Dr. Girdwood, a founding member of the Roentgen Society of the United States, delivered a paper on *Skiagraphy* at the Society's first meeting held at the Grand Central Palace, New York City, 13-14 December, 1900. The following year the organization's name was changed to the Roentgen Ray Society of America in order to include Canadians in an egalitarian manner. Dr. Girdwood was President of the society in 1902. He retired from his post at the Royal Victoria Hospital in 1911.

At the Montreal General Hospital, Dr. John L. Cox and his associate in physics, Dr. Hugh L. Calendar, served the increasing need for X-ray examination until W. P. Watson, who was also the apothecary and an amateur photographer, took over the work. Dr. Walter Ashley Wilkins, a McGill M.D. graduate of 1899, had the responsibility for the X-ray Department in 1900, at first as Registrar, which also included the usual work of a senior intern. In 1908 he became a part-time radiologist, replacing Mr. Watson who had been doing the work for ten years. Dr. Wilkins joined the American Roentgen Ray Society in 1908 and soon afterward became the first full-time physician-radiologist at the Montreal General Hospital. He retired from the hospital position in 1925 and established a private X-ray service in the new Medical Arts Building. When I entered private practice in 1926 my office was also in that building. I referred patients to Dr. Wilkins and, until I could afford to acquire a fluoroscope, I accompanied my patients to his laboratory and practised what I had learned from Hugo Roesler during my sojourn in Vienna.

I have fond memories of Dr. Wilkins. In 1920 during the fifth week of a severe illness which was diagnosed as Weil's disease by my teacher and devoted physician, Dr. Charles A. Peters, I was admitted to the Montreal General Hospital for investigation of my gastro-intestinal system because of persistent vomiting. When Dr. Wilkins handed me the barium sulphate mixture to drink, I told him of the danger that I might vomit and suggested he have an umbrella held over him. He assured me the liquid was too heavy to come up. He was right. The barium sulphate mixture was the first liquid I kept in my stomach since the beginning of the illness. This step initiated my recovery. I had a baked apple and toast when I returned to my room and have been eating ever since. Dr. Wilkins once said to me, as we looked at films of a patient who had carcinoma of the stomach, that if he should have this condition he would prefer not to be told and not to be treated surgically, because it's futile.

In 1895 a unique person occupied the post of Professor of Physics at Laval University in Quebec City. His name, Monseigneur J. C. K. Laflamme. His official title was Professor of Natural Sciences. He engaged in research and teaching of geology, botany, meteorology, astronomy, and physics with special emphasis on electricity. Laflamme had a number of Crookes tubes in his laboratory and in February 1896 began to assemble an X-ray apparatus. After a number of frustrating trials, on 2 April he finally succeeded in producing good X-ray pictures of the hand and the foot of a baby. In St. Hyacinthe, in 1896, Monseigneur Choquette, Professor of Physics at the Seminaire, used clinical radiology in his practice. In the June 1897 number of the *Union Médical du Canada*, Dr. Edouard Perron described a case of X-ray burn of the abdominal skin in a man who had had long exposure to X-rays, presumably during Mgr. Choquette's search for evidence of renal calculus; this burn is probably the earliest report of its kind in Canada.

The first two francophone physicians who pioneered radiology in Canada were in Paris in December 1895 when Roentgen's discovery was announced. Dr. Charles DeBlois (1867-1952) graduated M.D. at Laval University in 1892 and arrived in Europe for postgraduate education in 1895. He worked in Paris and in Munich to acquire expertise in medical electricity. In Paris the great pioneer of radiology, Antoine Béclère (1856-1939), was his teacher. He returned in 1900 and established a clinic in Trois Rivières which specialized in therapeutics with electrical instruments, in hydrotherapy and, to a rather modest extent, in the use of X-rays for diagnosis and treatment. DeBlois was an innovator in other spheres as well. He joined with Dr. Normand in founding the first school of nurses in Trois Rivières and he was a founding member of L'Association des Médecins de langue française de l'Amérique de Nord.

Dr. Henri Lasnier (1869-1936) graduated M.D. in 1895 and immediately sailed for Paris. He included the study in radiology with Béclère in his education in Paris. During his sojourn of two years at the London Hospital he probably found opportunities to study radiology. He returned to Montreal in 1900 and opened a private office at 143 St. Denis Street. He had bought a Gaiffe portable X-ray apparatus for thirty dollars and used it both in his private practice and also as the radiologist for the St. Justine Hospital. Dr. Lasnier published the first Canadian X-ray journal, *Les Rayons X.* Seven issues appeared in 1910. Only two sets are known to exist today.

Léo Pariseau (1882-1938), the brilliant innovator, perennial nonconformist and humanist, pioneered radiology as it evolved into the modern era. He graduated M.D. from Laval in Montreal in 1904. From 1906 to 1909 he was the radiologist of the Notre Dame Hospital in Montreal. From 1909 until he went overseas in the Canadian Army Medical Corps, he worked in Sherbrooke as the hygienist for the city, and also as the radiologist at St. Vincent Hospital. Pariseau served as radiologist at the Hôpital Laval de St. Claire during the war and on returning to Montreal in 1919 he became the first Chief of the Department of Electro-Radiologie at Hôtel-Dieu. He initiated electrocardiography at this hospital and was the founder president of the Société Canadienne-Française d'Electrologie et de Radiologie Médicales which came into existence on 22 May 1928 (Lipinski, 1983).

From the very beginning, Canadian radiologists became members of American radiological societies. From time to time, these societies held annual meetings in Canadian cities. Not until 1937 was a Canadian society formed with members from all parts of the country. The moving spirit in its founding was Gordon Earle Richards (1885-1949) (Lipinski, 1983). Richards was the radiotherapist at the Toronto General Hospital and at the Ontario Cancer Institute. He was joined and ably assisted by Howard Pirie and Léo Pariseau of Montreal. From the very beginning bilingualism was entrenched; the name of the organization was in both French and

English. The society began publishing the *Journal of the Canadian Association of Radiologists* in 1949; its head office was in Montreal.

In Canada, as in the United States, radiologists did not focus attention on the cardiovascular system to the same extent as Vaquez and Bordet, in Paris; Dietlen in Germany; or Roesler in Vienna and later in Philadelphia. During a visit to the National Heart Hospital in London in 1925, I saw John Parkinson routinely examine patients fluoroscopically. A few months later in Vienna I took the special course in cardiovascular roentgenology given by Hugo Roesler. David Baltzan had taken this course in about 1926. He brought his expertise to Saskatoon.

During my apprenticeship in cardiology at the Massachusetts General Hospital with Dr. Paul Dudley White we did not learn fluoroscopy of the thorax. We did not have the instrument in the department of cardiology. Patients were examined by the radiologist who reported to the clinician. When necessary, we visited the X-ray department to view and discuss the films. During his sabbatical year in 1928, Dr. White was in Europe. In his memoirs, he wrote of this time:

> There in Vienna we settled down for two months; there I studied pathology under the great Professor Erdheim and roentgenology under the brilliant young Hugo Roesler; these were weak spots in my own training but subjects in which the Viennese excelled (White, 1971).

Dr. White began to write his classic book on heart disease that year. The first of four editions appeared in 1931 and contains evidence of Dr. White's keen appreciation of the value of radiology. The chapter on this subject consists of 43 pages. The first few sentences reflect his excellent editorial judgement.

> Roentgenology has been sufficiently developed in technique and application to allow us to judge something of its real clinical value. It is not superfluous to examine fluoroscopically every individual with cardiac symptoms or signs. Sometimes surprising and frequently useful and interesting information results from such routine study (White, 1931).

In 1969 the following list of special radiological procedures for investigation of the cardiovascular system appeared in *The History of Radiology in Canada and the United States,* by Ruth and Edward Brecher (1969).

I. Circulatory System
   A. Heart and Great Vessels
      1. Intravenous angiocardiography
      2. Right-sided catheterization and selective cardiography
         a) Wedge arteriogram
      3. Retrograde catheterization into left ventricle
      4. Transbronchial auricular puncture
      5. Transthoracic left auricular puncture
      6. Transthoracic left ventricular puncture
      7. Retrograde brachial or subclavian aortography
      8. Coronary artery catheterization
      9. Injection of root of aorta through catheter
         a) Cardiac arrest and Valsalva maneuver
      10. CO_2 injection of right auricle
   B. Lumbar Aortography
      1. Catheterization
      2. Direct needle puncture
      3. Intravenous aortography (with dextran)
   C. Renal Angiography
      1. Selective catheterization or ring catheterization
      2. Direct lumbar aorta puncture
      3. Intravenous aortography and nephrotomography
   D. Peripheral Arteriography (extremities)
   E. Peripheral Venography
   F. Venacavography
   G. Splenoportography
      Needle or catheter technique
   H. Hepatic Angiography
   I. Intraosseous Venography
   J. Lymphography

Most of these procedures remain within the domain of radiologists, but a few, such as those associated with catheterization, are performed by cardiologists.

Grigg, in his excellent encyclopedic book on *The History of Roentgenology in the U.S.A. and Canada* has identified three stages in the evolution of radiology: 1) the era of the pioneers before World War I; 2) the golden age of radiology between the two wars, and 3) the atomic phase after World War II (Grigg, 1965). In Canada the golden age was fully developed. Canadian radiologists were well prepared to provide the cooperation required for cardiovascular catheterization which began immediately after World War II.

CHAPTER ELEVEN

Cardiac Catheterization

In the late 1920s, at about the time when electrocardiography had reached some degree of maturity as a widely used clinical method, clinical cardiac catheterization was born. Approximately two hundred years earlier, in 1733, Stephen Hales had published the results of his pioneering experiments in measuring arterial pressure. He inserted into the femoral artery of a horse a brass canula to which a glass tube was connected. This effort to measure a parameter of circulation, with a high degree of precision, is the first link in the chain of major achievements that brought forth clinical catheterization of the cardiovascular system. In 1963, Hoff, Geddes, and Guillemin published an exhaustive history of the earliest trials of cardiac catheterization that preceded the work of Claude Bernard, and they state: "Of the important and central position of Claude Bernard in the history of catheterization there can be no doubt" (Hoff, 1963).

Claude Bernard (1813-1878) invented intracardiac catheterization to solve the controversial problem related to comparing the temperature of the blood in the right and left ventricles. One school of interested people maintained that the temperature was higher in the right ventricle because it received blood from the tissues of the body where the process of metabolism raised its temperature. Those who followed the teaching of Lavoisier believed that "combustion" took place in the lungs and resulted in raising the temperature of the blood which left the lungs above that which entered them. In 1844, Bernard, at the age of 31, an assistant to Majendie (1783-1855), conceived the idea of measuring the temperature of the blood simultaneously in each ventricle by inserting one thermometer through the carotid artery and another through the jugular vein. The experimental subject was a horse. Repeated measurements revealed that the temperature was a few tenths of a degree higher on the right side. Bernard also studied intracardiac pressures and developed and described the technique of intracardiac catheterization so that it became a very useful tool for investigating cardiovascular physiology.

In the mid-nineteenth century, A. Chauveau (1827-1917), a professor of veterinary medicine and E. J. Marey (1830-1904), a physician, used catheterization to study the time relations of the apex-impulse and events of the cardiac cycle. Marey's invention of systems of graphic registration of pulses and pressures greatly extended Ludwig's kymographic method and greatly enhanced the method of Claude Bernard. By 1863, Chauveau and Marey had established for the first time such items as the duration of interval between atrial and ventricular contraction (0.2 sec.), duration of atrial systole (0.1 sec.), duration of ventricular systole (0.4 sec.), measurements which have been confirmed by subsequent more precise instruments.

The first trial of inserting a tube through a vein towards the heart of a human was made in 1905. The story of this event came to light about a month after Forssmann published his report on catheterization of his own heart in 1929. Forssmann himself wrote an addendum to his report in which he states, "Professor E. Unger informs me that Bleichroeder, Unger and Loeb carried out the same experiment in 1912" (Forssmann, 1929). Dr. A. J. Banatt of Berlin delved into this facet of the history of cardiovascular catheterization and wrote a note on the subject in 1949. He found that Bleichroeder read and published a paper in 1912 in which he mentioned that in 1905 he had passed catheters into the arteries and veins of dogs, and also into the veins of humans. He was interested at that time in cirrhosis of the liver and these experiments were designed to obtain blood from the vicinity of the hepatic blood vessels. Some years elapsed until in 1912 Bleichroeder resumed his work for the specific purpose of injecting medication as close as possible to the site at which the drug was to act. Chemotherapy was being introduced at that time. In that year he had treated four patients with puerperal sepsis by inserting a catheter into the femoral artery, moving it up to the bifurcation of the aorta and injecting the medication Collargol. He also reported that in 1912, on two occasions, Unger had passed a catheter through a vein in Bleichroeder's forearm up to the axilla. Similar experiments on three other subjects produced no side effects. On one occasion in 1905 a catheter was inserted into one of his own thigh veins and passed into the vena cava. Bleichroeder does not seem to have envisioned the great range of possible applications for venous and arterial catheterization. He did not live to learn about subsequent developments of the method. In 1912, and until he had to leave Germany, he was the Medical Director of a small hospital for women in Berlin. After the Nazis came to power he had to leave his home; he died while arrangements were being completed for his emigration to Australia (Banatt, 1949).

Forssmann's immediate purpose in exploring the introduction of a catheter into the right heart by passing it through a vein was the treatment of acute heart failure during surgical operation. The idea occurred to him after reading of Claude Bernard's use of intracardiac catheterization (Forssmann, 1956). Forssmann was 25 years old, an intern on the Urological service; he discussed the subject with a senior physician who emphatically discouraged him from undertaking such a procedure because at best, it might cause serious complications, and at worst, death. This information did not deter him. He first practised on a cadaver and found he could pass a ureteral catheter into the right ventricle by way of the brachial vein. Then, in secret, with the cooperation of a fellow intern, a well-oiled catheter was introduced through a large needle in his own right antecubital vein. When 35 cm had been passed in, the friend refused to insert it further, lest a catastrophe should occur. Forssmann was made of sterner stuff.

Soon afterwards he requested a nurse to prepare a ureteral catheter set as though it were for the usual purpose of treating a patient. The nurse, however, suspected something unusual and returned to the room to find him inserting a needle into his own right antecubital vein. She insisted that he try the procedure on her if he considered it harmless. He feigned acquiescence, strapped her down on a surgical table and with his back to her proceeded to expose his left cephalic vein and slipped a large needle into it. While he was passing the catheter through the needle, the nurse freed herself and eventually was of assistance to him. She held a mirror when he had placed himself behind a fluoroscopic screen to observe the progress of the catheter. As it passed through the brachial, axillary, and subclavian veins he became aware of a warmish feeling and the sensation of an impending cough. When 65 cms had entered, he noted that the tip had reached the right atrium.

In order to document the feat, he walked, accompanied by the nurse, through a long corridor and down two flights of stairs to the X-ray department where a technician photographed the chest. This picture appeared in his article entitled "Die Sondiering Des Rechten Herzens" (Forssmann, 1929). Instead of congratulating him on a signal achievement and encouraging him to carry on, his seniors regarded him as foolhardy and did not permit him to continue the project.

Nevertheless, in 1931, he performed an experiment which he

hoped would convince "The Establishment" of the important potentialities of his method. He passed a catheter into his heart under fluoroscopic control and injected a 25% solution of radio-opaque sodium iodide. He did experience a momentary blackout and had a bitter taste in his mouth but no other ill effects. He read a paper on the visualization of the right heart and pulmonary artery at a meeting of surgeons in Berlin (Forssmann, 1931). There was no applause and no discussion; consequently, he was discouraged. He entered general practice but continued to think of what might be achieved with his method (Forssmann, 1974). His town, Eberwalde, was severely bombed during World War II and his practice was dissipated. His wife, a physician, continued to practise in a rural region and he abandoned medicine and worked as a salesman. What a wonderful event when he was selected to share the Nobel Prize with Cournand and Richards in 1956!

André F. Cournand completed his medical education in Paris in 1925, after having served in the military forces of World War I between 1914 and 1919. He worked in Paris hospitals until 1930, when he came to the United States and joined the staff of the Columbia University Division at Bellevue Hospital, New York, as a resident in the Tuberculosis Service. Later, this service came to be known as the Chest Service. In 1931, he became Chief Resident and joined Dr. D. W. Richards in research on the physiology and physiopathology of respiration. He decided to settle in the United States and obtained his citizenship documents in 1941. Both Cournand and Richards were born in 1895. Richards served in World War I from 1917 to 1919 after having obtained his A.B. degree in languages at Yale. On returning from the war he studied medicine and graduated from Columbia University in 1923. After four years of internship at the New York Presbyterian Hospital, he spent a year in England with Sir Henry Dale. He then returned to New York and devoted himself to research in the Chest Service of the Columbia University Division of Bellevue Hospital. Thus, these two men worked together unravelling the physiology of the respiratory system. In his Nobel Lecture (11 December 1956), Dr. Richards stated:

> By the late nineteen-thirties, we were able to describe the ventilatory functions of the lungs, and with pulmonary measurements supplemented by arterial blood studies, in rest and exercise, define to some extent, the mixing and the diffusional aspects of pulmonary alveolar or alveolar-capillary functions. But we still could not measure blood flow through the lungs, and

> could not, therefore, move into those broader concepts of cardiopulmonary function which now began to be our goal. (Richards, 1956)

Cardiac catheterization could greatly facilitate their work at this stage. They knew about Forssmann's experiment and about the isolated instances of its use in Germany, Portugal, South America, and France. In 1940, Cournand and Dr. Helmert Ranges began to use the catheterization technique, and demonstrated its reliability and safety.

André Cournand delivered the Jimenez Diaz Memorial Lecture in 1970. He chose this occasion to compose the interesting story of the invention and evolution of cardiac catheterization from 1844 to 1945, which he relates in a fine literary style. The events are grouped into three phases: an initial period (1844 to 1900) begins with Claude Bernard's work and ends with the story of the Fick principle for measuring cardiac output and bloodflow. The second period, 1929 to 1936, begins with Forssmann's pioneering technique for introducing a catheter into the right side of the heart in humans and occasional use of the method by others, including Diaz and his colleague, Sanchez Cuenca who, in 1930, described their success in passing a ureteral catheter through an arm vein into the right atrium of a patient. In writing of the third phase (1936-1945) he states:

> In 1936 we (Cournand and Richards) considered whether the technique of right heart catheterization might provide help in obtaining the mixed venous blood needed for determination of respiratory gas concentrations, in accordance with our general plan. I arranged therefore, to visit with Dr. Ameuille, one of my former teachers, who had completed pulmonary angiography in 100 patients in his hospital in Paris. The protocols of these cases convinced me of the safety of the technique. Dick Richards and I, in collaboration with Robert Darling, then familiarized ourselves with the method, first in canine experiments and eventually in a chimpanzee. Meanwhile George Wright, a former student of Carl Wiggers, and then a resident in the Chest Service at Bellevue Hospital, offered to advance ureteral catheters, under fluoroscopic control, into the right atrium of human cadavers, in order to measure the distance between the catheter tip and a landmark on the anterior chest wall on lateral X-ray films; this datum would be needed to establish a reference point for measuring intracardiac pressures.

In 1940 our first attempt with a patient failed because the catheter was obstructed at the level of the axilla (due to a large lymph node, the seat of a metastatic carcinoma). Not long afterward, however, a new opportunity presented itself. Homer Smith, professor of physiology at New York University College of Medicine, with his collaborators, including Drs. William Goldring, Herbert Chasis, and Helmert Ranges at the Hypertension Clinic of Bellevue Hospital, was planning to measure cardiac output in hypertensive patients using a new model of ballistocardiograph. They had reached a stumbling block, however: to calibrate the ballistocardiograph curves, they needed reliable, independent values of cardiac output determined at the same time as the ballistocardiographic recording. For this purpose application of the direct Fick principle appealed to the brilliant physiologist, and there was little need for persuasion.

In a first report published in 1941 in collaboration with Ranges . . . we emphasized "*a.* the necessity that the patient be metabolically stable; *b.* the requirement for simultaneous and prolonged blood and air sampling; *c.* the value of the internal check provided by comparing results based on the application of the Fick principle to CO_2 and O_2 data (this resulted in rejection of at least half the experiments); *d.* the reproduceability of the results, and *e.* the acceptability to patients and innocuousness of the catheterization procedure."

Reflecting on the story of these events, it appears that the first opportunity for clinical application of the method bore very slender relationship to its ultimate use. As luck would have it, calibration of the Ballistocardiograph served to suggest the unreliability of the instrument for adequate measurement of cardiac output. But cardiac catheterization quite rapidly proved its very great importance as a clinical diagnostic tool and somewhat later as a therapeutic instrument in coronary angioplasty.

In his Diaz Memorial Lecture, Cournand tells a fascinating story of events spread over 101 years and the last sentence reads: "In a word, we were fortunate enough to achieve in some measure the fundamental association of experimental and clinical medicine of which Claude Bernard dreamed" (Cournand, 1970).

Cardiac Catheterization in Canada

The minibiographies of the three principal pioneers, Johnson in Montreal and Keith and Greenwood in Toronto, are followed by those who brought the new methods to the communities in which they settled. These are arranged geographically from the Atlantic to the Pacific and within each province chronologically according to the year in which they began their careers in these communities.

Dr. Arnold L. Johnson, M.D. McGill, 40; F.R.C.P.

The first Canadians who took an active interest in cardiac catheterization were Arnold Johnson of Montreal and John Keith of Toronto. By coincidence, both had served as medical officers in the Royal Canadian Navy during World War II. In 1945 Arnold Johnson, while still in the service, was given leave to engage in postgraduate studies with Dr. Paul D. White in Boston. A little later in the same year, he learned of the new developments in paediatric cardiology in the clinic headed by Dr. Helen Taussig. In 1968, he wrote to the archivist:

October 29, 1968

> This tardy letter is stimulated by my move out of my office at the Children's in September shortly before I went off on holiday and the finding among various papers your suggestion of a long time ago that you would like information relative to any historical points of cardiological interest in the local scene. This and the slight nostalgia of rifling through a number of old records in order to move, gives me cause to set forth a few points in this letter which might or might not be of interest to you.
>
> I was interested in checking back on the heart catheterization facilities which we set up in the Montreal Children's Hospital in the fall of 1946, and I did my first heart catheterization in October 1946 just twenty-two years ago. The catheterization laboratory has thus been in continuous operation at the Children's with the exception of a six-month period when I was with Doctor Taussig in 1947. I think that this catheterization laboratory has thus operated for a longer period than any in Canada.
>
> There are one or two features surrounding it which are of some interest in retrospect. As you know, at the time that I was invited to go to the Children's to start this work, I was working in the Department of Physiology under Hebbel Hoff during which time I was doing heart catheterization studies in dogs and eventually obtained my M.Sc., more particularly on the catheterization in the children. I am attaching a copy of the first paper about this heart catheterization in 1947 (Johnson, 1947). As you well know, since you were so helpful to him in his early days in Montreal, I had the privilege of starting work with Paul Sekelj. Although the first intra-cardiac pressure measurements were made with a

simple manometer giving us mean pressures, under Paul's guidance we started to use, in 1947, the Statham pressure gauges and photographic recording of pressures. The Hathaway camera which we used was a little unreliable and we sometimes ended up with not too much on a pressure tracing. Thus we were most pleased when eventually the direct writers came out. Had we been smarter, I suppose we would have got the company to really work away at our problem because, of course, now and for some years, everybody has been back at the photographic recording. It is also of interest, very old hat now, but then not too frequent, to have such close cooperation between a basic science university department and the hospital department, and such close liaison with a biophysics person. I presume that Paul's Department of Biophysics, which was established as a separate entity in 1957 at the Montreal Children's Hospital, must be one of the early ones if not the first in Canada.

Another heartwarming facet of those days which I have frequently reflected upon is the somewhat courageous stand taken by Drs. Alton Goldbloom (Goldbloom, 1959), John deBelle and D. E. Ross about allowing this procedure of catheterization to go forward.

The Department of Cardiology was recognized as such in 1947 at which time I became the Director. I have always been geographical full time in cardiology for good or ill, but in any case I suppose one of the few people in Canada at the time who started their career as a cardiac specialist and never improved his lot!

Relative to the Montreal Cardiac Society, I well remember the initial discussions which I was privileged to attend and in which you and Hebbel Hoff were so active. I guess I must have been one of the founding members and spent some time through the various executive positions. I recall also the many interesting sessions that we had in the setting up of the Association of Cardiologists, and similarly went through the executive ranks and happened to be the President at the time of the inception of Q.H.I.S. [Quebec Hospital Insurance Service] when Pierre Marion and I did the negotiating about the financial arrangements for the electrocardiograms with the government.

I still remember with interest the various meetings that we had with the women's groups prior to the final organization of the Quebec Heart Foundation, and always look back with pleasure at the skill which you and Al Grossman displayed in dealing with these very keen women who I thought also showed considerable generosity of spirit to get the Quebec Heart Foundation on its way.

I might add one or two other things with which I have been associated since 1958. In 1958 we set up the Joint Cardiorespiratory Service of the Royal Victoria Hospital and the Montreal Children's Hospital and I became the Director of the Cardiovascular Division. This has been an interesting experiment in inter-hospital department activity. It did a few things rather well. It was possible to set up a modern department of cardiology at the Royal Victoria Hospital rather quickly and a similar Respiratory Department at the Montreal Children's Hospital, and each have flourished since. It also provided a much wider use for the talents of Paul Sekelj. I had started helping him in a small way in his development of the ear oximeter back in 1947 and he made great progress with the dye dilution technique in the years since, but he subsequently required both adult and children's facilities. This joint operation provided a larger milieu for both clinical and research activity and for some interchange of fellows. There was an extremely large production of research work particularly under the direction of Maurice McGregor and David Bates. There were something like more than 100 papers published relative to cardiovascular things from our Joint Service between 1958 and the present.

Two items at the Royal Victoria that we were concerned with fairly early on was the application of the new knowledge regarding resuscitation techniques and electrical stimulation of the heart. You will recall that your friend, Mr. Trayst, was carried for thirteen months from the Spring of 1960 with an electrode catheter and subsequently had an implanted pacemaker put in. In 1960 also, we set up a resuscitation team which has persisted in its efforts to the present time. I'm sure that you've not reached this point in this long letter, but I felt that the initial parts must be of interest to you and refresh your mind about events in which you provided some strong support and empathy.

Dr. Arnold Johnson rose to the post of Associate Professor of Paediatrics and of Medicine at McGill. The first item in his bibliography is as co-author of a paper on "Electrocardiography in Hypertension," by William C. Bridges, Arnold L. Johnson, Reginald H. Smithwick, and Paul D. White, which was published in the 1946 *Journal of the American Medical Association,* volume 131, page 1476.

The very next item is the one which establishes his priority as a very early pioneer in the practice of cardiac catheterization in Canada, "Heart Catheterization in the Investigation of Congenital Heart Disease" (Johnson, 1947). In the 1940s and 1950s, rheumatic fever was still very prevalent. Dr. Johnson carried out extensive studies on its therapy with cortisone. His bibliography, naturally, contains many articles on congenital heart disease. He pioneered the application of implanted pacemakers for the treatment of complete A-V dissociation. His career has been unique for he directed the Department of Cardiology in the Children's Hospital and also in the Royal Victoria Hospital, where he was responsible for cardiology in adult patients. Dr. Johnson did not fill out the questionnaire, resulting in a paucity of information about his educational career.

Dr. John D. Keith, 23 February 1908, Winnipeg; University of Toronto, B.Sc. 26; M.D. 32.

Dr. John Keith, who was present at the founding meeting of the Canadian Cardiovascular Society in June 1947, was a charter member of the Society and served as its secretary from 1951 until 1956. He was a powerful catalyst in promoting the creation of the Ontario Heart Foundation and, soon afterwards, the Canadian Heart Foundation. On the death of the first President of the Canadian Heart Foundation, the late Dr. George F. Strong, the Board of Directors selected John Keith to take his place. He remained a member of the Board of Directors of the Foundation from its inception in 1957 until 1964, when he became a member of its Senior Advisory Council. In 1964, he also became a member of the Medical Advisory Board of the International Cardiology Foundation after having been a member of its Board from 1962 to 1964. In 1962, he took on the task of Treasurer of the International Cardiology Society. He served as a member of the Board of Directors of the American Heart Association during the year 1948-49. In the early 1950s he played a major role in founding the section of Cardiology of the Ontario Medical Association.

The work which John Keith performed in all these official capacities was one facet of his involvement in promoting the prevention and relief of cardiovascular disease. At what we may term the grass roots, he dealt with the problems of the individual patient. Working in the Sick Children's Hospital, he faced the challenges presented by infants and children, and concerned parents and relatives. He succeeded in convincing the administrators of his hospital, influential citizens, and the general public that heart disease can be controlled and prevented by adequate research. To this end, it was necessary to encourage men and women to dedicate their careers to this work. Money had to be provided to pay the cost of their research projects and their salaries. He led his colleagues in setting the example of dedication and in very significant achievements in the study and treatment of congenital and acquired heart disease in infants and children. A relatively brief summary of these developments appears in his response to our request for the story of the Department of Cardiology at the Hospital for Sick Children in Toronto, which he founded and developed. He wrote as follows in January 1967, in a letter which accompanied his curriculum vitae and bibliography:

> To add to the curriculum vitae so that it will appear a little more coherent, I might make a few additional comments. As far back as I can remember I had intended to go into Medicine. I suppose it is possible that because I had two uncles who were already doctors they had had some influence on this, but this was a subconscious effect and I always had the feeling that it was completely my own idea and not suggested from without. A decision at an early age in this matter makes it much easier to decide what subjects you take in either high school or university. When I see some of the problems the present generation face in trying to decide what to do, I think there is something to be said for singlemindedness.
>
> At the University I attended lectures, classes, clinics, etc., but did not thoroughly enjoy Medicine until I graduated. Perhaps the course that I enjoyed most at University was that given by Prof. Ned Pratt, the well-known Canadian poet. He lectured to us in English, which was an option during the first two years of Medicine and I took it during those two years. Then they switched it to the second and third so I was able to take a third year as an option as well. I don't think Dr. Pratt took the Medical group very seriously but he did present English Literature and Poetry in a most easy-going, fascinating way that made it very enjoyable and undoubtedly left a lasting impression on my mind as well as stimulating my reading into many new channels.
>
> I spent a fair amount of my time at university taking part in various athletics — particularly football — playing on the Senior Varsity Team from 1927-31. This was more enjoyable than the dull routine of lecturers, clinics, etc.
>
> On graduation I interned at the Rochester Strong Memorial Hospital in Paediatrics (Rochester, N.Y.) having decided some-

time before graduation that I wanted to do children's diseases and I also wanted to get away from Toronto for a while. This is a remarkably fine university and medical school with an excellent Paediatric Department under Professor Clausen. It had then and still has one of the best medical libraries in the world. The latter was so handy to the interns because you passed it continually in the hospital. Even at that time they had seven or eight hundred journals taken monthly and I am sure there is a much larger number at the present time [1967]. There was plenty of time to study each case leisurely and thoroughly and I found this one of my most rewarding years in Medicine.

The first year I was in intern, the second year assistant resident. In the second year I decided that I would like to go to England for a while and asked my professor [Clausen] which centre he would recommend. It is interesting that at the same time Dr. Harry Ebbs who was in New York asked his professor [Dr. Rusty McIntosh] the same question and both of them independently gave the same answer and recommended that we should go to Birmingham to study at the Birmingham Children's Hospital under Sir Leonard Parsons. This we both did and had an immensely rewarding time. I was the Assistant R.M.O. [Resident Medical Officer] for a period and then the Resident Medical Officer for a year. Following this I had a Research Fellowship known as the Athol-Moynihan in Research on Rheumatic Heart Disease. During the interval of holding the Fellowship, I made some original observations on the influence of the conduction time on heart sounds. They are still very valid and have been confirmed by many people since.

In my second year at Rochester, Dr. Albert Kaiser, who was the leading practising paediatrician, asked me if I would be interested in carrying out an investigation on the rheumatic patients in the hospital. This involved the evaluation of a streptococcal skin test in relation to the acute phase of the disease. Rheumatic Fever was so common then and I became quite interested in the disease. This led later to the Athol-Moynihan Fellowship, 1936-38 in England. A concern about all types of heart disease in childhood was a natural step. By this time in England I was doing a large number of autopsies at the Children's Hospital. Many of them had congenital heart defects which we attempted to diagnose during life. Thus when I returned to Canada in 1938, I had had considerable training and experience in the cardiac field.

On return in 1938 to the Hospital for Sick Children I was appointed to the Medical Staff and designated the Physician in Charge of the Cardiac Department. In 1938, as you are well aware, congenital heart disease was often a diagnosis in itself and little attempt was made to differentiate the various subdivisions. It was either congenital heart disease or rheumatic heart disease and that was that. Furthermore, the only people interested in the different types of congenital heart defects were a few pathologists such as Dr. Maude Abbott, but interest in specific diagnosis was awakened by Dr. Robert Gross's operation for the patent ductus arteriosus (1938). From then on it became extremely important to decide what specific lesion was present, so that my joining the staff of the Hospital for Sick Children coincided with a sort of renaissance in heart disease in childhood and the field has been advancing steadily ever since. Dr. D. E. Robertson operated on a number of children with patent ductus arteriosus in those days (1940) and I can remember the early operations were very bloody and difficult. Visitors looked over his shoulder in amazement to think that an operation could be done in or near the heart. As you are well aware, that operation is now the simplest of all and parallels some of the routine surgical procedures such as appendectomy.

At that time, 1939-40, I usually had 30 or 40 cases of rheumatic heart disease in the hospital at any one time and was beginning to use sulfonamides as prophylaxis. This was tested out on our wards with considerable success. We have never seen as many cases since the year of 1938, 1939 or 1940 because the incidence of rheumatic heart disease has fallen since. Although the population of Toronto has quadrupled in the intervening years, the incidence of rheumatic fever in the wards is about a tenth. This I am sure has been as dramatic a change for our generation as it was for those before us to see typhoid fever, diphtheria, etc. disappear from the hospital wards.

From 1942 to 1946 I was in the Canadian Navy and was attached to a North Atlantic convoy ship for nine months. Fortunately paediatric experience proved very useful in the Navy because so many young men were developing infectious diseases as well as rheumatic fever and I was able to study the use of large doses and small doses of salicylates in rheumatic fever and noted no difference in the incidence of heart disease or in severity. At the time, Coburn was recommending huge doses of salicylates intravenously in the United States military services and my study put a damper on this program of his. I think that experience since then has not shown any advantage of the large doses he was using, over modest amounts.

Before I returned to civilian life, in the early weeks of 1946, the Blalock-Taussig operation had been published (*J.A.M.A.*, 19 May, 1945) and I made arrangements while I was still in the Navy to go and visit Helen Taussig for long enough to acquaint myself with their techniques, surgical, medical and diagnostic. This was a most interesting visit. I always tell Helen that I regard myself as her first Fellow.

I then returned to Toronto and got deeply involved in diagnostic techniques, although we had no cardiovascular surgeon as such at that time. As you will recall, towards the end of the war Dr. Cournand in New York had developed the intra-cardiac catheter techniques in studying the haemodynamics and these became applicable to diagnosis as well. I visited in both New York and Boston in this regard and I think I was the first to introduce cardiac catheterization as well as angiocardiography into Canada in the year 1946-47.

Angiocardiography seemed a very obvious technique to apply to young infants and children. It was rarely used anywhere at that time, although work had been done on it by Dr. Castellanos in Cuba. I got hold of an X-ray engineering firm in town and we purchased a war-time American aerial photography machine that was able to take several pictures a second, and this was adapted for X-ray use in angiocardiography. Soon we were in business taking excellent pictures of contrast media going through infants' hearts. I think we were the first paediatric centre outside of Cuba to use this technique in studying infants and children. As you know, it has since proved very valuable and is now used universally.

When I started in cardiology at the Hospital for Sick Children, I had no office, no budget and was simply told to get on with it. I remember my first purchase was a stop-watch which cost about $25 and there was a lot of discussion whether or not this could be purchased by the hospital. However, they agreed and they have been increasingly generous over the years until at the present time we have thirty-eight people working full time in the department. This includes fifteen doctors, ten nurse technicians, an X-ray technician, electronics expert, secretaries and nursing aides.

A year or two after the war, I got my first Fellow attached to the Department. The Fellows, you will note, are listed along with my curriculum vitae. My first Fellow was Dr. Stephen Weyman of New Brunswick who went back to Saint John, New Brunswick, to practise paediatrics, which he did successfully for several years. Two or three years ago, he became Mayor of St. John and more recently is now the Minister of Health in the provincial government for New Brunswick. The others are scattered about different countries practising paediatrics, cardiology, whether as internists or paediatric cardiologists.

As indicated above, our chief investigations have been in the field of rheumatic heart disease and congenital heart disease. We have made a modest contribution in the field of prophylaxis of rheumatic heart disease and helped to spread this information to doctors across the country. Thus, from our studies and many similar ones, the prognosis has improved a great deal in rheumatic fever and rheumatic heart disease. We took part in the First International Control Study on the use of steroids and salicylates, and also in delineating the current trends of the natural history of Rheumatic Fever. Subsequent studies from this institution have shown that the greatest change in the past twenty-five years has been in the mortality in childhood.

Our group has been particularly interested in the haemodynamics of the newborn and a study of the changes that occur in the pulmonary artery following birth — the speed with which the pressure falls to post-natal normal levels — and also the mechanisms that bring about closure of the ductus arteriosus. These studies have been carried out in mongols (Down's Syndrome) during the newborn period, and in normal babies, and many similar studies were done in newborn pigs at the Ontario Agricultural College in Guelph, our group working in conjunction with staff there.

In 1946 we had no cardiovascular surgeon as such. An attempt was made on the part of the chief surgeon to do some heart surgery. Those doing chest surgery also did a little cardiovascular work. This did not prove satisfactory and the Chief of Surgery eventually suggested to Dr. W. T. Mustard that he take some special training in the heart field. This was done and later on a second cardiovascular surgeon was added to our group, Dr. George A. Trusler. This has led to a very excellent team both clinically and from an investigational point of view. I can remember immediately after the war having difficulty persuading the chief of surgery that we needed to have a cardiovascular surgeon, but eventually he agreed and this led to Dr. Mustard's appointment in this category. Since then we have seen successful surgical correction of coarctation of the aorta, pulmonary stenosis, atrial septal defect, ventricular septal defect, tricuspid atresias, etc. Our surgeons were in on the pioneer stage of many of these procedures. Dr. Bigelow at the Toronto General Hospital had developed a method of using hypothermia in permitting one to stop the heartbeat for an abbreviated interval and this was used by Dr. Mustard in correcting atrial septal defect and also relieving valvular pulmonary stenosis. This technique was also used in a limited degree in correcting coarctation of the aorta in order to avoid inadequate circulation of the lower part of the body and particularly the spine during the clamping of the aorta. All of these new procedures carried a relatively high surgical mortality when they were first introduced, but with considerable experience on the part of the surgeons, anaesthetists, postoperative nursing care, etc., the mortality has fallen to relatively low levels. I am sure you have had the same experience, but one would shudder to have to go through it a second time.

Perhaps the most exciting piece of work done in this institution has been that of Dr. Mustard's procedure for correcting transposition of the great vessels. Investigative work started on this soon after the war. Since this was one of the most uniformly fatal congenital heart defects, any procedure was justified that had any hope of success. Investigations were carried on in the lab and eventually transferred to the operating table but met with little or no success. The vessels were transposed on the operating table in elaborate procedures involving the shift of the left coronary from the venous ventricle side to the arterial side. These techniques seemed to come close to success but ultimately led to failure and death of the patient, or the animal if it was in the laboratory. It ultimately became clear that the transfer of transportation of the great arteries was not the answer and that the solution for correction must be reached at the venous end. Dr. Tom Baffes of Chicago introduced a method of partially correcting the venous return. This procedure was chiefly used on the few cases that survived to two years of age. After trying this and numerous techniques first experimentally, Bill Mustard devised an ingenious method of sewing in a baffle of pericardium in such a way that the superior vena caval and inferior vena caval blood is shunted into the left ventricle. At the same time, the arterialized blood returning from the lungs flows over such baffle into the right ventricle and thus out to the aorta. Since many infants had been kept alive with a palliative procedure by the creation of a large atrial septal defect, they have thus survived infancy in spite of the fact they are considerably cyanosed. It is this sort of case that is so suitable for the Mustard operation and many successful operations have been carried out here in Canada, England and in the United States. This has been a significant breakthrough, since 90% of cases with transposition of great vessels were dying in the first year of life and the majority of them in the first month. However, more needs to be done in this field since those with ventricular septal defect of significant size are developing pulmonary vascular disease and those with pulmonary stenosis cannot readily be treated with the Mustard procedure at the present time.

Over the years we have saved in jars a large number of hearts from children with congenital heart defects and this collection is somewhat unique. There is only one other that corresponds with it — that of Dr. Maurice Lev in Chicago. Dr. Richard Van Praagh and Dr. Shaher and others who have worked with us have taken particular advantage of this museum of specimens and have studied lesions that have been inadequately understood in the past, such as the complicated group of dextrocardia, corrected transposition of the great vessels, and all the anomalies that are associated with transposition of the great vessels. These have been classified, measured, investigated anatomically and pathologically, and written up for the literature. These studies have produced a great deal of clarity but further simplification of classifications is required in the future.

In the past ten years we have done a little pioneering in the data collecting field. We have recorded data on many heart defects — including material in the clinical, haemodynamic, surgical, pathological fields, putting it onto punch cards which can be transferred to tape and analyzed by modern computers. We have been doing this now for over ten years and have 12,000 cases on punch cards. In this way we have successfully analyzed a variety of defects and achieved figures that would have taken years by hand-to-hand methods. However, the accuracy of this data depends initially on a very carefully filled out form and this, of course, must be done by hand.

When I returned from the war it was difficult to get adequate funds for the support of cardiac research. There was some available through the National Health Grants but a very inadequate system of review of such applications existed. After several interviews with the Deputy Minister of Health in Ontario, he agreed to let me set up what we called a Committee on Cardiology in Ontario to carry out this function and we were then able to encourage numerous cardiologists to apply for funds through this channel. It soon became apparent that more funds and a better organization was required. I persuaded the Ontario Medical Association to let us develop a section on Cardiology. With this body functioning, we organized a small group who helped us create the Ontario Heart Foundation. This came into being in 1952. Funds were at first available only through the National Health Grants via the Ontario Department of Health but after many meetings and much persuasion the Ontario Provincial Government made an initial award that could be handled by the Ontario Heart Foundation for research grants in the province. At about the same time the British Columbia Heart Foundation was formed and with these two provinces and the help of outstanding physicians in Montreal and other parts of the country, the Canadian Heart Foundation was formed in 1956. You and I played a key part in this development and I think it is something we can look back on with considerable satisfaction since it has led to formation of similar bodies across the country, with public campaigns for funds.

Since 1954 and 1958 when I attended the World Congresses on Heart Disease, first in Washington, then in Brussels, I have been interested in Cardiology at this international level, and since 1962 have been Treasurer of the International Cardiology Society. This organization has been responsible for some international cooperation in the field, but its main duty has been to produce an International Cardiology Congress every four years. As you know, the Society is uniting its efforts with that of the International Cardiology Foundation and developing on a much wider basis in an effort to stimulate international research in cardiology, as well as to help with education and organization in the heart field to many countries around the world.

I should also say I was in at your organizational meeting of the Canadian Cardiovascular Society in June 1947 and you will recall I was its secretary from 1951 to 1956.

During the years 1935 to 1967, Dr. Keith's bibliography grew to 68 items, the majority co-authored with associates and pupils. Almost all deal with items of paediatric cardiology. In 1957, he wrote an article entitled "The Policy of the Canadian Heart Foundation," an element in his contribution to the vigorous development of this organization (Keith, 1957). The textbook on *Heart Disease in Infancy and Childhood* appeared in 1958. This text reflects the rapid rate of growth and progress made by the Department of Cardiology of the Hospital for Sick Children under John Keith's direction (Keith, Rowe, Vlad, 1958).

What we consider to be the crowning achievement of Dr. Keith's career is represented by the list of eighty-two Fellows who came to him from far and near to learn from him and his colleagues at the Hospital for Sick Children. This list was composed in 1972.

Name	*Country of Origin*	*Location in 1972*
Dr. Simon Munuz Armas	Venezuela	Caracas, Venezuela
Dr. Pierre Auger	Canada	Lèvis, P.Q.
Dr. D. S. Beanlands	Canada	Toronto, Ont.
Dr. Bjorn Bjarke	Sweden	Stockholm, Sweden
Dr. Iain F. S. Black	U.S.A.	Philadelphia, Pa.
Dr. Felipe C. Bolanos	Argentina	Buenos Aires, Argentina
Dr. Michael Braudo	S. Africa	Toronto, Ont.
Dr. Samuel Brew-Graves	U.S.A.	Baltimore, Md.
Dr. A. Louise Calder	Canada	Boston, Mass.
Dr. Alexander G. M. Campbell	Scotland	New Haven, Conn.
Dr. Su-Chiung Chen	Taiwan	Taipei, Taiwan
Dr. Anastasios Chrysothon	Greece	Salonika, Greece
Dr. Malcolm Clarke	England	London, England
Dr. T. Emmett Cleary	Canada	Orillia, Ont.
Dr. Joan Coggin	U.S.A.	Loma Linda, Cal.
Dr. George F. Collins	Scotland	Montreal, P.Q.
Dr. John F. Collins	Canada	St. John's, Nfld.
Dr. George Deslisle	Canada	Quebec City, P.Q.
Dr. R. N. Easthope	New Zealand	Wellington, N.Z.
Dr. Bachoo Edibam	India	Nagpur, India
Dr. George Emmanouilides	U.S.A.	Los Angeles, Cal.
Dr. Eshagh Eshaghpour	Iran	Philadelphia, Pa.
Dr. John R. Evans	Canada	Toronto, Ont.
Dr. Joel Fagan	Canada	Calgary, Alta.
Dr. John Fay	England	Kingston, Ont.
Dr. Ian Findlay	Australia	Melbourne, Australia
Dr. Eugene Fischmann	U.S.A.	Washington, D.C.
Dr. Peter Forbath	Hungary	Toronto, Ont.
Dr. Constance Forsyth	Scotland	Dundee, Scotland
Dr. Rodney S. Fowler	Canada	Toronto, Ont.
Dr. Hiroshi Fukuda	Japan	Fukuoka City, Japan
Dr. I.H. Glass	Canada	Toronto, Ont.
Dr. K. Hallidie-Smith	England	London, England
Dr. Richard Hawker	Australia	Baltimore, Md.
Dr. Hirohisa Kato	Japan	Fukuoka City, Japan

Dr. George Khoury	Egypt	Morgantown, W.Va.
Dr. Lins Lasso-Avalos	Mexico	Mexico
Dr. R. M. Lauer	U.S.A.	Iowa City, Iowa
Dr. Mock Dock Li	Taiwan	London, Ont.
Dr. Sahat M. Manoeroeng	Indonesia	Medan, Indonesia
Dr. Yves Marquis	Canada	Quebec City, P.Q.
Dr. Keith McKenzie	Jamaica	Kingston, Jamaica
Dr. Collin Miller	Jamaica	Kingston, Jamaica
Dr. Sheila Mitchell	U.S.A.	Bethesda, Md.
Dr. David Mymin	England	St. Boniface, Man.
Dr. Catherine A. Neill	France	Montreal, P.Q.
Dr. Aron Nordenberg	Israel	Harrisburg, Pa.
Dr. J. Hubert O'Hanley	Canada	Charlottetown, P.E.I.
Dr. Peter Olley	England	Toronto, Ont.
Dr. K. Ross Parker	Canada	Hamilton, Ont.
Dr. Gerald B. Peckham	Canada	St. John's, Nfld.
Dr. Akos Pereszlenyi	Hungary	Toronto, Ont.
Dr. Antonio Peschiera	Peru	Lima, Peru
Dr. Douglas Pickering	England	Oxford, England
Dr. Bennis Pittawa	S. Africa	Durban, S. Africa
Dr. L. K. Rathi	India	
Dr. Richard Rowe	U.S.A.	Baltimore, Md.
Dr. Paul Sawyer	England	Toronto, Ont.
Dr. Michael Scott	Ireland	Lurgan, N.Ireland
Dr. William Sears	U.S.A.	Toronto, Ont.
Dr. Frank Sellers	Canada	Ottawa, Ont.
Dr. Pravin Shah	India	Rochester, N.Y.
Dr. Reda Shaher	Egypt	Albany, N.Y.
Dr. Ali Shams	Iran	Toronto, Ont.
Dr. John Shone	Canada	Toronto, Ont.
Dr. Walter Singh	Guyana	Toronto, Ont.
Dr. R. J. Sommerville	Canada	Calgary, Alta.
Dr. J. R. Suarez-Arana	Central Amer.	San Salvador
Dr. Tadeusz Takrzewski	Poland	Tempe, Ariz.
Dr. Michael Tyrrell	England	Saskatoon, Sask.
Dr. Richard Van Praagh	Canada	Boston, Mass.
Dr. Stella Van Praagh	Greece	Boston, Mass.
Dr. Preecha Vichitbandha	Thailand	Dhonburi, Thailand
Dr. Dennis J. Vince	Canada	Vancouver, B.C.
Dr. Shyama Virmani	India	Nashville, Tenn.
Dr. Alfredo Vizcaino	Mexico	Mexico
Dr. Peter Vlad	Roumania	Buffalo, N.Y.
Dr. David Watson	U.S.A.	Jackson, Miss.
Dr. Geoffrey Watson	England	Manchester, England
Dr. Stephen Weyman	Canada	Saint John, N.B.
Dr. Warren S. Whelan	Canada	London, Ont.

One of the group of Fellows, Dr. Richard Rowe, not only co-authored the textbook on *Heart Disease in Infancy and Childhood* with John Keith and Peter Vlad, another Fellow, but at a critical stage of his career he represented the maturation of paediatric cardiology in Canada. An analogy exists between the process by which a given region of the world evolves into a mature industrial unit and the process which leads to maturity of a medical or other scientific discipline in a given region. In the first stage, needed knowledge and skills are imported from developed countries; in the next stage domestic industries and institutions are sufficiently advanced to provide training and education so that importation becomes unnecessary. The stage of maturity is reached when the skilled and educated workers create new methods and knowledge which attract students from the developed countries, and when one or more of the creative teachers is imported by the developed country from the previously underdeveloped region. This happened when William Osler (later Sir William) was invited to become Regius Professor of Medicine at Oxford. All his teachers, both in Toronto and at McGill, had studied and obtained degrees in Scotland (Edinburgh) or in England. He himself went to University College, London, for postgraduate studies immediately after obtaining his M.D. degree at McGill. Then after ten years (1874-1884) at McGill, five years at Philadelphia, and sixteen at Johns Hopkins Medical School in Baltimore, he accepted the post at Oxford. This activity symbolized maturity of medicine in North America. In a similar way John Keith, who learnt from Helen Taussig at Johns Hopkins, was Richard Rowe's teacher and when Rowe was appointed to fill the vacancy at Johns Hopkins because of Dr. Taussig's retirement, his career reflected the maturity of Canadian paediatric cardiology.

Dr. Keith's colleagues honoured him officially in several ways: The Canadian Heart Foundation presented him with the President's Award, in 1960. I had the pleasant task of making the presentation and spoke as follows:

> In his work at the Sick Children's Hospital, Dr. John Keith pioneered in applying and inventing new ideas and techniques for the control and prevention of heart disease. Among his confrères in the Canadian Heart Association as a member of its first council and later as secretary, he pioneered in bringing about the creation of the National Heart Foundation of Canada. Together with the late Dr. George Strong, he sought and obtained the sympathetic, indeed the enthusiastic sponsorship of the Hon. Mr. Paul Martin who, as Minister of Health and Welfare, invited

representatives from all parts of Canada to a meeting at which the Foundation was initiated. And when our founder president Dr. Strong himself became a victim of a fatal type of coronary heart disease, John Keith carried on the work and under his leadership the first Heart Fund Campaign became a successful reality. After relinquishing the presidency of the Foundation two years ago, he continued to serve as a member of the Board of Directors and also as a member of various committees including the Scientific Subcommittee.

On this great occasion, the National Heart Foundation wishes to express its grateful appreciation to Dr. John Keith and to present him, a pioneering president, with the President's Award.

Some years later, in 1972, the Canadian Heart Foundation gave Dr. Keith its highest honour, a gold medal, the Award of Merit.

In 1967 the Canadian Cardiovascular Society chose him for its Annual Lecturer and in the same year the Ontario Heart Foundation established "The John Keith Lecture" which has become an important feature of the Society's annual meeting; Dr. Keith himself delivered the first one.

Dr. William Frederick Greenwood, 18 May 1913, St. Catharines, Ont.; Trinity College, University of Toronto, B.A. 34; M.D. 37; F.R.C.P.(C); F.A.C.C.; F.A.H.A.

The letter which Dr. Greenwood wrote in responding to the special questions is here quoted at length:

> I suppose I came into cardiology by a series of accidents. I also came to Toronto by accident. Four members of my family graduated from McGill, and I always thought I would go to McGill except that my father died in 1923, and when it came time to go to university, my mother had married again, was living in Toronto, and there was no thought of spending extra money to have me board in Montreal. As an undergraduate and postgraduate student, I was awfully attracted to John Oille and his matter of fact and questioning method of approaching any problem. I had always thought that physiology helped me to understand patients better than any other of the basic sciences, including pathology, so that a good deal of my postgraduate training was spent in Departments of Physiology. The years of following medicine was really doing experimental work with Bob Cleghorn at the

Banting Institute with a minor clinical aspect to it. When I went to the Department of Physiology at the University of Toronto in 1938, I got interested in experimental hypertension and wanted to measure systolic and diastolic pressures in these animals, so got interested in other techniques and I suppose it was this early intensive reading that got me interested in cardiology. When I was in the army, Dr. Duncan Graham wrote me and asked me if I would like to come back and be his resident in medicine at the Toronto General Hospital. I was very anxious to do this and I think Dr. Graham exerted a bit of influence to get me out early in 1945, shortly after the war was over in Europe. I hadn't seen my wife for nearly four years and I cannot say whether this was an important factor in wanting to get home quick but certainly it all seemed very reasonable.

After a very fine year under Dr. Graham, he wanted somebody who would be able to know something about peripheral vascular disease and my training seemed to be along those lines, so I was sent to the Harvard Medical School under Dr. Eugene Landis whom Dr. Graham had known during the war. When I arrived there, there wasn't any work going on in peripheral vascular disease but Gene was interested in pathological physiology of cardiac failure and I was set to work on a problem having to do with the skin circulation in cardiac failure. While in Boston it was apparent that newer techniques of cardiac catheterization were teaching people an awful lot about heart disease and I spent a fair amount of time at the clinics of Sam Levine in addition to doing my own job in physiology. At rounds at the Brigham I saw a good deal of what could be accomplished by cardiac catheterization and special techniques in the diagnosis of heart disease. To me this seemed to be just applied physiology and consequently it seemed to be my meat.

On arriving back in Toronto I was given the responsibility of looking after patients on the ward and went to work trying to get the techniques of cardiac catheterization going and this kept me pretty busy. The techniques of doing blood oxygens by the Van Slyke method were not being done any place in Toronto and these damn machines drove me to distraction for some three or four years. There was no room in the X-ray department of the Toronto General Hospital, which was terribly over-crowded at those times, to do any of this work and there was no radiologist to give us a hand with it. Fortunately, the Wellesley Hospital went broke about this time and there was an operating room with an X-ray machine which had been bought for the ear, nose and throat people to locate foreign bodies in the trachea or bronchi. We took this over and did our cardiac catheterizations in the Wellesley Hospital until 1956 when a patient gave us some $36,000 to build a new cardiovascular unit. In the period from 1947 to 1956 we were very pushed for time, because no particular exemptions from teaching or ward responsibilities were allowed to do this special investigation. Consequently, I used to arrive at the hospital at seven, pick up the patient, take him in my own car to the Wellesley Hospital, catheterize him, bring him back to the Toronto General Hospital, take the bloods over to the Banting Institute, do the blood oxygens on the Van Slyke machines or else wrestle with an inexperienced technician. This gradually got sorted out so that technical help was better and this was particularly due to the fact that we could pay them on a grant that I had from the Ontario Heart Foundation. During these early years, at times the money from the Ontario Heart Foundation wouldn't come through and in order to keep my technician, who I thought was a wonderful person, I would pay her salary myself, and I have had her as much in debt to me as $1,000, at a time when I could ill-afford it. It was quite apparent that around Toronto the only source of money for anybody interested in heart disease was either the Heart Foundation which was then in its infancy, or through practice. Consequently about 1950, I started practising pretty hard and it was only this that enabled me to keep going. The university was never able to provide me with a living wage, and by the time 1956 came and the cardiovascular unit was opened and there was a chance for one person to have a full-time appointment with a reasonable salary from the Ontario Heart Foundation, it seemed apparent that my place in the scheme of things was to be a work-horse and do the clinical work which was necessary to keep the clinical material coming to the unit, in an increasing volume.

Since 1956, when Ramsay Gunton was given a full-time appointment, paid by the Ontario Heart Foundation, the cardiovascular unit has, I think, done a pretty fair job, and at the present time I think we can say that it is very unusual for our surgeons to be presented with a case of valvular disease or other types of acquired or congenital heart disease in which the diagnosis is not substantially correct. This, of course, just reflects the advances in the knowledge of heart disease that have occurred since 1947. It has been a wonderful time to live. We are all very proud of the people who have passed through the unit and gone on to make their contributions here and in other centres.

I think the year I bought my electrocardiograph was about 1950. . . . I think the association with other people from other centres in the Canadian Cardiovascular Society has been useful and a very happy association. I think the Canadian Cardiovascular Society meetings have provided a chance to present work that has been done, although the amount of time that has been left to look over what you have actually done due to the large volume of teaching and patients to be looked after and routine investigations that seem to pile up, has really been inadequate. We have often found ourselves here knowing that we had something that should be worked up and published, because it was of general interest and not yet known, and been unable to get around to it. I suppose we are just lazy.

I am thinking of old John Oille. He was really one of my most greatly loved and admired teachers. He seemed to have the ability to distinguish between what he knew and what he didn't know. He never seemed to explain things in any but a fairly simple manner which I could understand, and it seemed to me that his clinical acumen, his kindness and his personal honesty made him a most outstanding person.

John Hepburn to the younger men was a little more terrifying than John Oille, if such a thing is possible. Both of them I think were remarkable men, first-class teachers, and of their era first-class clinicians. Many of the things they taught are no longer true. However, I think that one can say that with the evidence available at the time their conclusions were as sound as could be, and they never really stopped teaching themselves or teaching others.

In 1965 Dr. Greenwood was Associate Professor of Medicine at the University of Toronto and Senior Physician at the Toronto General Hospital.

Dr. Greenwood represents the generation of physicians who became aware of the need for emphasizing the application of physiological principles and methods to clinical medicine. Their teachers had been schooled in morphology, pathological anatomy as the basis for understanding disease. Reading his letter provides a substantial impression of the struggle involved in the process of introducing physiological thinking and methods in clinical practice immediately after World War II.

Between 1939 and 1963, Dr. Greenwood's bibliography grew to 18 items. The first, entitled "Production of Hypertension by Prevention of Kidney Hypertrophy," was co-authored with R. Nassim and N.B. Taylor (*C.M.A.J.*, 1939: 41, 443). This item and the next five reflect that period of his career in which he worked in physiology first in Toronto, then at Harvard. The seventh item marks the beginning of his work in establishing the medical-surgical team at the Toronto General Hospital and the University — "Hypothermia, Its Possible Role in Cardiac Surgery: Investigation of Factors Governing Survival of Dogs at Low Body Temperature," co-authored with W. G. Bigelow and W. K. Lindsay (*Ann. Surg.*, 1950: 132, 849). One of his early papers, co-authored with J. K. Wilson, is "The Natural History of Mitral Stenosis" (*C.M.A.J.*, 1954: 71, 323), and in the same year there appeared "Mitral Stenosis With and Without Surgery," co-authored with W. G. Bigelow (*Surgical Clinics of North America*, 1954: 34, 875). These two very useful articles appeared early in the era of mitral commissureotomy. Acute interest in the subject was maintained; the eighteenth item is "The Effect of Mitral Commissureotomy on Duration of Life, Functional Capacity, Haemoptysis and Systemic Embolism," co-authored with H. L. Aldridge and A. D. McKelvey (*Am. J. Cardiol.*, 1963; 348). Beginning in 1954 all the articles stem from Dr. Greenwood's application of a dynamic physiological point of view to clinical problems.

Nova Scotia

Dr. Douglas Leonard Roy, 18 June 1923, North Sydney, N.S.; Mount Allison University, B.A. 43; Dalhousie, M.D. 48; F.R.C.P.(C) 52; F.A.H.A.

Immediately after graduation Dr. Roy began postgraduate training with internship and residency in internal medicine at the Royal Victoria Hospital in Montreal (1948-1950). In 1950-1951 he engaged in a special study of hypertension, and studied paediatric cardiology at the Montreal Children's Hospital with Dr. Arnold Johnson. During the year 1951-1952, he began his career in Halifax at the Victoria General Hospital with a study of the heart in thyroid disease supported by a grant from the National Research Council.

In 1971 when he updated his curriculum vitae he was Associate Professor of Paediatrics (Cardiology) at Dalhousie University, Head of the Division of Cardiology of the Isaac Walton Killam Hospital for Sick Children, Consultant in Paediatric Cardiology at the Victoria General Hospital, the Halifax Infirmary and the Grace Maternity Hospitals.

It is noteworthy that Dr. Roy obtained all his training in adult and paediatric cardiology in Canada, working with teachers who obtained their training in Europe and the United States. This is a good indication of the maturing of cardiology in Canada. Dr. Roy introduced catheterization in Halifax and served all the Maritime provinces. He did not submit his bibliography.

Quebec

Dr. Sydney Segall, 21 February 1917, Montreal; McGill University, B.A. 38; M.D., C.M. 42; F.A.C.P.; F.R.C.P.(C); F.A.C.C.; F.A.H.A.

In a letter which accompanied his curriculum vitae in 1968, Dr. Sydney Segall relates how he had the opportunity to learn the skills of cardiac catheterization in 1948 and was prepared to exercise them on his return to Montreal in 1950.

> After the war when I was retired from the army, I spent two years at the Queen Mary Veterans Hospital as senior intern and assistant resident in medicine. While working under Dr. Phil Hill I became interested in cardiology and I applied for a fellowship under Hebbel Hoff, who at this time was at McGill University and as you know was particularly interested in cardiovascular physiology. However, the particular year that I applied for, Dr. Hoff decided to leave McGill and accepted a position at Baylor University in Texas. However, Dr. J. S. L. Brown offered me, instead, a Caverhill Fellowship and a position with Dr. Louis Katz in Chicago where Dr. Louis Horlick was just finishing his fellowship and was about to return to Montreal. I was very gratified when Dr. Katz accepted me, being fully aware of his stature both as a physiologist and electrocardiographer.
>
> While at Michael Reese, I became one of the original members of the cardiac catheterization team when the unit was formed that particular year. In fact, my thesis for the diploma in internal medicine at McGill was on cardiac catheterization. Two papers of which I was co-author also stem from this work and appeared in *Circulation*.

The following year, with Dr. Katz's help, I was appointed chief resident in Medicine at City Hospital in Cleveland under Dr. Roy Scott.

After my year in Cleveland, I decided to return to practise in Montreal, primarily because of family ties in this city of my birth, and also as a Canadian, to practise in Canada, particularly after the help I had received from McGill University in obtaining my training.

Dr. Sydney Segall joined the medical staff of the Department of Medicine at the Jewish General Hospital. He was welcomed as a member of the Cardiac Clinic, but was frustrated by the absence of facilities for catheterization, as were the other members of the clinic. The institution lacked the space in which to establish a catheterization laboratory. Attempts to do the work in the crowded X-ray Department were unsatisfactory. About half a decade later when space and instruments were provided, Dr.Segall worked in the haemodynamic laboratory with colleagues whom he trained (Dr. Lyon Korenberg) all on a part-time voluntary basis. Eventually, a full-time worker was appointed, Dr. Rico Espinel.

When Dr. Segall updated his curriculum vitae in 1971,he was Assistant Professor of Medicine at McGill, Senior Physician at the Jewish General Hospital, Consultant Cardiologist at the Jewish Convalescent Hospital and the Mount Sinai Sanitarium.

Dr. Segall's bibliography begins in 1950 with two items related to the pioneer work in haemodynamics he did with colleagues under Dr. Louis Katz, "A Case of Marked Dilatation of the Pulmonary Arterial Tree Associated with Mitral Stenosis" (S. Segall, I.I. Ritter, and W. Hwang, *Circulation,* 1950: 1, 777); "Haemodynamic Study of a Case of Anomalous Pulmonary Venous Drainage" (W. Hwang, O. Prec, K. Kuramoto, S. Segall, and L. N. Katz, *Circulation*, 1950: 2, 553). The subsequent four items represent work done in Montreal related to the biochemistry of coronary artery disease, report of case of left bundle branch block of long duration with remission, and other such clinical subjects.

A valuable unpublished item of Dr. Segall's bibliography is his thesis, a requirement of the Diploma Course in Internal Medicine at McGill. He wrote about his experience in learning and exploring the usefulness of cardiac catheterization during his sojourn of a year (1948-1949) with Dr. Louis N. Katz at the Michael Reese Hospital in Chicago. The title of the 60-page essay is "Some Aspects of Intracardiac Catheterization in Diagnosis and Research." The bibliography lists 115 references. A brief review of the history of cardiac catheterization is followed by a meticulously detailed description of the technique, and a critical discussion of sources of error, in measuring pressures with the instruments then available. The major portion of the essay concerns results of studies on cases of congenital heart disease and extensive discussion of the haemodynamics. An interesting discussion of a rare combination concerns a case in which a ligated ductus arteriosus had recannalized. The patient had fared poorly immediately after ligation and improved with recannalization. The electrocardiograms before and after ligation of the ductus strongly suggested an aberrant coronary artery from the pulmonary artery. This made for a better supply of oxygen to the myocardium with ductus patent than when ligated.

Dr. Stewart E. A. Reid, 1917 Montreal; McGill, B.A. 38; M.D., C.M. 42; F.R.C.P.(C); F.A.C.P.; F.A.C.C.; F.A.C.C.P.; F.A.H.A.; C.P.S.Q. Cardiol. and Int. Med. 53.

Dr. Stewart Reid has an important place in the story of Montreal cardiology. He fully modernized the cardiac clinic at the Montreal General Hospital after World War II. His comments on the special questions tell the story succinctly.

> I was influenced in going into cardiology when I was an intern at the Montreal General Hospital and also, during the war, I came in close contact with Dr. C. C. Birchard, Dr. H. N. Segall and Dr. J. Palmer. They stimulated and interested me and I followed through in their footsteps.
>
> On returning from the war it was very difficult to obtain a postgraduate job. I was able to get an assistant residency in Medicine at the Montreal General Hospital in 1946 but planning further training in cardiology was very difficult. Finally, however, I went down to the Massachusetts General Hospital. I met Dr. Bland and applied to him for a job. It was amusing that he quizzed me about my war service and found that he had been stationed in the next hospital to the one to which I was attached in Italy. He knew John Palmer and the rest of the staff. He was good enough to give me a job for a year as one of their Fellows. From there I went to Hammersmith in London, England. Dr. Edward S. Mills, then Chairman of the Department of Medicine at the Montreal General Hospital suggested that I acquire the technique of cardiac catheterization so I spent a very happy time under Dr. (now Sir) John McMichael at Hammersmith. I was

closely associated with Dr. Garfield Kelly of Kingston and Dr. Richard Bayliss, now of Westminster Hospital, London. Following this I returned to the Montreal General Hospital where I set up the cardiac catheterization and the elements of a respiratory laboratory. I went into practice in cardiology in 1952 and bought my first ECG at this time.

In 1971 when Dr. Reid updated his curriculum vitae he was Associate Professor of Medicine at McGill, Director of the Division of Cardiology and Senior Physician at the Montreal General Hospital and Consultant Cardiologist of the Department of Veteran Affairs, the Huntington County, the Ormstown Memorial, the Brome Missisquoi Perkins and the Catherine Booth Hospitals.

Dr. Reid's bibliography begins with an article co-authored with colleagues at the Massachusetts General Hospital published in 1949. There follow thirteen items, all but one on subjects related to the cardiovascular system, all co-authored with colleagues of Boston, London, and Montreal. The first one which dealt with open heart surgery is also to be found in the bibliographies of Drs. A. R. C. Dobell, H. J. Scott, and R. F. P. Cronin — "Surgical Closure of Interventricular Septal Perforation Complicating Myocardial Infarction" *(J. Thor. & Cardiovasc. Surg.*, 1962: 43, 802). At the annual meeting of the Canadian Cardiovascular Society in 1962 he delivered a paper on "A Clinical Survey of 20 Patients Submitted to Aortic Valvuloplasty."

Dr. Osman P. Gialloreto, Padua, Italy, M.D. 46; F.A.C.C., C.C.P.S.Q. Cardiol.

A very good document about the introduction of cardiac catheterization in a hospital related to the University of Montreal has been contributed by Dr. Osman P. Gialloreto. The information was requested in November 1982, received on January 31, 1983, and is quoted in full, as translated by Dr. Osman P. Gialloreto.

Padova, July 29, 1946:
As for all experimental theses, the discussion of my doctoral thesis had been long and exhausting. Now I was leaning on the ramp of the elegant medieval portico gazing down on the interior court where Vesalius, Galileo, Acquapendente, Morgagni and many others had roamed in their academic gowns.

In the stillness of the warm July evening, in this "decor" still alive with conquests of the human intellect, I felt the dimension of what I had just accomplished.

The *magna cum laude* doctorate included the wreath of laurel decorated with tiny golden spheres — looking on this wreath poised next to my thesis I felt the still fresh scent of the laurel leaves and I realized that it was already part of the past. Slowly I became aware of a strange feeling of anxiety: what had been done seemed suddenly insignificant in the fact of what the future held in reserve in a country still echoing from the cries of a cruel war.

The university hospital was bare except for its beds and the school of specialization was receiving only the echo of the scientific advance of the New World. I could not wait!

A Rockefeller Foundation scholarship gave me the opportunity to visit countries untouched by war while at the same time revealing to me the plethora of research facilities by studying the histo-trophic cycle of malaria in South America and the Chagas myocarditis. Under the microscope the myocardium was fascinating: its functional capacity for survival astonishing despite the diffuse fibrotic invasion.

There existed a cult in South America for the Cardiology Institute of Mexico and I decided to visit it before my return to Europe. That stay proved to be decisive. Professor Ignacio Chavez impressed me with the concept of cardiology as a separate specialty. He also communicated to me his respect for the European clinical cardiology and his personal experience with Charles Laubry in Paris. Sodi Pallares and Enrique Cabrera, full of talent and enthusiasm easily transmitted, toyed with electrocardiography as a diagnostic method which seemed to provide all the answers, whereas Cordero showed me the anatomohistological ravages in acute rheumatic carditis. When leaving that country of proud and gracious people, my decision was taken: cardiology was "it." The situation in Padova had not changed and the tip of the wooden stethoscope could still be seen peeping out of my colleagues' white smocks.

Thanks to my anatomo-pathological training and to the rare interest of one of my professors, I was welcomed in the department of Professor Mahaim in Lausanne. It was incredible to find a country so calm and orderly with no sign of the recent war, only a few hours away from Padova! I greatly appreciated the clinical experience of Professor Mahaim. I had access to one of the most complete and documented files of cardiac tumours and I became aware that the 6000 microscopic slides for the study of the Bundle of His were a demanding reality.

When Professor Mahaim informed me that I was now ready for clinical training and that his friend Professor Jean Lenègre had just taken over the direction of the most complete service of cardiology in Europe at Boucicault Hospital in Paris, the next step of my training was decided.

One week later, Professor Lenègre, after reading the introductory letter of Professor Mahaim, promised to forget my histo-pathological ability although he was himself very much involved in the study of the cardiac conduction pathways. I was to follow the clinical activities of the service and work every morning in the new laboratory of cardiac catheterization.

The two years that followed were the most important and determining ones in my professional life.

André Cournand, who was to receive a few years later the Nobel Prize for his work on cardiac catheterization, had spent some time in Professor Lenègre's service and the enthusiasm he left behind was considerable. My first impression of the catheterization lab contained some kind of urological flavour between the sterilization techniques of the catheters and their bare-hand manipulation in the right heart. But the discussion of the new pressure curves and the spasmodic oscillation of the water column of the manometer were intriguing and fascinating. I was now exploring that myocardium whose morphology was so familiar to me and every day of work brought new experiences while the experimental physiological hypotheses were being confirmed in living man.

Wilson electrocardiography had been introduced in Paris by Enrique Cabrera just before my arrival and his well-known teaching talent was very much present and contagious in the service. The first case of coarctation of the aorta had been sent to Stockholm for surgical correction whereas I was busy learning electrocardiography monitoring in the tense atmosphere of Professor D'Allaine's operating room, treating mitral stenosis with azygos shunt.

The first World Congress of Cardiology was approaching and everybody was working hard to submit papers at such an historic event. I was also completing my thesis for the title of "Assistant Etranger à la Faculté de Médecin de Paris." In September 1950, I had the honour to present, with Professor Lenègre, two papers to the first World Congress of Cardiology on the electrocardiography of ventricular hypertrophy with bundle branch block. The same year I received the diploma of Foreign Assistant at the Faculty of Medicine of Paris.

The World Congress had raised a growing interest in cardiology judging from the number of visitors in the service. Meeting confrères from Canada, I came to know the country not only as a geographical entity.

A short visit to the universities of Padova, Bologna and Rome convinced me of the impossibility of continuing my work in these centres. The reorganization of services had started but could not outpace the slow economic recovery of the country. I was ready and eager to start so I remembered the invitation of my Canadian confrères and decided to visit this vast country.

1951: Montreal — Hôpital Notre-Dame — Rheaume Bursary of the Université de Montréal.

After visiting Quebec City and the Gaspesian Peninsula, I came to Montreal knowing that cardiac surgery had started at Notre-Dame Hospital with mitral commissureotomy and hoping that my experience in electrocardiography monitoring during surgery could be of some use.

I met Dr. A. de Guise, Chief of Cardiology, Dr. P. David of the same service and Dr. E. D. Gagnon, Chief of Cardiac Surgery and responsible for the first mitral commissureotomy in Canada. Through their interest I received the Rheaume Foundation bursary of the University of Montreal. My Canadian career began with the study of problems related to cardiac surgery.

Notre Dame Hospital was not yet equipped for cardiac catheterization, but we were able to start angiocardiography. Dr. P. Brodeur and Dr. J. L. Leger of the Radiology Department had conceived and created, with the cooperation of the Picker Company, a special device capable of taking six chest films in eight seconds, manually driven and in "visual" synchronization with the pressurized injection of the contrast material according to the Robb and Steinberg technique. A kind of selective angiocardiography was also done at this time with contrast material injected through a needle directly into the arch of the aorta!

In April 1953, our experience with angiocardiography illustrated by the study of five cases of congenital cardiopathies was published in the *Union Médicale du Canada.* At this time it became evident to me that cardiac catheterization and angiocardiography had to be used in an integrated way and that the equipment had to be concentrated in the same physical environment despite the division of two different departments, radiology and cardiology.

When I accepted Dr. P. David's invitation to join the team of the newly formed Montreal Heart Institute in 1953, I travelled to Stockholm where the new selective angiocardiography was making its debut. At the Karolinska Hospital with Professor Manneheimer, I used the revolutionary equipment of Elema and Schonander for the sequential orthodiagonal angiocardiography with an integrated electrocardiographic signal.

In the service of Professor Gustav Nylin, I familiarized myself with the technique of gas analysis, which upon my return proved to be quite handy for the training of our local technicians, and I used for the first time radio-isotopes for the determination of cardiac output.

When the Montreal Heart Institute opened its doors in January 1954, the concept of integrated facilities for heart catheterization and selective angiocardiography was a reality and we had the first bi-plane Schonander angiocardiograph functioning in North America.

In November 1959, the *Union Médicale du Canada* published our paper on the results of 840 haemodynamic investigations done in 789 patients with a mortality of 0.2%. This was our substantial beginning with the cardiac catheterization techniques.

Dr. Lucien Campeau, 20 June, 1927, Sudbury, Ontario; Laval, B.A. 48; M.D. 53; F.R.C.P.(C) 57; C.S.P.Q. 60; F.A.C.C.; F.A.H.A.

In June 1965, Dr. Campeau, one of the first to respond to the questionnaire, wrote a letter that defies summarizing, as it reflects so many facets of the education of a clinical cardiologist in his formative years in the early 1950s.

> I must say that I was oriented towards internal medicine since the beginning of my entrance to university. The first year of medicine was quite distressing for me. In fact, I considered changing from medicine to science, or engineering. I had the impression that it was mainly a cramming of the facts stuffed into memory; the study of anatomy had been disappointing. In the second year, however, I became more enthusiastic about the study of physiology and was especially interested in the study of the cardiovascular system. In 1950, we were fortunate in having Dr. Jean Lenègre [of Paris] as visiting professor at Laval University in Quebec. During the three months that he spent there, he gave two lectures a week on electrocardiography. Even though second year students were not always required to attend these lectures, I attended every one. I had acquired the Fateau-Rousseau volume

which I studied with great interest and attention. I maintained this interest during my training at the hospital. During the three clinical years, I sought every opportunity to attend demonstrations of the interpretation of electrocardiograms by either Dr. Drouin at St. Sacrement Hospital, or Dr. Jean Fortier, while I was training at the St. François d'Assise Hospital. At that time, electrocardiography was not part of the [clinical] curriculum; we had only heard about it during the course in electro-radiology. Neither interns nor even residents in medicine were expected to be able to read electrocardiograms. Only real specialists could do this and I remember at this time there were only four physicians in university hospitals who were qualified for reading electrocardiograms. In fact, Dr. Jean Beaudoin, at this time a resident at the Hôtel-Dieu in Quebec, created some excitement because of his knowledge of electrocardiography. I remember, too, that while I was a student in fourth year in the Department of Electrocardiography at the St. Sacrement Hospital, I was urgently called to interpret the electrocardiogram of a patient scheduled for surgery. Dr. Drouin was not present at the hospital. I mention these anecdotes to underline the fact that from the beginning of my medical studies, I had developed a special interest in electrocardiology. There was another student in my class interested in this subject and so we two had much pleasure discussing electrocardiography. It was Dr. Jacques Boulé, now a haemologist. Obviously, at present, it is quite common for an intern to have an elementary knowledge of electrocardiography and to be able to recognize an abnormal 'electro' or to diagnose a myocardial infarct. It is quite evident how much Dr. Jean Lenègre influenced me on this path.

Consequently, from the second year in medicine I was already more interested in diagnostic than in therapeutic medicine. Surgery did not interest me at all. When I decided to continue postgraduate studies rather than go into general practice, I was determined without hesitation to follow studies for internal medicine. At this time, I planned to establish myself at home in Sudbury in the practice of internal medicine. Several of my friends had chosen surgery and we planned to form a group. The tendency, at this period, was to go into general practice and I believe that about 60-75% of my colleagues followed this choice, though eventually some of them did become specialists. Because I did not consider myself sufficiently competent and still loved to study, I felt I could not yet go into practice.

It was very difficult to make this decision, since I had been financially on my own since the age of sixteen. I had managed to earn enough money to pay for my classical and university education by working in the summer for the International Nickel Co., and during the school term, as a school guard patrolling an intersection for a school adjoining the college, four times a day during the school year. I had also decided to get married. Because of limited funds, my choice of locale for postgraduate studies in internal medicine was limited. It was, of course, necessary that the remuneration be sufficient so that we could live on our income without having to borrow money for the next four to five years. I was not able to get a scholarship. There was no question of remaining in Canada, so I turned towards the U.S.A. I was fortunate in getting a post at the Harper Hospital in Detroit which paid me between $225 and $275 a month, which was a liberal sum for that period. We did not plan to have children, but we had one each year and so, of course, I had to find a way to increase my income. In addition to my regular work at Harper, I took night duties in a small private hospital facing the Harper Hospital. In spite of this, these years in Detroit were amongst the best years in my life. Though Harper was not a university hospital, it was affiliated with Wayne University and the postgraduate teaching was relatively well organized.

In the second year at Harper, I was drawn nearer to cardiology. Dr. Dodrill, a pioneer in heart surgery, with the help of engineers from General Motors, constructed an artificial heart giving a pulsatile flow. We performed about one catheterization a week and for two years, I assisted Dr. Robert Gerisch in these studies. It was a supplementary study and I was the only one among fifteen residents and assistants interested in this project. The catheterizations were performed in an X-ray room. On the day of a catheterization I, myself, carried the necessary electronic equipment to the experimental surgical room of Dr. Dodrill, in the Department of Radiology. In other words, I did the work of a technician, calibrated the manometers, and recorded pressure curves.

I was allowed to carry out a dozen right heart catheterizations during these two years. Because of this, I was able to observe all the interesting cases in cardiology. There is no doubt that cardiology was of greater interest to me than any other branch of internal medicine during those three years of training. I was especially impressed and motivated by Doctors Gordon Meyer and Jack Kaufman and Robert Gerisch. Dr. Gordon Meyer gave a series of lectures on electrocardiography each year.

During my third year at Harper, I spent four months in the research laboratory of Dr. Harper Hellams at Wayne State University. This was my introduction to research in physiology. There wasn't much research activity at Harper Hospital though there was a research unit, but it was mainly concerned with the study of the thyroid gland. Neither at the University nor during my successive hospital internships in Quebec did I hear any discussions on research projects except when there were visiting professors, or by Dr. Dugal who, I seem to remember, was the only full-time physician carrying on research in the Faculty of Medicine.

In the summer of 1955, at the suggestion of Dr. Maurice Dufresne, who was then a resident in radiology at Harper Hospital, I visited the Institute of Cardiology in Montreal. I met Dr. Paul David and was very much impressed by the organization in our French Canadian milieu at that time. At this point I decided to spend one or two more years, specializing in cardiology.

I was fortunate in being accepted at Johns Hopkins University as a teaching fellow attached to the Department of Cardiology. This year was spent mainly in teaching cardiac catheterization and electrocardiography as well as service in adult and paediatric clinics. I was supposed to remain another year in pure research with Dr. William Milnor, but I decided to return to Canada, having been offered a post as a junior associate at the Institute of Cardiology by Dr. Paul David. Since we already had three children at this time, it was becoming more and more difficult to balance our budget. Even if I had obtained a bursary from the American Heart Association or had agreed to replace a general practitioner every two weeks at Churville, it would not have been comfortable for my family. I admit that I did not realize the importance of training in pure research, since I had not come into contact with it until late in my training period. Looking back, I am convinced that I should have stayed at least another year at Johns Hopkins Hospital. It is my only regret as far as my postgraduate studies are concerned.

When I returned to Canada, after this stage, I received the certificate as Associate in Internal Medicine from the Royal College of Physicians and Surgeons. It was only after a year of practice at the Institute that I definitely decided to remain in this specialty. Probably if I had not been attached to the Institute of

Cardiology, but instead to a general hospital, I might have chosen to practise internal medicine. I had, however, acquired a special interest in cardiology during those years. My decision to remain in Montreal was the result of the desire to practise cardiology at the Institute. In the first four years at the Institute, I worked mostly in the clinic. Following this, for two years, most of my time was spent in the catheterization room and since then half time in the clinic and the other half in haemodynamics. I would have remained full time in haemodynamics, but in order to be closer to the public for financial reasons, I worked in the clinic too. Perhaps if I had spent more time in research, I might have remained in haemodynamics.

Concerning my avocations, they are rather limited. I must declare that I am father of four sons and I have to attend to them. I have had to discontinue golf because of this duty. However, I ski a good deal with my boys and my wife. In the summer I swim and we have camping holidays. During the past five years I have been active in gardening; I planted about twenty shrubs and trees. We have bought an old house in Lachine and I have had much fun and pleasure in restoring it. Needless to say I have done most of the work myself. So much for my sport activities.

When Dr. Campeau updated his curriculum vitae in 1972, he was Assistant Professor of Medicine at the Université de Montréal, Chief of the Department of Medicine and the Haemodynamic Service at the Montreal Institute of Cardiology. Between 1957 and 1972, his bibliography grew to 19 items. The first is on "Pregnancy in a Case of Tetralogy of Fallot," co-authored with Jack Kaufman, Paul Ruble, and Joseph Monsham, colleagues at the Harper Hospital (*Arch. Int. Med.*, March 1957). The first paper on work done at the Montreal Institute of Cardiology is "Maladie Ebstein" (*Un. Méd. Can.*, 1960: 89, 161). The last 17 are co-authored and reflect the excellent work in medical and surgical cardiology practised at the Montreal Institute of Cardiology.

Dr. Ghislaine Gilbert, 14 November 1924, Montreal; Collège Marie-Anne, B.A. 43; Université de Montréal, M.D. 49; C.S.P.Q. Int. Med. and Cardiol. 55; F.A.C.C.

Before the Montreal Institute of Cardiology was a gleam in anyone's eye, Miss Ghislaine Gilbert, a senior medical student at the Université de Montréal in 1949 chose to become a paediatric cardiologist with a special interest in congenital heart disease. It seemed appropriate that she should eventually settle in Montreal, which since 1907 has been known as a centre of knowledge in this field because of the late Dr. Maude E. Abbott's fame. Dr. Gilbert's career began about a decade after Dr. Abbott's death in 1940. Dr. Gilbert is one of those who made a serious effort in responding to the special questions; her comments, written in 1965, are quoted:

> Graduating in medicine in 1949, I decided to specialize in cardiology, more specifically in congenital heart disease. I was advised to acquire a solid foundation in general cardiology before specializing in congenital heart disease. To achieve this goal required a satisfactory plan for postgraduate study. In the organization of this program, I was advised and helped by Drs. Rodrigue Lefebvre, Hans Selye and Paul David. I spent two years in the Department of Cardiology at the Hôtel-Dieu under Dr. Rodrigue Lefebvre, where I learned auscultation, electrocardiography, and radiology. Then, recommended by Dr. Paul David, I was accepted for the postgraduate course in cardiology at the Massachusetts General Hospital given by Dr. Paul D. White. Because of my special interest in congenital heart disease, I was able to pursue my training jointly at the Children's Medical Center of Boston. For my research project, I chose phonocardiography with Drs. Sprague and Ongley. Recommended by Dr. Friedlich, who was in charge of the congenital heart disease department in Dr. Paul White's service, I was accepted for further study at Johns Hopkins Hospital under Dr. Helen Taussig. Finally I spent some time training with Dr. Pierre Soulié in Paris and Dr. Paul Wood in London.
>
> In 1954, a few months after the Institute of Cardiology was opened, I organized its paediatric service and in 1955 I took charge of it. The following year, because of the shortage of beds at the Institute, we took care of the subacute cases at the Marie Enfant Hospital. This helped to develop the Department of Paediatric Cardiology at the Institute. At present we have twenty beds for critical cases in the Department of Paediatric Cardiology and forty beds for less critical cases at the Marie Enfant Hospital. In the outdoor clinic we see twelve to fifteen new cases and about twenty old ones every week. Most of these young cardiacs have congenital cardiovascular malformations. In the clinic for rheumatic fever patients which we established at the Institute since its opening eleven years ago, we have followed three hundred young patients suffering from rheumatic heart

disease. Among the 3,370 children whom I examined at the Institute in the past ten years, 2,200 had heart disease. The incidence of cardiopathies in this group is as follows: Congenital malformations: 71%; Rheumatic: 22%; Other types of heart disease: 7%.

I have just completed a three-year research project for the study of the pathogenesis and prevention of rheumatic fever. My current project is concerned with the follow-up of surgically operated cases of interventricular septal defects.

The clinical study of congenital heart disease is of particular interest to me, it affords me the opportunity to make correlations with auscultation, electrocardiography, radiology, haemodynamics, and post-mortem examinations. The progress of the patients operated on is followed regularly and helps us to revise our surgical knowledge and methods continually. We also keep abreast of all publications in this field.

When Dr. Gilbert updated her curriculum vitae she was Assistant Professor at Université de Montréal. Between 1950 and 1971, Dr. Gilbert's bibliography grew to 50 items. True to her primary purpose, the study of both congenital and rheumatic heart disease, the first item is "Un Cas de Maladie de Lutembacher," co-authored with Leon Lebel (*Un. Méd. Can.*, 1950: 78, 902-907). At the beginning of her career at the Institute of Cardiology, she co-authored a general review article, with Claude Leonard and Paul David, titled "Maladies Congenitales Cardiovasculaires," (*Un. Méd. Can.*, 1954: 83, 1370-1377). Of the remaining 48 items, all but two are with co-authors. Nine of the 50 items are in English. All concern paediatric cardiology. By 1967, she could write about 440 cases of rheumatic fever in which prophylaxis had been practised. In 1957, she co-authored, with Edouard Gagnon and Leo Laflêche, an article on "Evaluation of Direct Surgical Relief of Pulmonary Obstruction in Fallot's Malformation," (*C.M.A.J.*, 1957: 77, 559-564).

Dr. Jean de L. Mignault, 3 February, 1924, Sherbrooke, Quebec; Université de Montréal, B.A. 45; M.D. 51; Cert. in Cardiol.; C.P.S.Q. 57; F.A.C.C.; F.A.C.C.P.; F.A.H.A.; F.A.C.P.

Dr. Jean de L. Mignault chose to become a cardiologist in a simple, logical, and unusual manner. Following is the story as he tells it:

I must admit I chose a career in cardiology by the back door. At the time that I decided to study internal medicine I intended to pay special attention to arterial hypertension. The courses I took at medical school left me with the impression that the problem was quite simple. The little experience which I acquired as an intern caused me to understand that the problem was more complex. Knowing the reputation of Dr. Irvine H. Page as an authority on hypertension, I sought further study in this field under him. During my stay with him I worked on the pharmacology of Serotonin in man. As my results were not in accordance with what he had found in animals, we arrived at a point at which we found it necessary to study the effects of infusion of Serotonin in man by determining the cardiac output and systemic resistance before and after infusion of Serotonin. Thus I was introduced to Dr. F. Mason Sones who was in charge of the cardiovascular laboratory. The earliest experience was somewhat arid because of my total ignorance of haemodynamics. I very soon appreciated that I had to have precise knowledge in this sphere if I wished to continue my studies of hypertension. I therefore spent a year in the service of Dr. Sones whose activist spirit and enthusiasm is well known. It is from him that I contracted the fever of cardiology and he gave a new orientation to my career, for which I shall always be truly grateful.

Dr. Mignault introduced cardiac catheterization and the study of haemodynamics in three hospitals. During the years 1957-1961 he was associated with Dr. Gialloreto at the Montreal Institute of Cardiology. From 1961-1968 he worked at the Hôtel-Dieu of Montreal and after initiating the haemodynamics laboratory he was Director of the Department of Cardiology from 1964-1968. His next appointment was that of Director of the Department of Medicine at the new medical school of the University of Sherbrooke. In 1971 when he updated his curriculum vitae he was Professor of Medicine and Dean of the Faculty of Medicine at the University of Sherbrooke. He exercised an important role in creating the Department of Cardiology at Sherbrooke which included a modern haemodynamic laboratory.

Between 1953 and 1969, his bibliography grew to twelve items. The fourth item is co-authored with Paul David, "Communication Inter-auriculaire chez l'Adulte" (*Rev. Lyon. Méd.*, 1950: 8, 803-805). Item 9 is "Cine-Angiographic Study in Intravenously Administered Isoptin" (*C.M.A.J.*, 1966: 95, 1252-1253). The 19th, co-authored with J. W. Ketelers, A. K. Amir-Jahed, and R. A. Nadeau, is "Modifications du Rhythme et de la Conduction au Cours de la Coronarographie Selective" (*Arch. des Maladies du Coeur,* 1967: 60, 792-805).

Dr. Yves Morin, 28 November 1929, Quebec City; Laval, B.A. (*magna cum laude*) 48; M.D. (*magna cum laude*) 53; F.R.C.P.(C); C.P.S.Q. Med. 58; C.P.S.Q. Cardio. 58; F.A.C.C.; F.A.H.A.

Dr. Yves Morin's postgraduate studies began with internship at the Hôtel-Dieu of Quebec during the year 1953-1954. He received a Rotary International Foundation Fellowship for the year 1954-1955 and devoted this year to study at the National Institute of Cardiology in London, England. During the following year he served as resident in Medicine at Sunnybrook Hospital, Toronto. During the year 1956-1957, he was senior resident in Medicine at the Toronto General Hospital and the following year, he returned to Quebec and served as medical resident at the Hôtel-Dieu. He was appointed as the first full-time cardiologist of this hospital and of the Medical Faculty of Laval University. He introduced the new points of view as well as the new techniques, including cardiac catheterization.

In the comments he made about the special questions he pays tribute to the teachers who stimulated and guided him during his undergraduate and graduate studies. Dr. Jean-Baptiste Jobin and Dr. Richard Lessard influenced him greatly before and after graduation at Laval University. Dr. Paul Wood of London, Dr. Jean Lenègre of Paris, Dr. Ray F. Farquharson, and Dr. Ramsey Gunton in Toronto contributed much to his postgraduate formation. Dr. Morin was well suited to the important task of creating the Medical Department of the Quebec Institute of Cardiology.

Between 1953 and 1972, Dr. Morin's bibliography grew to fifty articles, all on work done in Quebec. In 1959 he co-authored an article on "Physiological Studies in Beri-Beri Heart Disease by Injection of Radio-active Material," (Lessard, R., Bernier, J.P., and Morin, Y., *C.M.A.J.*, 1959: 80, 112). Quebec City was "visited" by an epidemic of myocardosis in 1966. Dr. Morin and his colleagues undertook the task of searching for the etiology and for appropriate methods of prevention and treatment. This work was fully described in a series of articles on "Beer Drinker's Cardiomyopathy," which appeared in 1966 and 1972. The work is summarized in a publication entitled "Alcohol, Coronary Haemodynamics and Cardiac Metabolism in Man" (*Am. Ht. J.*, 1972). By 1972, Dr. Morin and his colleagues had published 21 articles related to alcoholic cardiomyopathy. In 1962, Dr. Morin studied the "Application of Computer Technique to Reading Electrocardiograms" (*Laval Méd.*, 1962: 33, 702).

Dr. André Louis Davignon, 11 September 1930, Montreal; Université de Paris, Collège Stanislas, B.A. 48; Université de Montréal, P.C.B. 49, M.D. (*magna cum laude*) 54; F.R.C.P.(C) 58; C.S.P.Q. Cardiol. 62; F.A.A.P. 60; F.A.C.C. 71.

Dr. André Davignon's postgraduate education began with a year of research under Dr. Jacques Genest at the Hôtel-Dieu de Montréal, followed by residencies in paediatrics at St. Justine Hospital in Montreal and at the Boston City Hospital. He served as Fellow in Paediatric Cardiology at Johns Hopkins Hospital in 1958-1959 and at the Mayo Clinic, 1959-1960. Dr. Davignon pioneered paediatric cardiology in francophone Canada.

In 1972, when he filled in the questionnaire, he was Professeur Agrégé de Paediatrie, Plein Temps Geographique, Faculté de Medicine, Université de Montréal (1969-   ). At the St. Justine Hospital he was Chief of the Cardiopulmonary Laboratory.

Between 1955 and 1972, his bibliography grew to 43 items, all but one co-authored. The first eleven articles represent work done with Dr. Jacques Genest in the year 1955-1956. The last eleven are on work done between 1969 and 1972 on the medical and surgical management of Congenital Heart Disease. The one article he wrote without co-authors is "Le Rheumastisme Articulaire Aigu. Aspect Préventif et Therapeutique" (*Un. Méd. Can.*, 1966: 95).

Dr. Oswaldo Rico-Espinel, 11 September 1934, Sogamoso, Colombia; University of Saragosse, Espagne, M.D. (*magna cum laude*) 59; C.P.S.Q. Cardiol., F.A.C.C.

Dr. Rico Espinel brought his expertise in the study of respiration and of cardiodynamics from the Republic of Colombia and from Spain to Montreal, where he performed cardiac catheterization in three hospitals.

He was certified as a specialist in pulmonary physiology in France (1961), in Internal Medicine in Spain (1963), in Pneumology by Colombia (1964), and certified in Cardiology in Quebec (1968). At the time that he filled in the questionnaire in August 1972, he was Director of the Haemodynamics Laboratory at the Jewish General Hospital.

Dr. Rico's bibliography grew to 23 items between 1959 and 1967. The eighth item, co-authored with Y. Lessard, is "Coarctation Isthmique de l'Aorte; Etude et Commentaires à la Lumière de Huit Cas Personnels" (*Saguenay Méd.*, 1963: 10, 3). The 23rd, co-authored with L. Campeau, is "Modifications Hemodynamiques chez les Porteurs de Prothése Valvulaire Doubles, Aortique et Mitrale," a paper delivered at a meeting of the Montreal Cardiac Society on 24 April 1967.

Ontario

Dr. Ramsay Willis Gunton, 30 July 1922, Lexington, Kentucky; University of Western Ontario, M.D. 45; Rhodes Scholar 46; D.Phil. (Oxon) 49; F.R.C.P.(C) 52; F.A.C.P. 61; F.A.C.C.; F.A.H.A.

Dr. Gunton's postgraduate education began with internship at the Montreal General Hospital (1945-46). He returned to his alma mater in the Department of Medical Research in 1946, but soon after departed for Oxford as a Rhodes Scholar. His comments on the special questions summarize his activities and experience during these phases of his career.

> When I graduated from the University of Western Ontario Medical School I intended to specialize in surgery. My decision in favour of Internal Medicine was made during my year of junior internship in the Montreal General Hospital. I cannot define any single influence which directed me to Internal Medicine in place of surgery. It was, perhaps, the intellectual stimulation of medical cases and the fact that clinical research, which appealed to me, seemed at that time to be more applicable to medicine than to surgery. My primary interest in cardiology was probably formed in that year because when I went to Oxford in the following year, I looked around for some research project involving the cardiovascular system. In Montreal as a junior intern, I was on the service of Dr. Harold N. Segall and for some of the time, on the service of Dr. A. Shulman, whom I have not seen for a number of years but who seemed to have a dominant interest in cardiovascular problems. There I also knew C. C. Birchard, Montgomery, and McIver-Smith. Doug Cameron was then looking into the role of anti-coagulants in the treatment of coronary thrombosis.
>
> At Oxford my work was haemodynamic in nature and included studies on blood volume. When I returned to clinical medicine again at Victoria Hospital in London, I saw a great deal of Dr. George Manning who was, of course, interested in cardiology and, in particular, electrocardiography and I enjoyed my association with him. Bill Cameron was, at that time, back at Victoria Hospital as a staff physician. After completing senior

internship and residence at the Toronto General Hospital, I stayed on here as a Research Fellow and eventually as a staff member. I resumed my Oxford interest in blood volume determinations, doing a series of patients in heart failure. About that time haemodynamic investigations of patients considered for valvular heart surgery became a very important activity of medical cardiologists. I happened to be in Toronto, interested in this general field, at the time that this development occurred and so, rather naturally, I became involved in the development of the Cardiovascular Unit and investigative techniques in our hospital [Toronto General].

Dr. Wilfred Bigelow recalls that together with Dr. R. O. Heimbecker, Dr. Gunton pioneered left heart catherization in Canada in the course of their work in the cardiovascular unit of the Toronto General Hospital. Dr. Bigelow also noted that both their salaries and the maintenance of the unit were financed by the Ontario Heart Foundation.

When Dr. Gunton updated his curriculum vitae in 1971, he was the Richard Ivey Professor and Head of the Department of Medicine at the University of Western Ontario.

Dr. Gunton's bibliography between 1947 and 1965 grew to thirty-five items, in basic science, haemodynamics of the cardiovascular system, and pharmacology.

Dr. Howard Garfield Kelly, 16 August 1917, Kingston; Queen's University, M.D., C.M. 40; F.R.C.P.(C); F.A.C.P.; F.A.C.C.; F.A.H.A.

Dr. Kelly had a rotating internship at the Kingston General Hospital during his final undergraduate year (1939-1940). This period was followed by a year as senior in Medicine at the same hospital (1940-1941) and in 1941 he served a surgical internship at the Royal Victoria Hospital in Montreal. After military service he returned to Montreal and had an internship in neurology at the Montreal Neurological Institute. During 1946-47 he held a Fellowship in Medicine at the University of Toronto and in 1947-48 he was assistant resident at the Toronto General Hospital. He received a Nuffield Travelling Fellowship and spent the year 1948-49 at the Postgraduate Medical School at Hammersmith, England. In 1965 Dr. Kelly wrote the following comments on the special questions.

The decision to specialize in cardiology was reached in 1947, a full seven years after graduation, when I applied for a Nuffield Travelling Fellowship to do research work in cardiology at Professor McMichael's laboratory at the Postgraduate Medical School in London. In my case, as with many others of my vintage, graduate training was interrupted by the war, so that decisions in regard to specialty training were necessarily delayed and sometimes altered.

My decision in regard to my postgraduate training was largely self made, but I look fondly on the relatively few people who gave helpful advice and assistance in obtaining desirable appointments. They include: Dr. Stuart Townsend, Montreal General Hospital; Dr. Ray Farquharson, deceased, Professor of Medicine at the University of Toronto, and Dr. Duncan Graham, Professor of Medicine, University of Toronto. I suppose the major obstacle to my pursuit of graduate training was World War II.

My clinical interests are not exclusively cardiological. They are becoming increasingly slanted to the field of rheumatic disease. Because of my affiliation with Queen's University, and my position as Director Continuing Education, an increasing amount of time is taken up in the planning and development of graduate and postgraduate educational programs.

He received the status of Professor of Medicine at Queen's University in 1966 and was Attending Physician on the staff of the Kingston General Hospital and Consultant Physician to the Hôtel-Dieu and the Canadian Forces Hospital.

Dr. Kelly's bibliography grew to 24 items between 1944 and 1965. It includes one article, number 14, which suggests his involvement with cardiac catheterization: "The Haemodynamic Effects of Magnesium in Normal and Hypertensive Subjects, (abstract)" co-authored with H. Cross, J. D. Hatcher, and M. R. Turton (*Proc. Can. Soc. Clin. Invest.*, 22 January 1959). The majority of the articles are concerned with cardiovascular subjects, but there are several related to rheumatology and pharmacology.

Dr. S. Adrian Yaffe, Queen's University 36, M.R.C.P., A.A.C.P., F.A.C.C., F.R.C.P.(C)

The Medical School at McMaster University came into being in 1967. A member of the present staff should be able to recount the story of cardiac catheterization in Hamilton. Accordingly, I spoke with Dr. Ernest Fallen. He responded very generously and effectively as the letter dated November 26, 1982 quoted here demonstrates:

I had the opportunity of interviewing Dr. Adrian Yaffe who is the oldest living cardiologist in Hamilton and a rich source of information particularly regarding the early developments in Hamilton cardiology. Adrian graduated in medicine from Queen's University in 1936 and received his membership in the U.K. after having qualified at the Liverpool Infirmary (completely destroyed during World War II). He also studied in London with Schillingford and Paul Wood. In about 1948 he set up a practice in Internal Medicine in Hamilton. There were no subspecialties recognized as such in Hamilton (or anywhere else in Canada for that matter, I suppose). The only other individual in Hamilton who could be identified as a cardiologist was Dr. McGhie who practised as a consultant almost exclusively out of the McGregor Clinic downtown. His was primarily an office practice with only rare appearances in the hospital whereas Adrian set about developing certain diagnostic techniques in cardiology in the hospitals, mainly at the Hamilton General Hospital.

Dr. Yaffe performed the first heart catheterization in Hamilton in 1952. This is an interesting story. He managed to persuade the administration at St. Joseph's Hospital to raise about $3,500 for some capital equipment, particularly a two-channel Sanborn physiologic recorder, devices for measuring dilution, catheters, etc. He learned right heart catheterization from Bill Greenwood in Toronto. Curiously, Greenwood was only allowed to perform heart catheterization at the Wellesley Hospital since the Toronto General Hospital was not prepared to initiate this new technique. What is ironic is that the Wellesley Hospital now is probably the only central Toronto hospital without heart catheterization facilities. David Green from Buffalo was also helpful and, in fact, there was a close liaison between the cardiologists in Buffalo, Hamilton and Toronto. When one considers the longevity of the Montreal Cardiac Society, it may interest you to know that there was a tri-city meeting held annually made up of cardiologists from Rochester, Buffalo and Toronto-Hamilton. This society started in the early 50s and met annually almost continuously until 1979.

In any event Adrian returned to Hamilton ready to proceed with the first heart catheterization when he discovered that St. Joseph's Hospital was no longer interested in underwriting the costs for lab development. John Neilson, an assistant administrator of the Hamilton General Hospital and an army buddy of

Adrian, became interested and through various fund-raising measures, a small poorly ventilated basement laboratory was set aside in the Hamilton General Hospital. Together with Dr. Jack Sibley, Adrian began heart catheterizations. Most of the early cases were right heart catheterizations and most were rheumatic valvular disease. From David Green in Buffalo, he learned the rather horrendous technique of obtaining direct left atrial pressure by inserting a long 6- to 8-inch needle through the suprasternal notch and via the mediastinum puncturing the left atrial appendage. Adrian would then do a direct left ventricular puncture through the chest wall and obtain the pressure gradient. Dr. Yaffe and his associates began performing right sided angiography and it was now Buffalo's turn to learn from Hamilton. David Green came down and learned the techniques in angiography and went back to set it up in Buffalo in the mid 50s. Of interest is the fact that the radiologists at Hamilton General Hospital were completely uninterested in heart catheterization and therefore it was the sole property of Dr. Yaffe, Dr. Sibley and, a few years later, Dr. John Robinson. Dr. Robinson who is now the Chief of Cardiology at Hamilton General Hospital obtained his cardiological training at the Mayo Clinic. Although he had no formal catheterization experience he did learn cardiovascular physiology and mainly dilution curves.

The cases were largely those of rheumatic valvular disease with an increasing number of congenital heart lesions showing up in early adulthood.

Three important staff additions came during the 60s. Dr. Harold Stolberg arrived as a cardiovascular radiologist and immediately set about to develop a first-class laboratory with the assistance of Dr. Yaffe and Dr. John Robinson. In the early 70s, Drs. Robinson, Stolberg and Yaffe visited the Cleveland clinic to learn about coronary angiography. Dr. Eugene Biagioni who was a young general practitioner in Hamilton became interested in cardiology and spent several years with Mason Sones at the Cleveland clinic. He came back in about 1972. By this time the heart catheterization laboratory had moved to more presentable surroundings at the end of a corridor on the third floor of the Hamilton General Hospital adjoining the Intensive Care Unit and operating theatre.

It should be noted that the medical school started around 1967 and about three or four graduating classes occurred by the time the four horsemen of the apocalypse (Drs. Tanser, Holder,

Cairns and Fallen) arrived from the Royal Victoria Hospital to set up a university-based cardiology program in Hamilton. Prior to 1975, the only cardiologists in town to handle both a large clinical volume and student teaching were Dr. John Robinson, Adrian Yaffe, Eugene Biagioni and Brian Sealey (who was a half respirologist and half cardiologist). There were a number of internists who had a large cardiological practice. These included Dr. William Goldberg who was Chief of Medicine at St. Joseph's Hospital, Dr. Jack Sibley, Dr. John Eydt and Dr. David Leak.

Cardiac surgery developed slowly in Hamilton. Dr. Homer Beattie who is now Professor and Chairman of Surgery at McMaster University, performed the first mitral commissurotomy in Hamilton. There was someone named Dr. T. Fish who performed a few cardiac operations but then quit. The anaesthetists were not terribly happy supporting a cardiac program. However, eventually Dr. Beattie received support when Dr. Al Parisi arrived in town. Dr. Oliver Wesley-James, mainly a thoracic and vascular surgeon, came to assist in the development of coronary bypass surgery. Until the mid-70s, most patients who were catheterized in Hamilton either went to the Mayo Clinic or Toronto for cardiac surgery, particularly valve surgery. Dr. John Gunstensen then arrived in 1977 and a full-fledged cardiac surgical program was established.

Speaking to Dr. Yaffe, I came away with the impression that the early days of cardiology in Hamilton probably were no different than anywhere else in Canada. A few individuals who were interested in applying some of the newer diagnostic techniques were persuading hospitals to lend support. Radiology in general was rarely part of the picture as it is today. It is of interest that Hamilton was perhaps the first non-university community to perform heart catheterization in Canada. Electrocardiography was mainly carried out in the hospitals. Technical assistance at the time was extremely important and the technicians, by and large, were highly trained and had to do a good deal of troubleshooting when it came to repairing and maintaining the unwieldy equipment. Pressure measurements and dilution curves served the major measurements made during right heart catheterization. The Hamilton laboratories never really got into such diagnostic techniques as ballistocardiography although they did do some intracavitary phonocardiography at the time. There was no such thing as a full-time academic position. Physicians such as Drs. Yaffe, Robinson and Sibley had a growing consultant practice. It seemed that they developed techniques for cardiac investigation out of interest and curiosity as well as a need for techniques to more clearly define the state of certain cardiac disorders.

The above is more or less a capsule version of a history seen through the eyes of one individual. However, Dr. Yaffe does represent the most important source for the history of cardiology in Hamilton and I believe it is an accurate description.

Dr. E. Douglas Wigle, 30 October 1928, Windsor, Ontario; University of Toronto, M.D. 53; F.R.C.P.&S.(C); F.A.C.P.; F.A.H.A.

About a month after receiving the questionnaire in 1965, Dr. Wigle filled it in and dictated the following comments on the special questions. The spontaneous sentences and composition make for a sense of enthusiasm and freshness which merit being quoted without editing.

> I'm not just certain when I really decided to specialize in cardiology, I think during an assistant residency year in Vancouver. The year following my junior internship, I became a bit interested in it and interested in electrocardiography. The following year, I went to do pathology at Hammersmith Hospital, London, England, and Professor C. V. Harrison there put me to work on two projects in heart disease, which resulted in the first two publications in the bibliography. I think this is probably the stimulus to start with; however, I then came back to Canada and was thinking seriously of gastroenterology and particularly liver disease, and it was during my chief residency here at the Toronto General, when I looked after the medical aspects of all the cardiac surgical cases on the public service, that I really became interested in things. At this time, the late Professor Farquharson was most keen that I go into gastroenterology and, in fact, had a year planned for me with Chester Jones in Boston [at the Massachusetts General Hospital], but I backed down on this commitment in spite of the fact that there was no really well-trained gastroenterologist on the staff at the Toronto General at the time, and there were nine cardiologists. I must say that I pictured myself at sixty and I thought that I would much prefer using the stethoscope than a sigmoidoscope. I think my father perhaps had a bit of influence here too, when he said that if I did go into practice, which I never have, that people are much more willing to pay for an opinion on their heart than they would on their

tummy. I think there probably is some truth in this still. During my residency year I had my appendix out and had just previous to that been given Paul Wood's book on cardiology, and during my convalescence at home, I managed to read it, and as a result of reading it, on one occasion diagnosed I think probably the first Canadian case of a ruptured aneurysm of the sinus of valsalva, which was subsequently repaired, and was reported as the third article in the bibliography. I think by this time the course was set and then I got a McLaughlin Fellowship and went to England.

As far as planning any special training, Professor Farquharson obtained an Ontario Heart Foundation Scholarship for six months for me to work in the Cardiovascular Unit here at Toronto General, while I wrote my fellowship examinations, prior to going to England. I must confess that I didn't do much cardiology but mainly studied for my examinations during this period, but at least got a touch of cardiology. Then, I must say that I was very much influenced by Dr. Paul Wood, when I was at the Institute of Cardiology. One could not help but admire this man's direct approach to the problems in clinical cardiology and to stand very much in awe at his ability to make judgments on haemodynamic situations from the clinical findings. I think the time in England was well spent from a clinical cardiological sense, but as far as cardiovascular research, was probably not too rewarding. The time at the National Heart Hospital was very valuable from a clinical cardiological sense but as far as any research in cardiovascular disease, it was probably not that good. I then spent three months touring various cardiological centres in Europe, which was very pleasant and we got a few ideas from that, but this sort of travelling is probably not too good until one is well established, and has more specific enquiries to make when one travels to different centres. I then came back to North America and went to work in the Cardiovascular Research Institute at the University of California Medical Center in San Francisco under the direction of Dr. Julius Comroe. I chose to go there because when I was in England, and previously, I had been interested in pulmonary hypertension, that I thought it would be a good idea to get more training in pulmonary physiology. I was also, however, interested in cardiovascular disease very naturally, and I must say that I was disappointed and very much disappointed in fact, in the cardiovascular aspects of the Institute, and at the time I went, there was very little direction. The person with whom I was supposed to work, I am afraid proved a poor person to work with, and I, in fact, worked most of the time I was out there with a Swedish fellow, Dr. Al Holmgren. So I really arrived back in Toronto and aside from the clinical cardiological training in England, set about to train myself both in clinical, haemodynamic and research aspects of cardiovascular disease. I think I chose to come back to Toronto because I was offered a University position here, because I knew they had a good Cardiovascular Unit, with a large patient load, and this was the type of work that interested me. I have not yet bought an electrocardiograph, as I do not have an office outside the hospital.

I think membership in the Canadian Cardiovascular Society allowed me the first opportunities to present papers at scientific meetings, to get experience in this, and I think belonging to this Society has been a great help to me in getting to know cardiological colleagues across Canada and, of course, it has been a great help in experience in presenting papers.

Certainly from my own very brief and meagre career in cardiology, it seems to me that chance plays a very great part in what you end up doing and what your interests are. I came back to Toronto fully intending to work almost exclusively in pulmonary hypertension and the interrelationships between cardiopulmonary disease, but soon after I got back here, we saw our first case of muscular subaortic stenosis and since then it doesn't seem I've done very much other then that. However, there happens to be a large number of cases come here in Toronto, some fifty to sixty now, and it has been a fascinating time studying them. I suppose this is true of most things in life though, that one is wise to pick up a good opportunity when it comes along, but sometimes these opportunities end up moulding your lives.

I hope the above rambling account and the enclosed forms are of some value in compiling your archives. I am afraid I have been a little bit long-winded in dictating this, but this is as thoughts have come into my mind.

When Dr. Wigle updated his curriculum vitae in 1971, he was Associate Professor of Medicine at the University of Toronto and Director of the Cardiovascular Unit of the Toronto General Hospital.

In 1965, when his bibliography had reached eighteen items, many of which were indeed related to muscular subaortic stenosis, Dr. Wigle had also written on a considerable variety of other subjects, such as "Partial Anomalous Pulmonary Venous Drainage

With Intact Interatrial Septum Associated with Congenital Mitral Stenosis" (*C.M.A.J.* 1965: 31, 574), then the "Nature of the Disorder of Function in Chronic Post-infarction Aneurysm of the Left Ventricle" (*C.M.A.J.*, 1965: 92, 611).

In his comments on the special questions, he seems to regret having concentrated so much attention on that one subject, subaortic stenosis. A review of the bibliography that accumulated in the next six years, bringing it up in 51 items, plus 45 items published in the form of abstracts, reveals a wide variety of subjects related to all aspects of physiology and of medical and surgical management of cardiovascular disease.

Dr. Susan Mary Claire Lenkei, 24 November 1926, Budapest, Hungary; University of Zurich, M.D. 51; F.R.C.P.(C) 57; F.C.C.P.; F.A.C.C.P. 62; F.A.C.C.; F.A.C.P.; F.A.H.A.

Dr. Susan Mary Claire Lenkei is one of the earliest beneficiaries of the Ontario Heart Foundation.

Dr. William Greenwood refers to the installation of a well-equipped haemodynamic lab both with respect to personnel and instruments to replace the makeshift arrangements under which he worked. Dr. Susan C. Lenkei was one of the new young people who joined his team:

> In 1956 I became a Fellow in Cardiology at the Toronto General Hospital under Dr. R. W. Gunton. Under his most able guidance I became very interested in cardiology and decided to make it my specialty. I am quite sure that his teaching and interest in this subject was a deciding factor in my specialization. At that time I was an Ontario Heart Association Fellow and in the same year I wrote my Fellowship in Internal Medicine.
>
> Again, Dr. H. W. Gunton was most helpful in planning my special training and I have since then specialized in detail in cardiovascular physiology and in cardiac catheterization. I did not meet any obstacles in my training and since I came along at the right time, I got the job of running the Catheterization Unit at the Toronto Western Hospital.
>
> The Canadian Cardiovascular Society did not play any role in the development of my career.

In 1965 Dr. Lenkei was Assistant Professor of Medicine at the University of Toronto and Director of the Cardiovascular Laboratory at the Toronto Western Hospital.

Between 1951 and 1965, Dr. Lenkei's bibliography grew to eight items; all but the first are co-authored with medical and surgical colleagues and are on subjects related to the cardiovascular system. The fifth, a good example, is "Aortic Valve Homograft in the Treatment of Aortic Insufficiency," co-authored with A. J. Kerwin and Dr. R. Wilson (*N. Eng. J. Med.*, 1962; 266,852).

Dr. John Orval Parker, 13 November 1930, Hillington, Mich.; Queen's University, M.D., C.M. 54; F.R.C.P.(C); F.A.C.P.; F.A.C.C.; F.A.H.A.

Before going abroad in his program of postgraduate training, Dr. Parker had internship and residency in Medicine at the Kingston General Hospital (1954-56) and devoted a year to cardiovascular research in the Department of Physiology of Queen's University (1956-57). After this excellent preparation, he served as resident in the Cardiovascular Service of the Columbia University Department of Medicine (1958-60). He then enjoyed the privileges of the McLaughlin Travelling Fellowship in Paris (1960-61).

Dr. Parker wrote the following comment on the first two special questions.

> I made the decision to specialize in cardiology during my first year residency training. My period with Dr. Ford Connell was largely responsible for my decision to enter the field of cardiology. I was able to arrange my training period at Columbia [University] with the help of members of our Department of Physiology and Medicine. Funding at that time was a minor problem and I had to obtain financial support from the American College of Physicians and from the New York Heart Association. I bought my first electrocardiograph in 1962.

In 1972, he was Associate Professor of Medicine and Chairman of the Division of Cardiology at Queen's University. At the Kingston General Hospital he held the position of Attending Physician and he was Consultant Physician to the Hôtel-Dieu and the Canadian Forces Hospital.

The first five items on his list of publications concern work done during his training period. Number 4 is an example — "Quantitative Radiocardiography, 11. Technique and Analysis of Curves" (Donato, L., Rochester, D. P., Lewis, M. L., Durand, J., Parker, J. O., Harvey, R. M., *Circulation* 1962: 26, 183). After his return to Queen's in 1961 he published on a wide variety of subjects related to the study of haemodynamics and problems of therapy, both medical and surgical. His most recent article, Number 49 in the bibliography, "Effects of Quabain on Myocardial Potassium and Sodium Balance in Man" (Brennan, James F., McCans, John L., Chiong, M. A., and Parker, J. O., *Circulation,* 1972: 45, 107).

In 1982 Dr. Parker responded to our request for information concerning the introduction of cardiac catheterization in Kingston.

> I have been gathering information about the early development of cardiac catheterization at Queen's University. The laboratory at Queen's University was initially established in 1952 and was supported in part by a grant from the Bickell Foundation. This laboratory was established by Dr. H. G. Kelly, who was the original director. Dr. Kelly had received his early cardiologic training at the Hammersmith Hospital in London,where he trained under Dr. John McMichael. His contemporaries at the Hammersmith Hospital included Dr. Stewart Reid of Montreal and Dr. Richard Bayliss who later became physician to Queen Elizabeth II.
>
> The first right heart catheterizations were carried out in 1952 by Drs. Garfield Kelly and Donald Hatcher. Dr. Roxroy O. West joined the laboratory in July of 1959 as research fellow and has been an active member of the cardiovascular laboratory since that time.
>
> In 1959, the laboratory was moved from the hospital to new facilities in Etherington Hall adjacent to the Kingston General Hospital. The laboratory was funded through provincial funds and by the Ontario Heart Foundation. The new laboratory was under the co-direction of Dr. H. G. Kelly of the Department of Medicine and Dr. R. B. Lynn, Director of the Division of Cardiovascular and Thoracic Surgery at Queen's University.
>
> [Dr. John Parker returned to Queen's University in 1961 and shortly thereafter became Director of the cardiovascular laboratory.] In 1962, we carried out our first coronary angiogram. These were initially done through aortic root injections but in the spring of 1963, we first embarked on selective coronary angiography using the Sones technique. At that time there had been approximately 20 of these procedures carried out at the Toronto General Hospital and we became the second centre in Canada to embark on the technique of selective coronary angiography.
>
> As one looks back at these early procedures, one can recall using, not an image intensifier, but the old fluoroscopy units. These required long periods of accommodation with glasses and

angiography and coronary catheterizations proved to be extremely difficult. By 1964, image intensification became available and our initial studies were carried out using a mirror to view the image. This later gave way to the use of closed circuit television and progressive improvements in technology which greatly simplified these catheterization and angiographic facilities.

Dr. Frank Berkman, Queen's University M.D. 49, F.R.C.P.(C).

Cardiac catheterization was introduced in Ottawa at a relatively early time. This information has been supplied by Dr. Frank Berkman in a letter which he wrote November 1, 1982 in response to my request.

After graduation from Queen's in Medicine in 1949, I took a rotating internship, a year in pathology and two years in internal medicine before starting my formal cardiological training in Washington, D.C. The first year was as a resident in cardiology and the second year as a research fellow. During this time I had training in heart catheterization.

On returning to Ottawa in 1955, I joined the Department of Medicine of the University of Ottawa and had joint appointments at the Ottawa Civic and Ottawa General Hospitals. Shortly thereafter I organized a Heart Catheterization Unit at the Ottawa General Hospital. A wide spectrum of both congenital and acquired (paediatric and adult) types of heart problems were studied by myself, and most of the surgery at that time was done by Dr. David Hooper. There was gradual expansion in volume of cases and with the passage of time, additional cardiologists, both paediatric and adult, joined the unit. Because of the volume of cases, a second lab was subsequently developed at the Ottawa Civic Hospital.

With increasing volume and advancing technology, it was clear that new laboratory facilities would have to be built. The very large expense involved made it clear that this facility would have to be developed in one hospital in Ottawa. This facility was eventually developed at the Ottawa Civic Hospital under my direction as Chief of Cardiology.

At the present time, under the direction of Dr. Brian Morton as Head of Haemodynamics, there is an exceptionally fine Catheterization Unit with all modern facilities and it is fully integrated, functionally and geographically, with the coronary care area, cardiac surgery, and nuclear medicine. There are now 7 cardiologists (6 geographically full-time) doing catheter studies and one cardiac radiologist. It has been very gratifying to see this grow over the years.

Dr. Donald Stewart Beanlands, 27 December 1932, Halifax; Dalhousie, M.D., Ch. B. (Gold Medal) 58; F.R.C.P.(C) 62; F.A.C.P. 69; F.A.C.C. 71; F.A.H.A.

Dr. Beanlands omitted details of his postgraduate training on the questionnaire but alludes to the most important elements in two letters he wrote in 1968. The relevant excerpts are quoted.

> I am not absolutely sure how I arrived at the decision to specialize in cardiology. I would suspect that it was due to the fact that I was intimately involved with the establishment of a new Cardiac Catheterization Laboratory in Halifax and was stimulated by this scientific approach in the investigation of patients. This experience arrived during my second year of residency training.
>
> As far as experience in planning my training is concerned, Professor R. C. Dixon, at Dalhousie University, was most helpful in advising me and in assisting me to obtain adequate training in cardiology. I found no particular obstacle in my way in obtaining training. However, it was very frustrating indeed not to have some guidelines to go by as far as the Royal College was concerned. In one's junior training one does not meet influential people in the field and this makes a great difficulty in assessing adequate training facilities.
>
> With regard to influences which led me to choose my present practice in cardiology are concerned, I have always been interested in academic medicine and had planned to establish myself in a university centre when my training was finished. Dr. Ramsay Gunton influenced my final decision on this and instead of going back to Halifax as I originally planned, I stayed in Toronto.
>
> I would think that the one person in Canada who has influenced me most is Dr. Ramsay Gunton. I was his Fellow at the Toronto General Hospital for one year and his interest in cardiology sparked me and kept my enthusiasm high. Dr. John Keith also influenced my career as I spent a year with him. As far as the Society is concerned, I have attended the annual meetings on a regular basis and the presentation of papers has given me an opportunity to present material and become known. This opportunity would not have afforded itself if the Canadian Cardiovas-

cular Society did not exist. I think that the Canadian Cardiovascular Society, itself, is well worth while as it does allow those interested in cardiology in Canada to come together and to exchange ideas for the benefit of Medicine in Canada.

When Dr. Beanlands updated his curriculum vitae in 1971, he was Assistant Professor of Medicine, University of Toronto, on the Attending Staff of the Toronto Western Hospital and Director of its acute coronary care unit. Dr. Beanlands did not submit his bibliography.

Dr. John Edward Morch, 28 July 1931, Port Credit, Ontario; McGill, B.Sc. 56; M.D., C.M. 56; F.R.C.P.(C); C.S.P.Q.; F.A.H.A.

Following graduation and two years of internship (1956-1958) at the Royal Victoria Hospital (Montreal), Dr. Morch engaged in general practice until 1960 when he resumed post-graduate training. He began with one year of cardiology under Dr. Greenwood in Toronto, after which he worked with Dr. Maurice McGregor and Dr. Arnold Johnson in the cardiopulmonary unit of the Royal Victoria Hospital in Montreal (1961-65). He then joined the staff of the University of Toronto and in 1972 was Assistant Professor of Medicine and Assistant Director of the Cardiovascular Unit at the Toronto General Hospital.

Between the years 1966 and 1972 Dr. Morch published alone or as a co-author, fourteen articles which reflect his training in cardiodynamics and his wide interest in many aspects of clinical cardiology. The first article is on "Rupture of the Sinus of Valsalva: A Study of Eight Cases with Discussion on the Differential Diagnosis of Continuous Murmurs" (*Am. J. Cardiol.*, Vol. 18, No. 6, 1966: 827-836). In 1972, together with Drs. G. Froggatt and A. Trimble, he wrote "The Adult Cyanotic Tetralogy of Fallot: Late Haemodynamic Studies After Total Intracardiac Repair" (*Circulation,* Vol. XLVI, No. 4, October 1972).

Dr. Shahid Ulla Mecci, 2 February 1941, Bangalore; University of Bangalore Medical School, M.B., B.S. 62; F.R.C.P.(C) 69.

In 1972 Dr. Mecci wrote the following replies to the special questions:

During my last years of residency in internal medicine, I worked for six months with the cardiologist at the Rochester General Hospital, Dr. Sidney Goldstein, and this influenced me into taking up cardiology as my career.

I really did not have to worry about my special training particularly in the Cardiovascular Unit at the Toronto General Hospital for there was enough exposure to cardiology and the study of cardiovascular dynamics.

My inability to practise my field in my home country made me decide to practise the same in Canada and I chose Sudbury because there was a real need for a cardiologist here and also this place was recommended to me by my former chief.

I have been a member of the Canadian Cardiovascular Society only for the past year or so although I have been attending the meetings for the past two years and I find the association with the other practising cardiologists in the country stimulating and it gives me a good opportunity to exchange ideas and information.

I do wish to take part in the extra curricular activities and community services but so much of my time is taken up by the practice and also because of my being the Chief of Medicine at one of the hospitals in the city, I find very little time to devote to other activities. History of Medicine in particular fascinates me and I hope to devote more time to its study in the future.

Dr. Mecci filled the need for a medical cardiologist to work with Dr. Field in his project of establishing a cardio-thoracic unit. In contrast with cardiologists in centres with a medical school, who tend not to mention the Canadian Cardiovascular Society as of much significance in their careers, these two men stress its importance to them.

Dr. John Buchanan Armstrong, 19 October 1918, Toronto; University of Toronto, M.D. 43; F.A.C.C.; L.M.C.C.; Manitoba and Ontario, 43; F.R.C.P.(C) 50; M.R.S.H.; F.A.H.A.; F.A.C.C.

In 1965, Dr. Armstrong wrote the following summary of his career:

In the summer of 1940 and 1941, I worked at the Banting Institute in Toronto, under Dr. R. A. Cleghorn, then a member of the Department of Medicine at the University of Toronto and an authority on adrenal cortex. These studies were concerned with a standardized method of producing haemorrhagic shock in dogs, and were later published in the *C.M.A. Journal,* as indicated in the bibliography.

This work brought me in contact with both Sir Frederick Banting and Dr. Gordon Murray, and by the time of graduation I was convinced that I wished to engage in research in the cardiovascular system.

During my service in the Army I had the good fortune to be associated in Italy with No. 1 Research Lab, R.C.A.M.C., which was studying resuscitation in the acutely injured. This very stimulating group was of considerable influence in my deciding in favour of clinical physiology of the cardiovascular system.

Before leaving the service in 1946, I decided in favour of clinical training first, in order that I would establish the necessary rapport with the clinicians in teaching hospitals (to do clinical physiology, it was clear I had to have my clinical union card). Accordingly, I applied and was accepted in the Diploma Course in Internal Medicine at McGill, spending two years in Medicine at the Royal Victoria Hospital with a most interesting ex-military service group from many parts of Canada. I was particularly interested in the backward, as against the forward, theories for the mechanism of congestive heart failure, and accordingly spent one year with each of Dr. Eugene Stead at Duke University and Sir John McMichael, Postgraduate Medical School, London, Hammersmith Hospital.

When I returned to Canada in 1950 I was offered a position in the Department of Medicine in Toronto at $2,400. I accepted an invitation to join the staff of the Department of Physiology and Medical Research, under Professor J. Doupe, at the University of Manitoba and was a Canadian Life Insurance Officers Association Fellow for two years. During the years 1952-1956 I was a Markle Scholar.

Before returning to Canada in September, 1950 I attended the Physiology Course in Copenhagen, and within the next three months wrote the Fellowship examinations for the Royal College and presented my first paper to the Canadian Heart Association, to which I was elected a member.

During the next two or three years I gained the impression that the Canadian Heart Association was dominated by a small group, and voiced my objection by letter to some of the proposals that were made. The result of this correspondence would seem that I was appointed to the Council very suddenly, but never had the privilege of attending a Council meeting.

It was through the Canadian Heart Association membership that I first learned of the plans to form a Heart Foundation and responded to the notice sent to the membership regarding the need of an Executive Secretary. The remainder is quite well documented.

The original suggestion that the Heart Foundation be called the Canadian Heart Foundation was not acceptable to the Secretary of State because of the possible confusion with the Canadian Heart Association. This name however did become acceptable and the change was made in January 1962 on condition that the Canadian Heart Association changed its name.

Dr. R. S. Fraser and myself were signatories to the application to have the name of the Canadian Heart Association changed to Canadian Cardiovascular Society.

Not long after John Armstrong became a member of the Society (then the Canadian Heart Association), he had the urge to disagree with some of the ways in which the Society was managed. He did not hesitate to write to the proper members of the Executive about these things. Thus, in addition to being a highly trained cardiologist engaged in research and teaching, he was quite prepared to take an active interest in the development of the fledgling organization of Canadian cardiologists. Little did he know then, nor did anyone else know, what a great role he would play in organizing the work of promoting cardiology in Canada.

The task of Executive Secretary of the Heart Foundation since its inception calls for many skills, in addition to a wide range of knowledge. John Armstrong discovered that he had all the skills and the ability to acquire the knowledge. He proved to be the ideal person for the job. He was as much at home among administrators and those dealing with problems of finance, as he was in the physiological laboratory or a hospital ward. It is rare for one man to acquire expertise in so many fields of knowledge and skills. This accounts for the signal achievements he has accomplished in carrying out programs of work to promote the prevention and relief of heart disease here and everywhere in the world. In 1965 he resigned from his post in the Canadian Heart Foundation and resumed his career in research as Associate Professor of Pharmacology at the University of Toronto.

Dr. Armstrong published his first paper during his military service. Its title "Mental Disorders in the Armed Forces" (*U. of T. Med. J.*, 1942: 19, 147) suggests that he might have been led into the road of adopting psychiatry as a career. His next paper, however, which was published in 1943 with associates (*C.M.A.J.*, 1943: 49, 355-362) was concerned with "A Standardized Method for Producing Shock in Dogs by Bleeding." All subsequent articles deal with matters somatic, and include a series of articles on bronchial circulation which appeared in *Thorax* between 1951 and 1953. His article on "Cardiac Catheterization in Congenital Heart Disease" (*Univ. Manitoba Med. J.*, 1955: 27, 65) indicates that he began this work in Winnipeg and would have continued it if he had not chosen to become the first executive secretary to the Canadian Heart Foundation in 1956. With L. Cudkowicz, he co-authored a chapter in a German book, *Die Pathologische Anatomie der Bronchial-Arterien. Ergebrisse der Gesamten Tuberkulose- Und Lungenforschung:* Band XIV, 1958: 191-206.

Saskatchewan

Max Israels wrote about his career in Regina in June 1965. In the story of electrocardiography's beginnings in Saskatchewan (page 116) he appears as the pioneer in Regina. In this letter, he also describes performing cardiac catheterization in 1952:

> I did the first catheterization in this city (possibly the province) in 1952. Dr. David Stein, now a cardiologist in Winnipeg, was my resident at the Regina General Hospital. He later worked with Hans Hecht at Salt Lake City.

Apparently, his experience with cardiac catheterization was rather brief.

Dr. Louis Horlick, 2 December 1921, Montreal; McGill, B.Sc. 44; M.D., C.M. 45; Dip. Int. Med. McGill 50; F.R.C.P.(C) 52; A.O.A. 45; F.A.H.A.

After a brilliant career, winning many prizes as a student, Dr. Horlick began postgraduate education with a rotating internship at the Montreal General Hospital (1945-1946). During the next two years he worked at the Michael Reese Hospital in Chicago as resident and Fellow in Cardiovascular Diseases. During 1950-1952 he was a Research Fellow of the American Heart Association, working with Professor Lyman Duff on atherosclerosis at McGill. In 1951 he was appointed to the staff of McGill Medical School as Demonstrator. In 1953 he was appointed Associate in Medicine at the Montreal Jewish General Hospital and the Hospital of Hope. In 1954 he moved to Saskatchewan where he rose to the position of Professor and Head of the Department of Medicine at the University of Saskatchewan in 1968.

Cardiac catheterization became firmly established in Saskatchewan with the advent of Louis Horlick to the University Hospital in Saskatoon. I made my request by long distance telephone and received the following letter:

November 12, 1982

Dear Harold:

Thank you for your telephone call of November 9, 1982. I decided to sit down and dictate this letter immediately after your call, so that you could receive this information as quickly as possible. I will restrict myself to events which occurred in Saskatchewan only.

I arrived in Saskatoon in April of 1954 and my mandate was to create a proper cardiovascular centre. This involved setting up an electrocardiographic non-invasive laboratory and a haemodynamics laboratory. I was joined by Dr. John E. Merriman in the fall of 1954. Dr. Merriman had had experience in an invasive laboratory in Boston working with Dr. C. S. Burwell, and he also had a considerable amount of training in pulmonary medicine. The two of us worked together to establish both the electrocardiographic and haemodynamics laboratory and carried out the first cardiac catheterization sometime in 1955. It was, by modern standards, a very primitive affair. We used a standard fluoroscope in a darkened room. I was the person who inserted and manipulated the catheter, and John stood by to obtain the blood samples and run down the hall to the Physiology Department where Dr. Louis Jacques had lent us a Van Slyke apparatus. There John tediously Van Slyke'd samples and obtained the blood gas determinations. It was not until the next day that we were able to inspect the data and determine what the diagnosis actually was. The techniques of course improved very rapidly after that and within a year or two we had all of the necessary modern paraphernalia for carrying out cardiac catheterization. Simultaneous with the institution of cardiac catheterization of course was the development of cardiac surgery in our centre. Dr. E. M. Nanson, a New Zealander who had been very well trained at Johns Hopkins and in England joined us as Head of Surgery, and began doing a fairly wide variety of cardiac procedures including Blalock-Taussig shunts, closure of atrial septal defects under hypothermia, and mitral valvotomies closed. In 1956 or 57 we were joined by Beverly Lynn, a Canadian from Ontario, who had trained in England and was widely recognized for his skills as a peripheral vascular and thoracic surgeon. While in England at the British post-graduate hospital, he had become acquainted with Dennis Melrose who had developed one of the first effective pumps for open-heart surgery, and he brought some of the pieces of the Melrose pump with him when he came to Saskatoon. In the course of the next two years he assembled the Melrose pump and did some experimental work in animals, and in 1957 or 58 carried out the first closure of a ventricular septal defect in a patient in Saskatchewan. Unfortunately, Lynn left us shortly thereafter to go to Kingston, and open-heart cardiac surgery suffered a severe setback in our centre.

Another item of some historical interest was the fact that Dr. Nanson introduced the Allison technique for obtaining left-sided cardiac pressures. This involved passing the bronchoscope and piercing the left main bronchus with a very long needle. The needle entered the left atrium and a fine polythene tube was passed through the needle into the left atrium and left ventricle. It was a rather barbaric procedure but it did open up the left side of the heart to physiologic investigation in man. I reported some of Dr. Nanson's results at a meeting in San Francisco in 1957 or 58 and I remember Dr. John Sampson listening to me incredulously. He could not believe that someone coming from a remote centre in Canada had been able to accomplish something which was not being done in San Francisco.

Additional firsts in Saskatchewan really included the introduction of a formal hospital-based exercise rehabilitation program by Dr. John Merriman in 1969. In many respects John was a pioneer in this field and was widely known by exercise physiologists and rehabilitationists around the world. The program was intended from its inception to be a research program to determine the effects of cardiac rehabilitation on longevity but was unfortunately never completed when John left us in 1977 to go to Tulsa, Oklahoma.

Other firsts included the work done here by Dr. Rudolf Altschul in the late 50s and early 60s on experimental atherosclerosis and the effects of nicotinic acid on cholesterol levels. My own work on the biosynthesis of cholesterol and the effect of dietary changes on plasma cholesterol levels was begun in the mid 50s and with the collaboration of Dr. H. S. Sodhi was expanded to include cholesterol balance studies and the effect of various drugs on cholesterol metabolism in the mid-60s and 70s. It represented the first time that anyone in Canada had attempted to do this type of very complex biochemical work. The success of this work was largely due to Dr. Sodhi who was both an M.D. and Ph.D. biochemist and who unfortunately died two years ago of a nasopharyngeal sarcoma, thus terminating a very promising, indeed brilliant career.

There were many other interesting firsts, some of which I have now forgotten. In the area of technological development we were assisted by our biomedical group to produce the first simple prototype transmitter for transmitting electrocardiograms from Canora, Saskatchewan to Saskatoon and sending the responses back immediately. Subsequently, numerous commercially developed devices became available but this may well have been the first device of its kind to be used in Canada.

I hope that the above is essentially what you wanted and if you have any further questions please do not hesitate to call or write me. With best personal regards, I am

Yours sincerely,

L. Horlick, M.D., F.R.C.P.(C).

Between 1948 and 1971 Dr. Horlick published fifty articles, the majority on subjects related to the pathology and biochemistry of atherosclerosis. The first nine appeared in the years 1948 to 1950 and stemmed from work done in the laboratory of Dr. Louis N. Katz. There follow five important articles, the result of work in the laboratory of the late Dr. Lyman Duff at McGill. The remainder of his bibliography consists of articles published on work done at the University of Saskatchewan.

Dr. John Edward Merriman, 12 October 1924, Hamilton; Queen's University, M.D., C.M. 47; F.R.C.P.(C) 53; F.A.C.P.; F.A.C.C.P.; F.A.H.A.

Dr. Merriman began his postgraduate training with a rotating internship at the Kingston General Hospital. There followed a senior internship in Medicine 1948-49 and senior internship in Pathology 1949-50, at the Ottawa Civic Hospital; assistant resident in Medicine at Sunnybrook Hospital, Toronto 1950-51; Research Fellow in Medicine at Harvard Medical School, Boston, 1951-52; Graduate Medical Research Fellow in Physiology, University of Western Ontario, 1952-53 and Instructor in Physiology at this University, 1953-54.

In 1971, when Dr. Merriman updated his curriculum vitae, he was Professor of Medicine at the University of Saskatchewan, having begun as a Lecturer at this University in 1954. He was on the active staff of the University Hospital and Director of the Exercise and Pulmonary Function Laboratory. He also held the post of Visiting Consultant at the Saskatoon City Hospital and the St. Paul Hospital.

Dr. Merriman's response to the special questions adds significantly to the description of his preparation for a distinguished career as a pioneer of cardiopulmonary research in Saskatchewan.

In my second year of postgraduate training, while a senior intern in Medicine at the Ottawa Civic Hospital, 1948-49, Dr. James H. Graham, now secretary of the Royal College, was one of the enthusiastic and able teachers on the ward service. He had just returned from his position as resident in Medicine at the Peter Bent Brigham Hospital. In his teaching he would quote George Thorn in endocrinology and Sam Levine in cardiology. Thus, this teacher played a major role in my decision to go on into cardiology. He subsequently arranged an interview with Dr. Thorn who subsequently had me see Dr. Sidney Burwell. This gentleman stressed to me that God made the blood go from the right heart through the lungs to the left heart. Thus, you could not truly separate cardiac disease from pulmonary disease as far as the major symptom dyspnoea is concerned. Thus, with this year in Boston, I became interested in being an internist first but a cardiologist second, and working in academic medicine — and in Canada.

My own university, Queen's, had no organized training program in Internal Medicine. Initially it was a family friend and former academic internist, Dr. Gordon Cornett of Hamilton, who influenced me during my final year to consider the subspecialty of medicine. Thus, my early years in postgraduate training were along the fields of Internal Medicine but on a year-to-year basis. No long-term plan was organized and it was a matter of where could I get accepted and for how long.

When I returned from Boston, I was convinced that I wanted to do academic medicine — cardiology in Canada, but that to better prepare myself, I should be firmly grounded in physiology. Thus, the two years were spent at the University of Western Ontario. There were definite economic as well as other problems in this first year in London, Ontario. Things did not 'pan out' as had been originally planned. It was at this stage that I nearly threw the chips in and said, 'I will go out and practise medicine so that I can feed my family and not see them starve and suffer.' Again, it was Dr. James Graham who suggested that I hold off this decision for at least a few months. The second year in London, Ontario was at a slightly increased stipend — such that I could comfortably feed my family. This supporting grant was from the Ontario Heart Foundation. The first year had been supported by an N.R.C. Fellowship. It was during this year that I began looking around for a position in academic medicine in Canada. At that stage in 1953, there were few places which were considering full-time positions and especially in clinical medicine. This was a trend that began in the United States about seven years ago and, as remains in many other trends, Canada was behind a good five to ten years.

I believe that I had heard from some source that the University of Saskatchewan was starting a new medical school and thought that I would get another inquiry letter off. Much to my surprise, I did receive a very encouraging reply from Dean Wendell MacLeod in the Fall of 1953. We continued corresponding and I subsequently went out to Saskatchewan, site unseen, in the summer of 1954.

It was after I had been in Saskatoon that I joined the Canadian Cardiovascular Society.

Between 1954 and 1957 I had a joint appointment at the University of Saskatchewan with the major appointment in the Department of Physiology and a minor appointment in Medicine. At that time we were just beginning the teaching of the new Second Year. In 1957 I switched over so that I was more in the Department of Medicine than in the Department of Physiology, since after all I had my Fellowship and did consider myself at least a cardiologist. My main activities in these early years was the setting up of the Cardiopulmonary Laboratory in the University Hospital and University of Saskatchewan.

In 1961-62 Dr. Lou Horlick, my colleague, took his sabbatical leave. During this year I had all the responsibility for all cardiac catheterizations — adults and children — all electrocardiography, all cardiopulmonary teaching and the majority of the electrocardiograms. This I could not have accomplished without a superb cardiac resident, Dr. R. C. Hayton.

1962 did bring its stressful moments with the Saskatchewan Medicare crisis. In the Fall of 1962 I began looking into my future and where I wanted to move. I became convinced that we had to put more objectivity into the practice of medicine and especially into the practice of cardiology. I had been involved in biomedical engineering and had been impressed with the usefulness of this discipline. Thus, in the winter of 1962 I took university night classes in elementary mathematics to supplement my very meagre Ontario high school mathematics.

I applied for, and subsequently was granted, a year's sabbatical leave to study in the Department of Computer Science, Birkbeck College, University of London, England. This was only half-salary and I did have a small travelling grant from the Canadian Heart Foundation. This was a very educational experience for the whole Merriman family, but it definitely did have its trying moments. There were problems in changing from one standard of living to another. I purposely had my base in a non-medical department. One can learn a great deal about medical care by keeping one's mouth closed and eyes and ears open.

Following my return from sabbatical leave I was convinced about two things — (1) that computers could play a role in medicine and especially in cardiology, in both patient care, teaching, and research, and (2) that exercise, a side interest of mine for many, many years, could be both a useful diagnostic and therapeutic tool.

In the fall of 1964 I was invited to visit Australia by the Queensland Division of the Australian Heart Foundation. This, again, was a wonderful experience and I hope was as profitable to Australia as it was to me.

Since then I have continued my interest in both computers and in exercise. Which is the winning horse? I sometimes wonder, for I have recently married these two interests. If I fail as a teacher or a cardiologist, I can probably go on the market as a scientific programmer and certainly make much more than I am now making in an academic institution.

However, one should be happy in his work.

Dr. Merriman's first publication dealt with his experimental work at Queen's University, "Cardiovascular Effects of Hexamathonium in Acutely-produced Experimental Anaemia in the Dog" (Sunahara, F. A., Merriman, J. E., and Gowdey, G. W., *Federation Proceedings,* Vol. 12, No. 1, March, 1953). The first item which represents work done at the University of Saskatchewan is an article with Dr. L. Horlick on "Congenital Valvular Stenosis of Pulmonary and Aortic Valves with Atrial Septal Defect" (*Am. Ht. J.*, Vol. 54, No. 4, October, 1957). Many of his papers are related to respiratory physiology. However, there are various other items which reflect a wide range of interest, e.g., "A Historical Review of the Canadian

Association of Sports Sciences," 1967, and several articles on the application of computers to medicine.

Dr. John Michael Tyrrell, 14 April 1936, Oxford, England; University of London, M.B., B.S. 59; F.R.C.P. (London) 62; F.R.C.P.(C) 70.

Before it became an officially recognized subspecialty, Dr. Tyrrell chose to become a paediatric cardiologist. He obtained training in England, in Boston, and in Toronto during the ten years after graduation and before he chose to develop his career in Saskatchewan. He describes his experiences in making these choices in his comments on the special questions.

> I first became interested in cardiology during my first exposure to internal medicine at St. Bartholomew's Hospital, London, England where I was taught by the late Dr. Geoffrey Bourne. After graduating I obtained some general experience in internal medicine before returning to St. Bartholomew's Hospital and having some further exposure to cardiology while working for Dr. Graham Hayward. I then spent three years in a regional cardiac unit near Cambridge, England, which dealt with both adults and children, and learned how to perform cardiac catheterizations under the guidance of Dr. Hugh Fleming who had in turn been trained by the late Dr. Paul Wood. During this time I became more interested in congenital heart disease and the treatment of children which caused me to go to the Children's Hospital in Boston and spend two years with Dr. A. S. Nadas taking further training in paediatric cardiology. I spent a further year in Toronto with Dr. John Keith gaining more experience in paediatric cardiology and performing some research projects.
>
> To practise paediatric cardiology, one is obliged to stay in a large centre of population or a University Centre which receives patients from a large area. The University Hospital, University of Saskatchewan where I am now, is a referral centre for almost all of the children with cardiac disease in this province and has an active Cardiac Surgical Service which can deal with a wide range of congenital heart defects.
>
> Since taking up this appointment I have been pleased to be a member of the Canadian Cardiovascular Society and have enjoyed attending the last few annual meetings.

In 1972 when Dr. Tyrrell responded, he held the post of Paediatric Cardiologist at the University Hospital and also Visiting Consultant to St. Paul's Hospital and the City Hospital in Saskatoon, and Assistant Professor of Paediatrics.

His bibliography of six items published in the years 1969 to 1972 reflects work done with teachers and associates during his years of postgraduate training.

Alberta

Dr. Robert Stewart Fraser, 14 February 1922, Nelson, B.C.; University of Alberta, B.Sc. 44; M.D. 46; M.Sc. Biochemistry 50; F.R.C.P.(C) Cert.; F.A.C.P.; F.A.C.C.; F.A.H.A.

During his final undergraduate year, Dr. Fraser served an internship at the Royal Alexandra Hospital in Edmonton. Following graduation he had an internship at the University of Alberta Hospital during 1946. The next year he worked at St. Paul's Hospital, Vancouver. In 1948, he worked again at the University of Alberta Hospital and in 1949 at the Royal Alexandra Hospital. During the years 1950-1953 he worked in the Department of Cardiology at the University of Minnesota. He returned to the University of Alberta in 1953, was awarded a Markle Fellowship, and pioneered the creation of a haemodynamic laboratory.

When he updated his curriculum vitae in 1971, Dr. Fraser was Director of the Division of Cardiology and a member of the Attending Staff of the University of Alberta Hospital, as well as Professor of Medicine at the University of Alberta.

In responding to the special questions, he tells the story of his choice of cardiology and of his postgraduate training in preparation for pioneering modern cardiology in Alberta.

> I am not sure when I reached my decision to specialize in cardiology. It was obviously one of the more challenging and exciting new fields about 1950 to 1953 when I was taking my postgraduate education. I think it also provided a challenge to a person who was interested in orderly thinking and the opportunity to correlate clinical findings with special types of investigation which became possible about that time. Having obtained a Masters degree in biochemistry from a rather generous university I was faced with suggestions from Dr. C. J. Watson in Minneapolis that I became interested in the porphyrins. Because his whole department revolved around porphyrins it was a reasonable suggestion but the field seemed crowded. I was then approached by Dr. Carl Chapman about taking a year in clinical research in cardiology and I think it was at this time that the

University of Alberta was also interested in having someone come back and set up a diagnostic unit. The University of Alberta then asked me if I would accept their nomination as a Markle Scholar and this appealed to me when I had no other definite commitments for the future. I was successful in obtaining the Markle Scholarship which began in July of 1953 and it was under this arrangement that I came back to Alberta to set up the diagnostic unit.

My experiences in Minneapolis during the years 1952 and 1953 were somewhat hit and miss as far as learning the diagnostic techniques of cardiac investigation was concerned. The year I spent with Carl resulted in two or three papers which dealt with our project in evaluating some of the haemodynamic affects of healed myocardial infarctions as they may have affected the performance of subjects on the treadmill. I managed to work in attendance at a hypertensive clinic for the year and also attended the regular cardiac rounds. In addition, it became obvious that I would have to know a bit about cardiac catheterization and I spent some time in the laboratory although I did not actually do more than a handful of catheterizations myself.

When I returned to Alberta I came armed with the information I needed concerning equipment, a good deal of enthusiasm and a youthful disregard for the difficulties and hazards of setting up a catheterization laboratory.

The first year was indeed a pioneer one and I owe much to Dr. Joe Dvorkin who supported me in so many ways. He not only helped with the procedures but provided most of the early patients for catheterization. We worked with a two-channel Sanborn machine to record pressures, and the electrocardiogram, and had a large oscilloscope which did a reasonable job of monitoring the electrocardiogram. Because we were only able to get into the X-ray room after all the regular work for the day had been done, we frequently started catheterizations at 3 o'clock in the afternoon and a technician on loan from the Department of Laboratories worked with me while we both did Van Slykes until approximately 10 o'clock at night. This was a far cry from our present organization in every respect. We now have an image intensifier, a room of our own in the X-ray Department, three full-time technicians, some four Electronics for Medicine Recorders and all the other trappings that go with such an organization.

One of the appreciable obstacles was convincing the Attending Staff of internists that cardiac catheterization did indeed have a place in the diagnostic investigation of certain patients with heart disease. It took several years before some of the more conservative members of the staff felt that this was anything other than a dangerous research procedure which really had no place in the investigation of the ordinary patient.

As regards the Canadian Cardiovascular Society and the part that it may have played in the development of my career, although I may not have voiced this opinion very widely I have told my friends that my membership in the Canadian Cardiovascular Society has been something for which I have always been most grateful. It enabled me to form lasting friendships with people across the country who have not only been a stimulus in my own work but have also been a great help in proffering advice and encouragement. To add a personal note, I would think that it would have been very doubtful that I would have had the privilege and pleasure of Dr. Segall's friendship over the last ten years if we both had not belonged to the Society. I am sure that any of the middle-aged and younger people in our Society have treasured the friendship of those who were the real pioneers in cardiology in Canada.

Dr. Fraser was among those who attended the meeting in Ottawa, called by the Hon. Mr. Paul Martin, at which the Canadian Heart Foundation was organized. He was the Founding President of the Alberta Heart Foundation and has maintained a sustained active interest in both organizations.

The first ten items in Dr. Fraser's list of publications deal with subjects which reflect the stages of his period of training between 1950 and 1954. By 1965 another twenty-seven items joined the list. These are usually co-authored and deal with a wide variety of subjects. There are of course titles concerned with the diagnosis of cardiovascular disease using cardiac catheterization and reports about cardiac surgery. But there are a number of editorial type articles by Dr. Fraser which reflect his active participation in the education of his confrères and the explosive progress in knowledge related to the cardiovascular system.

Dr. Neil Fraser Duncan, 2 October 1925, Edmonton; University of Alberta, B.Sc. 47; M.D. 49; Cert. R.C.P.(C) 53; Cert. in Paediatrics 53; F.A.A.P. 53; F.A.C.C. 66; F.A.H.A.

Dr. Duncan began postgraduate training with internships at the Royal Alexandra Hospital (1949-51) followed by a year at the Hospital for Sick Children, Toronto, and a year as resident at the Children's Hospital and the University of Alberta Medical School.

When he updated his curriculum vitae in 1971, he was Associate Clinical Professor of Paediatrics at the University of Alberta and on the Attending Staff of the University Hospital. After having practised general paediatrics for several years, he resumed postgraduate studies to acquire expertise in paediatric cardiology, including cardiac catheterization. He is among the early pioneers in this field.

Dr. Duncan did not provide a bibliography.

Dr. John Colvin Morgan, 6 November, 1926, Fort William, Ont.; Queen's University, M.D., C.M. 50; F.R.C.P.(C); F.A.C.P., F.C.C.P., F.A.H.A.

Dr. Scarlett (page 117) depicted the status of cardiology in Calgary before World War II; Dr. Morgan depicts the introduction of postwar cardiology by men who had special training in the United States.

> After completing my training in internal medicine and pathology I thought it wise to take extra time in a medical subspecialty. Accordingly, I spent the next fourteen months at the Johns Hopkins Hospital in Baltimore as an American Heart Association Fellow in cardiology. This was followed by some time in the Cardiovascular Investigation Laboratory which, at that time, was attached to the surgical division at Johns Hopkins. This also entailed some attendance at Dr. Taussig's clinic at the Harriet Lane in Baltimore. I think I began considering cardiology seriously at that time back in 1954 with the great surge of interest in specific cardiac diagnosis leading to surgery.
>
> I found the work in Baltimore under Dr. Coles Andrus extremely stimulating and Dr. William Milnor, with his scientific approach to the diagnosis of heart conditions, also was very helpful. The group in Baltimore in cardiology consisted of six or seven people at that time and there was a free interchange of ideas as well as intense interest in the postgraduate student. Dr. George Mirick, who was our Chief in Medicine at the Baltimore City Hospital at that time, had a considerable influence on me with his intense interest in the plans of his house staff as far as postgraduate training was concerned and he, more than anyone else, helped direct me along these lines.
>
> I came to Calgary in 1956 because at that time no one in this area was doing cardiology. I had the good fortune to come here at the same time as Dr. George Miller who had been trained as a cardiovascular surgeon and he and I were able to set up our dog

lab and investigative unit at the Holy Cross Hospital. We were on the ground floor in this area and beginning in 1958 had our catheterization unit going and were doing closed heart surgery. We developed our five-man team on the heart-lung machine and have been doing open-heart cases since 1961.

I would judge that I spend anywhere from twelve to fourteen hours a day in the subspecialty of cardiology in a consulting capacity. This gives very little time for other interests.

I suppose that I should tell you that cardiology has been my opportunity to gradually build a senior consulting practice which I doubt would have been possible in the general field of internal medicine.

In 1965, Dr. Morgan's bibliography consisted of four items. The first is on "Pericardial Tamponade, a Complication of Staphylococcus Pericarditis" (*C.M.A.J.*, 1964). The fourth item is "Coarctation of Aorta in Identical Twins," presented at the 1965 meeting of the Canadian Cardiovascular Society in Toronto.

Dr. Simon Jong Koo Lee, 21 July 1932, Seoul, Korea; Seoul National University, M.D. 57; F.R.C.P.(C) 63; F.A.C.P. 71; F.A.C.C. 71; F.A.H.A.

Dr. Lee followed an excellent program of preparation for his career in research, teaching, and practice of cardiology. Beginning with a rotating internship at Victoria Hospital, London, Ontario, in 1958, there followed senior internship in Pathology at the New Mount Sinai Hospital, Toronto (1959), senior intern in Medicine at the Victoria Hospital (1968), and at Westminster Hospital, London, Ontario (1961), resident in Medicine (1962), and Fellow in Cardiology (1962-64) at the Montreal General Hospital. In 1964-65, he worked at the Carolinska Institute, Stockholm as a Merck, Sharp, and Dohme Travelling Fellow.

In 1966, he settled in Edmonton. During 1966-69, he was Canadian Heart Foundation Senior Research Fellow in the Department of Medicine University of Alberta. In 1971, he was Associate Professor of Medicine and a member of the Active Staff of the University of Alberta Hospital.

Dr. Lee's bibliography grew to ten items between 1961 and 1971. All are on medical and surgical aspects of cardiovascular disease. In addition, between 1968 and 1971, he co-authored six published abstracts, the last of these with Dr. M. Harophongse on "The Effects of Nitroglycerine on the Coronary Sinus Flow in Man and Experimental Animals" (*Ann. R.C.P.S.C.*, 1970).

Dr. Lawther Logan, Yale University, B.S. 46; McGill, M.D., C.M. 50; M.R.C.P.(E); F.R.C.P.(C); F.A.C.P.; F.A.C.C.; F.C.C.P.; F.I.C.A.; F.R.C.P. (Edin.); F.A.H.A.

Dr. Lawther (Pat) Logan partially completed the questionnaire. After internships at the Montreal General and the Queen Mary Veterans hospitals, he obtained a British Council Fellowship and worked at the National Heart Hospital, London, England, 1953-55. This period was followed by a year as clinical associate in the Cardiac Department at the London Hospital. Before returning to Canada, he spent some time in Edinburgh. His postgraduate studies were completed with a year (1955-56) as Fellow in Cardiology at the University of Saskatchewan.

In 1965, he was Director of the Division of Cardiology at the Calgary General Hospital and Consultant to three other hospitals in Calgary. Dr. Logan did not comment on the special questions, nor provide his bibliography.

British Columbia

Dr. George Millington Woodwark, 27 April 1923, London, England; University of Cambridge, M.A.; Westminster Med. Sch. M.B., B.Ch. 47; M.R.C.P. (Lon) 53; Cert. Int. Med. R.C.P.(C) 60; F.A.C.C. 66.

After graduation in medicine, Dr. Woodwark had postgraduate training in several London hospitals, namely the Westminster, the Brompton, the Westminster Children's, and the National Heart Hospital. Of his career in cardiology he wrote a few laconic sentences in 1968.

> Cardiology entered by mistake. I took a job in chest diseases and as an after-thought the hospital also assigned me to Dr. Paul Wood's patients. I pioneered heart catheterization labs in four centres and was happiest away from research institutes, so I found Victoria ideal for my interest in community practice while working in a lab.

Before settling in Victoria in 1959, Dr. Woodwark practised cardiology in Salisbury, Rhodesia for five years and while there set up the first haemodynamic laboratory in Central Africa. He worked for one year at the University of Colorado before going to Victoria. His war experience included service with the Red Cross related to the liberation of Nazi victims in the Belsen Concentration Camp in 1945.

Through the good offices of Dr. Dennis Vince, additional information about his achievements in Victoria were obtained from Dr. Woodwark in 1983. Again he composed laconically:

> In 1958, three open-heart operations carried out under hypothermia by Dr. C. Whiteside (formerly Professor, University of Alberta).
>
> March 1960, heart catheterization laboratories opened at Royal Jubilee Hospital and St. Joseph's Hospital, Victoria, by Dr. G. M. Woodwark.
>
> 1967, coronary angiography begins on regular basis at Royal Jubilee Hospital.
>
> 1971, coronary ambulance manned by paramedics with radio telemetry of ECGS to both Victoria hospitals initiated using Saanich ambulance system.
>
> July 1973, first open-heart operation carried out in new unit under the direction of Dr. Richard T. Brownlee. A total of 2753 open-heart operations have been carried out in Victoria up to 28 February 1983.
>
> 1983, a second heart catherterization laboratory is under construction for Victoria General Hospital at Helmcken Road.
>
> Dennis, I would be happy to fill in any stories or details behind these rather bleak facts and dates but this may be all the basis that Dr. Segall needs for his historical account.

Dr. Donald Munroe added this comment about him. "Dr. Woodwark has made a major contribution to cardiology on Vancouver Island. In spite of the fact that there was no surgical capability there at the time, Dr. Woodwark developed a laboratory for cardiac investigation. His patients were referred to Vancouver for required surgery."

Dr. John Alan Osborne, 22 April 1922, Medicine Hat, Alta.; University of Alberta, B.Sc. 44; M.D. 48; Cert. in Int. Med. R.C.P.&S.(C) 51; F.A.C.C. 64; F.A.H.A. 66.

Dr. Osborne experienced rotation internship during his final undergraduate year, at the Royal Alexandra and the University of Alberta hospitals and at the latter hospital during 1948-49. He remained at the University Hospital the following year for internship in Medicine. In 1950-51 he began his career of training for cardiology with an appointment at the Institute for Medical Research at the Cedars of Lebanon Hospital in Los Angeles. In responding to the special questions he relates the story of the years 1950-53 in California and in England. In 1953-54 he was Assistant Chief of Medicine for Medical Education at Baylor University Hospital. He became Assistant Director of the Cardiology Department of Vancouver General Hospital in 1956 and Director in 1962. In 1968 he was Clinical Instructor at the University of British Columbia.

Osborne made the following comments about the special questions.

> My specialization in cardiology was determined primarily by opportunity rather than a clear-cut decision at some particular point. There were several aspects of internal medicine which I found appealing, but when I had an opportunity to spend a year with Dr. Myron Prinzmetal in Los Angeles ... the course towards cardiology was pretty well determined.
>
> I had very little difficulty in planning my specialized training since for the most part this was done for me, first of all by Dr. Kenneth Hamilton, who arranged the year with Dr. Prinzmetal. While with the Cedars of Lebanon group, Sir George Pickering visited Los Angeles and offered me a position with him for the following year, which I was able to accept when I received the Nuffield Travelling Fellowship in Medicine. While with Sir George at St. Mary's, I then had an offer to spend a year with Dr. George Griffith back in Los Angeles through a contact made with an American from Los Angeles who was also working at St. Mary's. Considering the difficulties many of my contemporaries had in obtaining the training they desired, I had a remarkably smooth course and at no time was I subject to the uncertainties as to where I would be the following year. As you can tell from my history, I have not engaged in private practice of cardiology so that I have never bought an electrocardiograph for myself. I have, however, been involved in the purchase of electrocardiographs for institutions, or hospitals actually since my year with Dr. Prinzmetal, and my participation was due to my interest in instrumentation.
>
> While I value the Canadian Cardiovascular Society as important in the medical community, I cannot honestly say that my membership has knowingly played any significant role in my career. I think it is true to say, however, that one has associations which can contribute to one's activities in a meaningful fashion without any particular knowledge that this influence actually exists.

Between 1946 and 1967 Dr. Osborne's bibliography grew to nineteen items, including co-authorship in two books, *The Auricular Arrhythmias* (Charles C. Thomas and Company, Springfield, Illinois, 1952), and *Accelerated Conduction: Wolff-Parkinson-White Syndrome and Related Conditions* (Grune and Stratton, Inc., New York, 1952). A considerable number of the articles are concerned with the biophysics of electrocardiography. Not many physicians can write authoritatively on this subject.

Dr. Doris Kavanagh-Gray, 15 September 1930, Carleton, Que.; University of Ottawa, M.D. 54; F.R.C.P.(C); F.A.C.P.; F.A.C.C.

Dr. Kavanagh-Gray did less travelling in acquiring her postgraduate training than her peers. Immediately after graduation she entered the Henry Ford Hospital where she had residencies in Medicine and Cardiology, in both Adult and Paediatric Departments, during the years 1954-1959. She then joined the staff of St. Paul's Hospital in Vancouver, and in 1971 when she updated her curriculum vitae, she was Chief of Cardiology at St. Paul's Hospital and the Children's Hospital, as well as Clinical Instructor at the University of British Columbia. She installed the haemodynamic laboratory and pioneered cardiac catheterization in these two hospitals. Dr. Kavanagh-Gray did not offer any comments on the special questions.

Early in her career as an expert in the study of haemodynamics, Dr. Kavanagh-Gray showed her awareness of the risks involved. The first article she published on haemodynamics is entitled "Complications of Left Heart Catheterization Using the Right Trans-Thoracic Approach" (*Am. Ht. J.*, July, 1958). The remainder of her bibliography which reached the number of 25 by 1970 contains a wide variety of subjects related to congenital and acquired cardiovascular disease.

Dr. Dwight Irving Peretz, 16 February 1931, Shanghai, China; University of British Columbia, M.D. 56, McGill, M.Sc. Exper. Med.; F.R.C.P.(C); F.A.C.P.; F.A.C.C.

Dr. Peretz had all his postgraduate training in Canada. He offers the major details in his response to the special questions.

> I was born in Shanghai, China and took my primary education there, moving to California where I took two years of high school and finished up my final year of high school in West Vancouver. I then attended the University of British Columbia,

taking three years of pre-medical training and entered the Medical School at that university, graduating with the M.D. degree in 1956. Following that, I went into general practice for four years with my father in West Vancouver. My father practises exclusively Internal Medicine although he is not certified and this gave me a great deal of interest in Internal Medicine as I had had even before going into medical school. I think that cardiology came into my mind about half way through medical school since I was particularly fascinated by the relative exactness of the diagnosis available in this specialty and also the tremendous advances coming about at the time I was training which allowed one to give a considerable amount of benefit to many of the patients with cardiovascular disease. Following the four years of General Practice I returned to train specifically in cardiology and since it was going to be a very expensive venture, I decided to take ten days off and fly to several of the major centres in the East. I was very impressed by the Royal Victoria Hospital, Montreal, and particularly with some of the personalities there, Dr. Arnold Johnson, Dr. Maurice McGregor and his wife, Margot Becklake, and Dr. Philip Hill. I think that this clinched it even over Boston, New York, Philadelphia and Toronto where I also visited. I spent two years (1962-64) at the Royal Victoria Hospital on the Cardiopulmonary Service, one year as a resident and one year as a Fellow doing catheterization and pulmonary function laboratory techniques, only to return to Vancouver for my fourth year which was divided between Pathology and Internal Medicine under Dr. Harold Taylor and Dr. R. B. Kerr. I then wrote the Fellowship in Internal Medicine. About this time I also wrote the American Board Examinations. It was fortuitous that just as I returned back to Vancouver, the Mr. and Mrs. P. A. Woodward Foundation was offering a considerable amount of money for the construction of a first-class Intensive Care and Coronary Care Unit and Dr. F. W. B. Hurlburt of St. Paul's Hospital asked me if I would get together with the architects to construct the Unit, equip it and run it and I have remained the Medical Director of the Unit since 1966 when it was built. We have published a number of papers out of this Intensive Care area in scientific journals.

When Dr. Peretz updated his curriculum vitae in 1972, he was Assistant Clinical Professor of Medicine at the University of British Columbia, Director of the Intensive and Coronary Care Unit at St.

Paul's Hospital, and Consultant in Cardiology at the Lions Gate Hospital.

The first item in Dr. Peretz's bibliography (25 items, 1955-72) is concerned with cardiology, entitled "Variant Angina Pectoris of Prinzmetal" (*C.M.A.J.*, 1961: 35, 1101). During his studies at the Montreal General Hospital, the Royal Victoria Hospital, and McGill University, he was involved in a number of projects related to the investigation of shock and resuscitation. He has also written a number of papers on the management of pacemakers and on clinical pharmacology.

In response to a request for information about the introduction of cardiac catheterization in British Columbia, Dr. Peretz wrote the following in November 1983.

> In 1954 Dr. John Osborne came to Vancouver and set up the first cardiac catheterization laboratory at the Vancouver General Hospital. Shortly after that he was joined by Dr. Max Walters. Cardiac surgery was carried on but without benefit of the open-heart technique. Dr. Harold Rice came to Vancouver from his position as a professor of physiology both at the University of Alberta in Edmonton and prior to that at the University of Manitoba in Winnipeg. He built the first heart-lung machine used in the lower mainland and that machine continued to be used until about ten years ago. Open-heart surgery was started at St. Paul's Hospital in 1957 after Dr. Doris Kavanagh-Gray came to that institution and set up a cardiac catheterization laboratory. It may interest you to know that she had to catheterize a dog with the medical advisory committee in attendance in order to convince them that such a procedure could actually be done! Doris carried the ball at St. Paul's for four years when I joined her as the second cardiologist on the staff at St. Paul's Hospital. In the meantime, the Vancouver General Hospital had acquired Dr. Mel Shaw and a host of other practising cardiologists and recently the staff of the University of British Columbia, Division of Cardiology, set up with Dr. Henry Mizgala as chief, brought in Dr. Harry Henning, Dr. Donald Ricci and Dr. Victor Huckell as research associates as well as consultants in cardiology.
>
> I started the first Coronary Care and Intensive Care Unit west of Winnipeg at St. Paul's Hospital in 1965. The doors actually opened in 1966. This unit was funded by the Mr. and Mrs. P. A. Woodward Foundation and has operated ever since that time, in 1983, separating into a separate Coronary Care and Intensive Care area.

After St. Paul's and the General Hospital had their cardiac catheterization and open-heart surgical units going, Shaughnessy Hospital, then the local military hospital, also established these same facilities. About 15 years ago, Dr. Tom Godwin opened a catheterization laboratory at the Royal Columbian Hospital but they have never done any kind of cardiac surgery there, all the surgery being referred either to St. Paul's or to the Vancouver General Hospital. You already have information about the set-up in the Victoria area.

About six years ago Dr. Denton Corrigall and then later Dr. Burt Brossuek joined Dr. Dorrance Bowers in Kelowna and set up a cardiac catheterization unit there as well. They do no cardiac surgical procedures.

I am sure that you do not wish me to go back to the era when cardiology essentially started in Vancouver with Dr. Fritz Strong, Dr. Jacob Freundlich, etc., since I am sure that you know far more about them than I do.

There are now about 30 procedural cardiologists in British Columbia with six cardiac catheterization laboratories and three centres for open-heart surgical procedures.

St. Paul's Hospital does more cardiovascular surgical work than any other hospital in Canada, quite an accomplishment for a 550-bed institution. We are largely oriented towards cardiological problems.

There is a very well set up network of continuing medical education in cardiology in this province with cardiologists going out to communities at their request through the University Continued Medical Education Division.

Ten or eleven cardiac surgeons perform about 30 open-heart surgical procedures a week.

Dr. Ronald John Forth, 28 October 1930, Toronto; McMaster University and University of Manitoba, B.Sc. 53; University of Manitoba, M.D. 60; F.R.C.P. C) 67; F.A.C.C. 70; F.A.H.A.

Before settling in Victoria Dr. Forth spent the years 1961 to 1968 at the Mayo Clinic. The first 56 months were spent in internship and residency in Internal Medicine and Cardiology and the remainder as Assistant to the Staff in 1964-65, and Consultant in Cardiology 1966-68. He joined the staff of St. Joseph's Hospital in Victoria in 1968 and held the post of Director of the Coronary Care Unit when he submitted his curriculum vitae in 1972. He was also Consultant to the Veterans Hospital in Victoria.

Dr. Forth made cogent and unique comments on the special questions.

I had an early interest in cardiology, but my goal initially was to be well trained in the entire field of internal medicine. Accordingly I took extra training in haematology and was considering joining the Mayo Clinic Staff in the section of pulmonary diseases when exposure to further cardiology training crystallized my interest in this field. I was then presented with the option at the Mayo Clinic of pursuing a career as a chest physician or taking more prolonged training with the object of joining the staff in cardiology. I selected the latter course, although it was involvement with more prolonged training and economic cost to myself.

I was fortunately given the opportunity to have a large say in the course of my training both in the field of internal medicine and subsequently in cardiology, perhaps because I was fortunate enough to be strongly considered for a permanent position on the Mayo Clinic Staff. I was given unusual leeway in obtaining such training as heart catheterization experience.

The influences that have led me to leave the Mayo Clinic practice of cardiology and come to Victoria, British Columbia, Canada are probably varied and my rationalization for this move involved the following factors. I was concerned about being too highly compartmentalized into a niche of cardiology practice in a big institution without continued experience in a broader type of cardiology practice. This was a particular concern to me as a young cardiologist recently out of training. I would have been more content to be compartmentalized into a specialized niche of cardiology after having a much broader clinical experience. It is a personal feeling that I have that there is a trend toward too early subspecialization both within the field of internal medicine and subsequently even within the subspecialty fields and in fact in large postgraduate training institutions it is hard not to be pressured into a highly specialized area very early in one's training.

Victoria, British Columbia offered an environment with a large patient population and it seemed to be an environment where cardiology practice could be developed without bureaucratic regimentation frequently found in large university hospitals and postgraduate training centres. This has been the case in Victoria and under the influence of my partner, Dr. George Woodwark, who started specialized cardiology practice in this area, heart catheterization was underway and coronary care units had been opened prior to my arrival, and I have been delighted that in this area we have been able to go ahead with full support from the medical community and financial backing from the business community to do the things in cardiology which we feel should be done. This has led to the development of very capable coronary care units in our two major hospitals. We have been able to bring about a concept of progressive coronary care using radio telemetry monitoring of ambulatory patients, a telephone monitoring system is used for following some 200 or more pacemaker patients, and I enjoy what I expected would be the practice here of doing a full range practice of consulting cardiology including office practice, hospital consultations, coronary care unit management, heart catheterization, coronary angiography, pacemaker installation. We are this year opening our open-heart surgery unit so that I have been very pleased with the development of cardiology practice in Victoria. I would say that for someone of my own personality, I appreciate the freedom to develop a cardiology practice, take part in fund raising, bring about the introduction of new technology, etc., without being involved in what I visualized to be problems of university politics.

The role of membership in the Canadian Cardiovascular Society has not influenced the development of my career to this point as my postgraduate training and professional contacts concerning new technology, etc., are largely in the United States.

The only item I miss in the location and type of practice that I am involved in is my former involvement with resident training. I thoroughly enjoyed this while I was a staff member of the Mayo Clinic. Here we are involved with intern training and we train our own Coronary Care Nurses. I enjoy this kind of work and it has taught me to have a high degree of regard for the capacities of nurses to engage in a much more responsible activity of medical care than would have been considered proper a few years ago.

I still miss the contact that I formerly had with residents in Internal Medicine and Fellows in the Cardiology Training Program. I found that very stimulating and of course it isn't available in this practice.

Dr. William Glenn Peter Friesen, 27 June 1937, Hague, Saskatchewan; University of British Columbia, M.D. 61; L.M.C.C. 62; F.R.C.P.(C) Int. Med. 68; F.A.C.C. 69.

Dr. Friesen began postgraduate training with an internship at the Detroit Memorial Hospital (1961-62), followed with two years of general practice. He then spent three years training in cardiology at the University of Oregon. In 1969 to 1972 he was on the staff of the University Hospital in Edmonton. In 1972 he was Assistant Professor of Medicine at the University of Alberta. In that year he moved to Victoria. These "bare bones" descriptions of his career after graduation acquire interesting flesh in his comments on the special questions.

In third year medicine at U.B.C. at the bedside teaching sessions, I found that I could hear the low pitched mitral diastolic murmurs and time the cardiac events better than my peers. I liked the diagnostic problem-solving in cardiac patients. Cardiologists were in a fast-developing and aggressive field and I loved dealing with emergency situations. I decided, however, to take two years of general practice before specializing so that I could be sure of this interest before making the commitment. The commitment was difficult because I knew it would involve having to take the F.R.C.P. Internal Medicine Exams, which is formidable.

After one year of general practice, I consulted with local internists in New Westminster, B.C. and my former teachers at U.B.C., then made application to the University of Washington in Seattle and the University of Oregon in Portland. My interview in Seattle was devastating. "You have three strikes against you, first, you didn't intern in a University Hospital, second, you didn't take a straight medical internship, and third, you went into the backwoods of medicine (general practice) where you could have forgotten all the good habits and learned bad habits." I then went to Portland and spoke with the Chairman of the Department of Medicine, Howard P. Lewis, a famous diagnostician who was a giant of a man in medicine and physically. He was most receptive and had received my excellent references and was a real gentleman during the interview. A few weeks later I received notice that I had been accepted into their program in Internal Medicine. That year I was one of three first-year residents accepted. Two years later I was accepted with two others into the Cardiology Program (Herb Griswold, Melvin Judkins and Albert Starr, the surgeon, were prominent teachers in the program).

I wanted to come back to the West Coast of Canada and do research cardiology but Vancouver was in a difficult position so I accepted a good position at the University of Alberta in Edmonton. With the recession, difficulties in obtaining research funds on a continuing basis, and restrictions in research facilities, I decided to leave the University of Alberta to practice cardiology in Victoria with Doctors G. M. Woodwark and R. J. Forth, both progressive cardiologists who have served the Island community in an excellent manner. An open-heart surgical centre is being planned for Victoria next year and having had experience with such centres I feel my contribution could be valuable to them. We hope to carry on some ongoing research in cardiac isotopes.

Dr. Friesen delivered his first paper at the meeting of the American Heart Association in San Francisco in 1967 on "Haemodynamic Comparison of Atrial and Ventricular Pacing in Postoperative Cardiac Surgical Patients." Between 1968 and 1972 he published eight papers on items such as Atrial and Ventricular Pacing, Right Atrial Electrocardiography, the Effect of Sublingual Nitroglycerine on Left Ventricular Volume, and Performance in Supine Patients with Coronary Artery Disease. This last item was the subject of a paper delivered at the meeting of the Canadian Cardiovascular Society in Saskatoon, October 1971.

CHAPTER TWELVE

Cardiovascular Surgery

The introduction of general anaesthesia and asepsis in the latter half of the 19th century initiated the present era in the practice of surgery. Vascular surgery began in the physiological laboratory of Professor Ivan Pavlov at the Imperial Academy of Medicine in St. Petersburg (Guthrie, 1912). There in 1877, Nicholai I. Eck performed the operation establishing a direct communication between the portal vein and the inferior vena cava which has come to be known as Eck's Fistula. This made possible eliminating the liver by next ligating the hepatic artery, in experiments designed to study metabolism with the liver functioning normally or with the liver excluded. Eck also suggested that such a fistula might be used to divert blood in cases of portal obstruction. However, this procedure came into use only in 1945 when Blakemore devised an efficient technique for establishing a sutureless communication using a vitallium tube. Thus, an end-to-end, intima-to-intima, approximation of the two veins made over the vitallium tube was fixed in place by tying a ligature around the veins at the points where there were ridges on the tube.

In 1897, John B. Murphy of Chicago had described a method of uniting a divided blood-vessel by invagination. In 1900, Carrel repaired a carotid artery which had been traumatized during removal of a tumour. In 1902, Floresco began experimental grafting of organs; in 1905, he reported that one animal lived for a month after one of its kidneys was removed and replaced by a kidney of another dog. Between 1900 and 1910, Alexis Carrel, Charles D. Guthrie, and their associates laid the foundation for effective vascular surgery which later came to be applied in cardiovascular surgery as other problems were solved, mainly those of maintaining normal respiration during thoracic surgery, those of anaesthesia, and of extracorporeal circulation. In his book on *Bloodvessel Surgery and Its Applications* (1912), Guthrie alludes to this work.

> In 1905, Carrel and the writer began experimenting with the anastamosis of bloodvessels in the Hull Physiological Laboratory of the University of Chicago, with a view, among others, of

making a complete study of transplantation of veins. Several series of experiments were undertaken in order to study the results of uniterminal and biterminal transplantations, and they were thoroughly successful. The technique previously studied by Bedard and Carrel, and by Carrel and Morrow in 1902, was first tried but very soon the endeavour to avoid penetrating the intima was discontinued, and its inclusion in the stitches as recommended by Dorfer was practised. Other modifications were developed until finally we developed a technique which is equally well adapted for arterio-arterial, veno-venous, or arterio-venous anastamosis and which gives uniformly successful results.... In 1907, both Carrel and the writer reported successful results from repairing divided bloodvessels with segments of bloodvessels from different species of animals. Carrel transplanted segments of dog's arteries into cats, two of five such operations being successful.

In the first decade of the twentieth century, the arterio-venous anastamosis technique devised by Carrel and Guthrie served to perform direct blood transfusions. C. W. Crile of Cleveland reported on the application of this technique in seven patients with good results, although no blood matching tests had been done; none were known at that time. Such tests were first suggested by Hektoen of Chicago in 1907, but the methods were first devised and used by Ottenberg of New York in 1911. This greatly reduced the frequency of post-transfusion reactions. The next forward step occurred on 27 March 1914 when Dr. A. Hustin, of Brussels, demonstrated citrate to be the appropriate anticoagulant, making possible indirect transfusions and establishing what is essentially the current method.

Thus, before the beginning of World War I, the technique for the treatment of vascular traumatic lesions and of performing blood transfusions with a high degree of safety existed. Yet neither came into use during that war, famous for the massive casualties related to the period of trench warfare. The management of vascular wounds in that war did not differ from what Korotkoff experienced in the diagnosis and treatment of such wounds during the Russian-Japanese War (1904-1905) (Korotkoff, 1910). Moreover, things were not much better during World War II. In 1946, DeBakey and Simione analyzed their experience with 2471 cases of battle injuries to arteries and declared:

> It is clear that no procedure other than ligation is applicable to the majority of vascular injuries which come under the military

> surgeon's observations. It is not a procedure of choice, it is a procedure of stern necessity for the basic purpose of controlling haemorrhage because of the location, type, size, and character of most battle injuries.

Suture repair was performed in only 81 cases; of these, only three were end-to-end anastamoses.

In 1974, Julius H. Comroe and Robert D. Dripps published their article entitled *Ben Franklin and Open Heart Surgery*. They sought to draw attention to the fact that basic science, in the course of which important discoveries are not infrequently made by serendipity, contributes greatly to progress in knowledge and technology. They reported on a poll conducted among the physicians and surgeons on the question, "What are the ten most important advances in cardiovascular and pulmonary medicine and surgery since 1945?" The list is headed by open-heart surgery. It is followed by 2) cardiac resuscitation, 3) intensive cardiovascular and respiratory care, 4) chemotherapy and antibiotics, 5) vascular surgery, 6) medical treatment of coronary insufficiency, 7) oral diuretics, 8) new diagnostic methods, 9) drug treatment of hypertension, and 10) prevention of poliomyelitis. They make the story of the evolution of open-heart surgery very interesting by tracing the discoveries, many by serendipity, retrospectively.

Once the pump oxygenator was constructed and used effectively by Gibbon, open-heart surgery took off. But Gibbon had enjoyed the availability of knowledge and techniques concerning anticoagulants, blood groups, blood storage (blood banks), basic knowledge about the diffusion of oxygen and carbon dioxide, synthesis of new materials which provided plastic tubes, bags, valves; knowledge which permitted arresting and restarting the heart beat, closed circuit anaesthesia, and muscle relaxants necessary for thoracic surgery, X-rays, electrocardiography, methods of measuring arterial and venous pressure, microbiology, etc. They composed a list of twenty-five bodies of knowledge essential for the full development of open-heart surgery. As for the instruments and apparatus required for cardiac catheterization in 1974, there were 12 different types of catheters, 11 items related to X-ray equipment, 9 electronic instruments, 5 items related to sterile equipment, 3 types of calculators, 11 drugs and chemicals, 5 instruments related to biochemistry, and 8 unique items from micro-syringes to gas sample collectors. The story of the origin and evolution of all these techniques and instruments, told in depth, would make for several interesting volumes.

His experience with a patient who died of pulmonary embolism led John Gibbon to undertake research for an apparatus which would permit him to by-pass the lung and thus make possible removal of the embolus (1931). It would appear he did not have open-heart surgery in mind. The birth of mirco-vascular surgery grew out of the experience of Julius Jacobson (1960). Two fellow members of the Faculty of Medicine of the University of Vermont asked him to perform a "guaranteed total denervation" of the carotid arteries of the dog, so that they could test the responses to drugs of completely denervated vascular smooth muscle. He cut the artery in two and then stitched it together again. This procedure required the use of a dissection microscope and thus led to the development of micro-vascular surgery. Carrel worked at the problem of suturing blood vessels because he wanted to transplant organs in order to study their metabolism, one at a time. These are a few of the illustrations which Comroe and Dripps mentioned to underline the fact that many of the basic requirements for open-heart surgery were discovered without this type of surgery being on the minds of the workers.

The following anecdote reflects the point of departure early in the twentieth century from which the new specialty of cardiovascular surgery developed. New technology in skilful hands performed operations which previously seemed impossible. Courageous pioneer patients accepted the risks. Those who died, as well as those who survived, made sacrifices which benefited the patients who followed. In the winter of 1926, as a postgraduate student in Paris, I frequently attended medical rounds, seminars, and lectures at the Hôpital de la Pitié because Professor Henri Vaquez, one of the leading cardiologists in France, was the chief there. His books were the most widely used French monographs on the cardiovascular system. At 11:00 o'clock one morning, Dr. Vaquez presided over a meeting attended by his staff and some foreign students. He had prepared an hour's talk on cardiac surgery, an unusual subject for 1926. He approached his comments about Cutler and Levine's recent work on mitral valve surgery, the main subject of the lecture, with a broad, friendly smile and remarked, "Les Américains osent tout" (the Americans will dare to do anything). On 24 May 1923, Drs. Cutler and Levine had demonstrated their first case of mitral valve surgery and made history. Cutler and Levine were in their early thirties — Levine was actually thirty-two. The occasion was a special meeting at the Peter Bent Brigham Hospital in the course of the celebration of the hospital's tenth anniversary. On 20 May, Cutler had performed the operation; four days later he and Levine brought the patient into the amphitheatre, and in the presence of visiting dignitaries, they demonstrated this patient, a little girl of twelve who had severe mitral stenosis, with severe shortness of breath, haemoptysis up to 300 cc's at a time. In the second paragraph of their published report of this case we find,

> It so happened that Professor Wenckebach of Vienna was visiting our clinic just at this time. The great enthusiasm and approval of the method of attack of the problem that he manifested and the considerable discussion and general interest that the presentation of the case aroused made it appear advisable to us to detail as exact a preliminary report as it is possible at the present time. So far as we can determine this is the only case on record of such a surgical attack upon mitral stenosis being complete.

Actually, Allen and Graham had performed a similar operation in 1922; the patient died at the time of the operation. Before doing the surgery on this child, Cutler and Levine had worked for two years in an attempt to produce mitral stenosis and test which operation would be the best one for its treatment, but they failed to produce mitral stenosis.

> None of these methods proved successful in our hands. The experience gained, however, proved of great value chiefly in educating us in the ability of the heart muscle to stand trauma, in the methods of restoring an injured heart to renewed function, and in our ability to locate and feel valves in a writhing, pulsating organ.

The anaesthesia was with a nasal catheter; intubation was not yet in vogue at the time. Following are some details of the actual surgical procedure:

> 0.5 cc of 1 to 1000 adrenalin solution was allowed to drip over the heart followed by some hot salt solution. At once the heart responded with vigorous and full contraction. This moment was seen as our most propitious one and rolling the heart out and to the right with the left hand the valvulotome, an instrument somewhat similar to a tenotome, or a slightly curved tonsil knife, and the one which we were most familiar with in our experimental work, was taken in the right hand and plunged into the left ventricle at a point of about one inch above the apex and away from the branches of the descending coronary artery where two mattress sutures had already been placed. The knife was pushed upwards about 2½ inches until it encountered what seemed to us

> must be the mitral orifice. It was then turned mesially and a cut made in what we thought was the aortic leaflet, the resistance encountered being very considerable. The knife was quickly turned and a cut made in the opposite side of the opening. The knife was then withdrawn and mattress sutures already in place were tied over the point at which the knife had been inserted. There was absolutely no bleeding.

On the second post-operative day there was pneumonia in the right upper lobe:

> In view of the severity of this complication the outlook at this stage looked very dubious, but the child responded well to digitalis and oxygen therapy and was greatly helped and comforted by her faith in the affection of her nurses, on whom the chief burden fell.

Such was the treatment of pneumonia in the absence of antibiotics. In the last paragraph of the report they state,

> The experience with this case, however, is of importance in that it does show that surgical intervention in cases of mitral stenosis bears no special risk and should give us further courage and support in our desire to attempt to alleviate a chronic condition for which there is now not only no treatment but one which carries a terrible prognosis. Unquestionably, further attempts would be made and our own experience in this instance has shown us technical improvements that should render a subsequent attempt both less hazardous as well as more hopeful for success.

About six weeks after this operation, Dr. Levine phoned us at the Massachusetts General Hospital, to ask if we could find a case of severe mitral stenosis that would be suitable for this operation. Dr. Paul White was in Europe, and as the one Cardiac Fellow, I was given the responsibility of responding. We had at that time a young girl of about twenty-one who had immigrated from Ireland and worked as a servant in one of the tall houses with four sets of stairs. She "broke down" and she too had haemoptysis with severe mitral stenosis. Dr. Levine came to see her and found her to be the right kind of case. She was transferred to the Peter Bent Brigham Hospital and was the fourth and last of this series of patients who had the operation. The first little girl lived for four and a half years; all three that followed died soon after the operation.

Professor Vaquez' attitude towards the mitral valve surgery at that time accentuated my sense of guilt in determining the fate of that young woman. Among the facts that were weighed in the balance before the decision to operate was made were those relating to the ethics of the choice. The social service worker reported that the patient had recently immigrated from Ireland to work as a house-maid. She served a family in a four-storey house: those stairs! She had been raised in an orphanage and had had no next of kin. This intensified my own sense of responsibility; was I substituting for her family? I could not clearly answer that question. What decision would I make if the entire responsibility were mine alone? The obvious fact was that the authoritative seniors were confident that she had a reasonable chance to enjoy better health after the operation. Nevertheless, her death has remained an event which has affected my judgement in the selection of "pioneer patients" who accept the great risks to their lives as the medical and surgical researchers, by trial and error, do their very best for these courageous self-sacrificing people and for humanity in general.

An analogous experience had a happier ending twenty-seven years later. In February 1950, Dr. Paul David and Dr. Edouard Gagnon of the Notre Dame Hospital in Montreal had made all the necessary preparations for performing their first mitral commissureotomy. They invited me to function as a consultant. I examined the patient, an orphan boy of seventeen without next of kin, who had the clinical signs of tight mitral stenosis and pulmonary hypertension with haemoptysis. In the light of the recent work of Dr. Charles Bailey (1946) and his colleagues in Philadelphia, I agreed that this patient should have the mitral commissureotomy done. I attended the operation and again admired the pioneer surgeon, Dr. Edouard Gagnon. The kaleidoscopic arrhythmias which appeared in the electrocardiograms during the operation caused me considerable anxiety. The patient had a somewhat stormy post-operative course; he made a good recovery, led an active life until he died at the Montreal Heart Institute on 5 March 1963, after reoperation for replacement of a Starr-Edwards mitral valve prosthesis which had been inserted in 1960 (Segall, 1970).

The operation which has gained the reputation as the first in the history of modern cardiac surgery belongs rather to thoracic surgery plus ligation of an artery, the patent ductus arteriosus. Cardiac surgery implies procedures related to acquired disease of pericardium, myocardium, valves, coronary arteries, and a wide variety of congenital cardiac anomalies. Richard H. Mead has assembled an interesting series of references about wounds of the heart throughout recorded history (Mead, 1961). They are mentioned in records of Egyptian history (3000 B.C.) and there are references to wounds of the heart in the Bible as well as in Homeric stories. Among these is one attributed to William Harvey. The patient was the eldest son of Viscount Montgomery in Ireland. When he was a boy he fell and hurt his chest, fracturing some ribs of the left chest. An abscess formed and discharged profusely. This discharge continued for some time. At the age of 18 or 19 he travelled in France and Italy and came to London. During all of this time a very large and open space "continued in his breast so that the lungs, as it was supposed, could therein be both seen and touched." Harvey was commissioned by King Charles I to examine the boy and bring him to be seen by the king. Harvey found that the heart itself was exposed and covered with a membrane. He "carried the young man to the king and both of them found the heart to be devoid of sensation as the boy was not aware when his heart was touched. The boy kept the area clean and covered and led a normal life." Coxe, who relates this story, then adds that Galen had pointed out the insensibility of the heart and included in his article Galen's account of that observation in Latin. Finally, Coxe stated that Cabriolus "had found in the heart of the thief that was hanged the remaining scar of the wound that had been cured, about two fingers long and about the thickness of a sixpence."

The achievements of progress in anaesthesia and in thoracic surgery after World War I made possible direct surgical procedures on pericardium and myocardium in the open chest during World War II. A convenient point of departure for tracing the evolution of modern surgical intervention in the interior of the heart is the article by Sir Lauder Brunton published in the *Lancet* in 1902 on "Surgical Operation for Mitral Stenosis." As it is an historical landmark it is here quoted in part.

> Mitral stenosis is not only one of the most distressing forms of cardiac disease but in its severe form it resists all treatment by medicine. On looking on at the contracted mitral orifice in a severe case of this disease, one is impressed by the hopelessness of ever finding a remedy which will enable the auricle to drive the blood in sufficient stream through the small mitral orifice, and the wish unconsciously arises that one could divide the obstruction as easily during life as one can after death. The risk which such an operation would entail naturally makes one shrink from it but, in some cases, it might be worthwhile for the patient to balance the risk of a shortened life against the certainty of a prolonged period of existence which could hardly be called life,

as the only condition under which it could be continued might to them be worse than death. But no one would be justified in attempting such a dangerous operation as dividing a mitral stenosis on a fellow creature without having first tested its practicability and perfected its technique by previous trials on animals. Accordingly I obtained a license and certificate a year ago in order to make the necessary experiments, but unfortunately other calls upon my time had not allowed me to do more than make trial experiments of dividing stenosed valves in diseased hearts from the post-mortem theatre and on healthy valves in the hearts of cats and also to try the proposed operation in the dead animals. It may be some months longer before I can get anything more done and I therefore think that it may be worthwhile to write this preliminary note especially as, after all, if the operation is to be done on man, it will be surgeons who will do it and they must, of course, make their own preliminary experiments, however fully the operation may be described by others, and each must find out for himself the method which he will employ in each particular case.

Brunton was then 58 years old. He had been a fertile source of new ideas and methods since 1867, the year before he wrote his graduation thesis on digitalis. At the age of 23, when he attended a man suffering from angina pectoris who also had a high systolic pressure, the idea occurred to him that by administering amyl nitrite the pressure would be lowered and this should relieve the pain. Thus this drug and nitroglycerine came to be introduced for the relief of angina pectoris; how it produces the relief remains a controversial subject of ongoing research. In the course of his long career Brunton devoted much attention to the physiology and pharmacology of the cardiovascular system. A week after the appearance of that article, Sir Arbuthnot Lane, a famous surgeon in London of that period, wrote a letter stating that some years previously Dr. Lawrison Shaw had suggested an operation for widening the valves in mitral stenosis and that he was still waiting for someone to refer a case to him. This letter brought forth a strongly worded letter from Dr. Shaw, in which he dubbed the procedure suggested by Brunton a useless operation, adding, "It is possible to do many things that are useless and some that are harmful." Some years later, Brunton recalled that he had intended to pursue that experimental work further but illness (blood poisoning) had interrupted his schedule. Twenty years elapsed before another important item appeared in the literature on this subject.

In 1922, Allen and Graham recorded their experimental work in search of a method of surgical treatment for mitral stenosis. They demonstrated that the best surgical approach to the mitral valve was through the left auricle. They were also committed to the technique of seeing the valves in order to see what they were doing. They invented a cardioscope whose efficiency Harken later referred to as very weak. None of their confrères would refer a patient to them for the operation. But eventually a country physician did refer a rather sick patient with mitral stenosis. Unfortunately, when they reached the point at which the cardioscope was being introduced, the patient suddenly died. It is important to note that in the course of his experimental work Allan found that where normal valves of the experimental animal were cut they did not "heal." He followed them for 11 months and at that time it was seen that the edges had become epithelialized but that no fusion had occurred.

The clinical notion that patients tolerate mitral insufficiency better than mitral stenosis received some support from the experimental observation of McCallum, Cushing, Branch, and Bernheim (1907-1909). Their experimental work at Johns Hopkins consisted of producing mitral insufficiency by using a cardiotome to cut away segments of the mitral valve. Their contribution consisted of demonstrating that if the size of the segment that was cut away was not too large, the animals made good recoveries and so were able to tolerate mitral insufficiency. They did not succeed in creating experimental mitral stenosis. In the 1920s the teaching of Sir James Mackenzie exercised great influence especially in the English speaking world. He believed that the principal determining factor in cardiac function in cases of valvular disease was not the degree of impairment in valve function but rather the degree of impairment in myocardial function. It required considerable courage of conviction to disagree with this generally held principle and to adopt rather the principle that in cases of mitral stenosis, if, as suggested by Brunton, the opening were widened, the function of the heart would be improved. Samuel Levine believed this and encouraged Cutler, the surgeon, to devise a procedure which would be effective. They decided to transform mitral stenosis into a certain degree of mitral insufficiency. Their first patient was referred to them by Dr. Maurice Fremont-Smith, the girl of twelve with mitral stenosis and insufficiency (see page 347). She made a good recovery but the operation did not appear to have improved her general condition. She died four and a half years later.

An interval of about a quarter of a century elapsed between the early abortive attempts at treating mitral stenosis surgically and the later successful operations which were performed in all parts of the world on large numbers of patients. Dr. Maurice Campbell studied the history of this era in search of an explanation for the long hiatus (1965). He drew attention to the important experimental work of Allen and Graham of St. Louis (1922). They identified the important fact that the approach to the mitral valve through the left atrium was the best and safest. Moreover, they concluded that this applied to man as well as to their experimental animal, the dog. Allen mentioned only the one operation on a patient referred to above. This rarely mentioned article is alluded to by Cutler and Beck (1929). In 1925, Soutar of London performed an operation on a fifteen-year-old girl who was referred to him by his medical colleague, Dr. Otto Leyton. He used the left atrial approach to the mitral valve and commented on the relative smoothness of the operation. Dr. Maurice Campbell qualified this by adding, "which may have been due to the skill of John Challis, the young anaesthetist at the London Hospital" (Campbell, 1965). Dr. Soutar found that the mitral orifice admitted his finger. He felt the regurgitation which he later described as resembling the jet of a fire hose playing on his finger. Because he wished to avoid the increasing degree of the regurgitation, he only broke down the adhesions which tethered the cusps. This patient lived for seven years but the operation did not have much beneficial effect. These surgical experiences in the 1920s could not have encouraged the physicians and the surgeons to persist in their trials. At that time the significance of the mechanical element *per se* was obscured by the general acceptance of Sir James Mackenzie's teaching which blamed the myocardium almost entirely for cardiac failure. Campbell states that up to the time of his death (1946), Sir Thomas Lewis, a leading authority in his time, still wrote about surgical treatment as follows: "I think it will continue to fail not only because the interference is too drastic but because the attempt is based upon what usually, at all events, is an erroneous idea that the valve is the chief source of trouble." Lewis marshalled clinical and experimental studies which rendered this plausible.

If history were to move smoothly then the next step, after Soutar, should have been made by John H. Powers, a young man who worked with Elliott Cutler as resident in surgery. Between 1929 and 1932 he published four papers in which he described the successful production of mitral stenosis in dogs, the surgical treatment by removing segments of the stenosed valve, as Elliott Cutler and Claude Beck did in six human cases after that first successful one. The six all died as a result of the operation. Powers (1929-1932) demonstrated experimentally very conclusively that the procedure was unphysiological and wrong. The experience of Soutar and the demonstration by Allen that cutting the mitral valve leads to persistence of the slit, prepared the ground for trying commissureotomy. This eventually was done by Charles P. Bailey in 1946, not as the result of a premeditated plan, as the following quotation from Richard H. Mead's book reveals.

> In 1945, Bailey operated on a patient with mitral stenosis expecting to bite out a piece of the mitral valve, but he tore the auricle and lost the patient from haemorrhage. In 1946, he operated on his next patient with the same object in view. He was planning to use a backward cutting instrument which he would pass through the left auricular appendage. During the operation the stenosis was found to be so severe that he could not pass his instrument through the valve. Quoting from Bailey's letter to me, "At that moment my medical men became a great help to me because they urged me to go ahead to make further efforts to relieve the valvular obstruction because the rapid deterioration of the patient on the operating room table augured ill for a survival.... In desperation, remembering Soutar's report, I inserted my finger through the auricular appendage, palpated the valve and pushed my finger through the diminished slit. Although the leaflets were calcified both commissures split well and I immediately appreciated three things. One was that there was now an opening many times larger than that which had existed previously. Second, the diastolic thrill which in this particular case was very prominent in the region of the valvular structure itself immediately disappeared. At the same time I was unable to recognize any regurgitant jet of blood from the valve. I was quite familiar with the digital feel of the regurgitant jet from my animal experimentation. I was, therefore, convinced that I had both relieved the stenosis and failed to produce any regurgitation. For about twenty-four hours postoperatively, the patient's condition improved remarkably and steadily. There was no clinical evidence of regurgitation; however, one day later she suddenly collapsed and died. From the post mortem examination it was clearly evident that both commissures had been split and considerable mobility of the leaflets had been accomplished. It was evident from the intact suspension of the valve leaflets that regurgitation had not been produced."

In 1949, I attended the annual meeting of the American Heart Association and among the scientific exhibits I stopped to see Charles Bailey demonstrating a patient on whom he had performed commissureotomy, on June 10, 1948. She was a mother of two children, a healthy-looking slender woman in her thirties who had benefited greatly from the operation. This convinced not only Bailey but many cardiologists and their surgical colleagues. Russell Brock (later Lord Brock) performed the operation of commissureotomy by the Soutar technique in September 1948 without knowing of Bailey's or Harken's experiences. Very soon the operation was being performed wherever there were thoracic surgeons.

Two surgical procedures drew universal enthusiastic acceptance from the very beginning — that is, after the first successful case was reported. The surgical ligation of a patent ductus arteriosus recorded by Gross and Hubbard in 1938 changed Dr. Maude Abbott's opinion, because it removed her fear that the operation might cause the development of bacterial endocarditis. Indeed, soon afterwards (1943) Touroff reported a case in which ligation of a ductus which was a site of bacterial endocarditis (streptococcus viridans) resulted in the cure of the patient; this, before the use of penicillin. The other procedure, the Blalock-Taussig operation, a more complex and daring surgical effort, met no adverse criticism. When Dr. Blalock delivered a lecture on this subject at the Royal College of Surgeons in London (1946) the hall was packed and he repeated the lecture within the hour to a similarly packed hall. This operation could not have been performed successfully without the relatively recent advances in the art and science of anaesthesia. The Blalock-Taussig operation set the stage for the explosive growth of cardiovascular surgery of the current era. Cases of patent ductus arteriosus and cyanotic congenital heart disease quite suddenly ceased to be the rarities that they had been when no specific therapy existed. The cyanosed patients taxed the diagnostic skills of the physicians. Cardiac catheterization and angiography joined the other methods of routine clinical examination to aid in sharpening diagnosis and the measurement of therapeutic results.

Cardiovascular Surgery in Canada

Wheresoever thoracic surgery was being done in Canada, there the foundation for the specialty of cardiovascular surgery was being laid down. In Montreal, the late Dr. Edward W. Archibald (1872-1945) pioneered both thoracic surgery and neurosurgery. He was born and educated in Montreal, graduating M.D. at McGill in 1896. In his third undergraduate year he went to Europe for a year; he spent one semester at the Medical School in Freiberg. Thus he learnt French and German while studying medicine. He spent three years of internship and residency at the Royal Victoria Hospital in Montreal and then a year in Europe mainly studying pathology with Ludwig Aschoff and general surgery with Von Mikulicz-Radecki. In 1886 Mikulicz had made surgical history when he was the first to perform resection of cancer of the esophagus and plastic transplantation of the esophagus. This revealed his interest in thoracic surgery which led him to suggest to his newly appointed assistant, Frederick Sauerbruch, in 1903, the prevention of pneumathorax in the course of thoracic surgery as a subject for research. Contact with Mikulicz may have influenced Archibald in choosing this field as one of special interest. In 1914 he published a paper on the role of surgery in the treatment of pulmonary tuberculosis. He spent the years 1915-1917 in France in the Canadian Army Medical Corps and in 1916-1917 published four papers on war surgery, one of which dealt with the employment of blood transfusion in war surgery and one with wounds of the lungs in World War I. He was a charter member of the American Association of Thoracic Surgery which was formed in 1917, and in 1931, when the *Journal of Thoracic Surgery* was started, he was appointed a member of the advisory editorial board. Archibald played an important role in the creation of the Montreal Neurological Institute. The late Dr. Wilder Penfield wrote a biographical sketch of Dr. Archibald in which he quoted the following excerpt from the address which Dr. Archibald gave in the opening exercises of the Montreal Neurological Institute in 1934.

> To gather knowledge and to find out new knowledge, is the noblest occupation of the physician. To apply the knowledge with understanding and with the sympathy born of understanding to the relief of human suffering is his loveliest occupation and to do both with an unassuming faithfulness sets the seal on the whole.

He was appointed Professor of Surgery in 1923 and Chief of Surgery at the Royal Victoria Hospital in 1928. Working in close harmony with Dr. Charles F. Martin, the Dean of the McGill Medical Faculty and the greatest catalyst for growth in McGill Medical School in the twentieth century, he promoted the education and development of young men and women who became leaders in thoracic and cardiovascular surgery while he continued his own special interest in surgery of the pancreas and the gastro-intestinal system with the assistance of another group of young professionals. Dr. Penfield also quoted a jingle which Dr. William Howell, the Anaesthetist-in-Chief of the Royal Victoria Hospital, wrote in celebration of the event when Archibald had just received an honorary degree from the University of Paris. It is quoted here to offer some clue to the character of the man.

You never published balderdash
You never sold your soul for cash
You never bragged and bluffed or lied
You never were puffed with pride

When I consider your career
It seems to me it's rather clear
Without those aids I don't see how
You ever got where you are now.

You've only brains and industry
Good breeding, kindness, modesty
The faculty of making friends
With ne'er a thought to serve your ends.

Sound judgement, sympathy and skill
To comfort and heal the ill.
Oh, Edward, you would be sublime
If you only could be on time.

(Penfield, 1958)

When Dr. Archibald retired in 1936, Dr. Francis A. C. Scrimger (1878-1937) succeeded him. Dr. Scrimger, the son of the Reverend John Scrimger, principal of the Montreal Presbyterian College, was educated at McGill, obtaining the degree B.A. in 1901 and M.D. in 1905 at the age of 27. After serving as house surgeon at the Royal Victoria Hospital he spent the year 1909 in Europe studying pathology in Dresden, and surgery with Professor Bier in Berlin. On his return to Montreal he joined the surgical staff at the Royal Victoria Hospital and McGill. He was closely associated with Dr. Archibald in experimental research. They co-authored a number of papers. In World War I he served at the front and for his heroic performance as a frontline medical officer which included saving the life of Captain (later Brigadier General) F. H. MacDonald, he was decorated with the Victoria Cross. The story of this event is well told in the obituary of Dr. Scrimger which appeared in the *Canadian Medical Associa-*

tion Journal of March 1937. He died very prematurely at the age of 57 (Lewis, 1969, p. 193).

Scrimger did make a significant contribution to early cardiac surgery in Montreal. In June 1932 he removed a 7 cm long darning needle which accidentally pierced through a young woman's chest during a fall and transfixed the heart. He exposed the heart with the same midline incision which Cutler used in 1923 to avoid entry into the pleura. The electrocardiogram was recorded before, during, and after the operation. In reporting this experience, Scrimger drew attention to what he learnt about cardiac surgery. "That the heart could tolerate compression of the auricle for five or six seconds and recover its rhythm." Manoeuvring the heart elicited ventricular ectopic tachycardia and also ventricular fibrillation with spontaneous return to sinus rhythm (Scrimger, 1933).

Louis Gross (1895-1937) and **Mercier Fauteux** (1898-1950)

The earliest Canadian pioneers of surgical therapy for coronary heart disease, both Louis Gross and Mercier Fauteux began to study the feasibility of bringing coronary heart disease within the range of surgical therapy in 1935, but from different points of departure, with different concepts of how to achieve the objective. During the three years from 1935 to 1937, Louis Gross and his colleagues published ten articles on the subject. Mercier Fauteux also published ten papers about his work: they appeared between 1940 and 1948. Both men died very prematurely, Louis Gross in the crash of the airplane "Mainliner," 17 October 1937, and Mercier Fauteux on 28 April 1950.

A brief profile of Louis Gross's career appears on page 59. Our search for information about Mercier Fauteux was rewarded by a brief obituary in the *Canadian Medical Association Journal* and a eulogy in the *Union Médicale du Canada*. The obituary in *C.M.A.J.*, June 1950: 62, 622 states:

> Dr. Mercier Fauteux, aged 53, internationally known for his research work on heart disease, died at his home early on April 28, following a brief illness. Dr. Fauteux was a brother of the Hon. Gaspard Fauteux, former speaker in the House of Commons and Mr. Justice Gerald Fauteux of the Supreme Court of Canada.

Dr. Edouard Desjardins (1897-1983) was a student at the same time as Fauteux, only one year ahead as he was indeed one year older. Dr. Desjardins practised as a general surgeon and exercised his fine literary talents in his spare time. He wrote on the history of nursing and of medicine and many necrologies of Quebec confrères. Archivist of the Royal College of Physicians and Surgeons of Canada, he became the Editor-in-Chief of the *Union Médicale du Canada* in 1970 and retired in 1978. His eulogy of Mercier Fauteux appeared in the *Union Médicale du Canada,* 1950: 79, 1506-08:

> Mercier Fauteux, 1898-1950
> Not many of his contemporaries could rejoice that at birth they had received so many generous gifts and magnificent attributes from Heaven. Mercier Fauteux is, in effect, from a very remarkable family; a grandchild of a premier of the province of Quebec, Honoré Mercier, and nephew of Lomer Gouin, who also served in that high office.
>
> Marvellously endowed, he showed his quick wit early in his career. When quite young, he manifested his keen powers of observation and also a taste for elocution. In 1918, he obtained the degree Bachelor of Science at Laval University. Together with his brothers, Gaspard and Aimé, he joined the C.O.T.C. [Canadian Officers Training Corps] and as his brothers registered in the Faculty of Dentistry, he matriculated into the Faculty of Medicine at the University on Saint Denis Street [Laval University of Montreal].
>
> As a medical student, he amuses his pals by imitating their professors so well that he fools them at times. He is so popular that he can afford the adventure of seeking election as vice president of the medical students. But in spite of his inherited talent for eloquence in public speaking he does not succeed in winning the honours after an epic campaign. In fact, if he had won, he would have allowed himself to be snapped up, as so many of his relatives did, by the passion for public service and he would have been lost to medicine.
>
> He obtained his medical doctorate with distinction in 1923, and he continued the internship which he began in the autumn of 1922 at the Hôtel Dieu of Montréal.
>
> He was especially interested in the periods he spent on the surgical service with Professors Amédée Marien and Eugène Saint Jacques. The latter, like Mercier Fauteux, is from St. Hyacinthe. The relationship of place created a strong bond between teacher and student. The teacher facilitated his getting a grant to study in Paris and promised him an appointment on his service when he would return.

The two years spent in France provided Fauteux with the opportunity to study anatomy with Rouvière, histology with Prenant, pathological anatomy with Roussy, cancerology with Regaud, and surgery under the tutelage of Pierre Duval and Ernest Desmarets.

On his return to the Hôtel-Dieu, the field of action seemed limited for him. A new hospital had just been opened. He applied and in 1928, he was appointed Surgeon-in-Chief of the Hôpital de Montréal Est. His duties were not very heavy, allowing him to continue his activities at the Hôtel-Dieu, including teaching. He made a favourable impression, so that at the age of 34, Mercier Fauteux moved from the Hôtel-Dieu to the Hôpital de Verdun of which he became the first Surgeon-in-Chief.

It is glorious that by 1932, less than ten years after graduation, Fauteux acquired a reputation and honours which were not usually met with at such a young age. To have arrived, almost effortlessly, with a prodigous dash, might have resulted, in many another, in arrest of ambition.

Mercier Fauteux was not content with this rise, so sought after by the majority of his colleagues; he needed something else. Fluent speaker, audacious operator, this was not enough! And from this moment, dated the entry of Fauteux into the experimental domain.

After witnessing a tragic event, a death from coronary artery thrombosis, he felt a keen desire to find an effective remedy for this condition. He gradually forsook the operating room and visited the pathology laboratory, approached cardiologists, familiarized himself with the electrocardiogram, got into contact with Boris Babkin [Professor of Experimental Physiology at McGill] and began to operate on dogs.

McGill opened its doors to him. First Archibald, then Gavin Miller [Professors of Surgery] encouraged him. His researches were prolonged, the experiments were difficult, the results collected at the beginning were difficult to apply to humans. Fauteux searched, he tried, he repeated until the day when all was ready for application to the patient.

Rumour outran events. Patients came full of hope. The results did not satisfy to a maximum degree; there remained many points to clarify. Elliott Cutler invited Fauteux to Harvard. He opened his laboratories to him, appointed him Research Fellow in Surgery and also Assistant in Surgery at the Peter Bent Brigham Hospital in Boston, titles and functions which he retained from 1942 to 1946.

Harvard is the sanctuary of medical science; researchers have a special, choice place there; they are well understood. They are not asked to produce quickly, but to do the job well. It did not matter whether the thesis was difficult to develop or whether it was finished promptly,the chiefs have confidence in their disciple.

The Surgeon-in-Chief Fauteux became a member of the unit on Cutler's surgical team. He devoted to pure science the long years of his sojourn in Boston, but he continued his own research on pericoronary neurectomy associated with ligature of the main coronary vein. He was searching for ventricular fibrillation problems associated with coronary artery disease. In short, he did not alienate himself from the original problem he tackled, namely, the surgical treatment of angina pectoris.

In 1946, he returned to McGill and the Royal Victoria Hospital for a rather brief stay.

The Université de Montréal opened a competition for a Fellowship in the Department of Cardiac Surgery, a section of general surgery. Fauteux presented himself and was appointed. He participated in teaching in the Department of Pathologie Medicale.

The transfer of his laboratory from McGill to the Université de Montréal took place gradually, and not without sorrow. In the meantime, Fauteux was invited to lecture abroad.

The Academie de Chirurgie de Paris put him on the program of its meetings. He was also invited by the Société de Chrirurgie de Lyons, in which he became a foreign corresponding member.

Those who heard him were greatly impressed, as the French surgeons who listened to him in Paris or Lyons reported, and as soon as they arrived in Montreal, they lost no time in seeking to meet him. Professor Réné Fontaine of Strasbourg, very much interested, attended many operations Fauteux performed in 1945 and took an active part in some.

The Société Médicale des Hôpitaux Universitaires de Quebec, the Association des Médicins de Langues Française, the great majority of our scientific associations did not look down upon our compatriot researcher. The name of Mercier Fauteux is inscribed everywhere. It would have been strange if one who was invited by American universities and the principal French surgical society, would be ignored in his home territory.

On the contrary, he was well received by the Royal College of Surgeons of Canada, who granted him a Diploma of Honorary Lecturer.

The passage of time is required in order to assess the value of a therapeutic procedure. Beck and his associates are better able than I am to appreciate the capital work of Mercier Fauteux.

But even if he made a minuscule contribution to cardiac surgery, this would be a great deal, especially since very few of us achieved fame as pioneers, initiators or precursors in Medicine or Surgery.

To reach a new height, Mercier Fauteux, of his own accord, chose the arid road, the difficult way, the route seeded with traps; at 34, he could have considered himself as having arrived at the destination of his career, and proceeded to accumulate money, but he preferred to start again and he left us on 28 April at the age of 52, on the eve of a future which would bring gratitude, too late for him but early enough to compensate his family for the sacrifices he imposed on them for the benefit of science.

May Madame Mercier Fauteux and her sons find here the expression of our deep sympathy.

EDOUARD DESJARDINS

When Louis Gross began to study surgical therapy of heart disease, he was Director of Laboratories at the Mount Sinai Hospital in New York City. The experimental procedure reported by Robertson (1935), ligating coronary veins in stages to produce vascular anastomoses which render the heart less vulnerable to coronary artery occlusion, led Gross and Blum to raise some questions (Gross, 1937). As the coronary artery occlusion was also performed in stages, was this gradualness responsible for widening arterial anastamoses? Secondly, would another method of widening anastamoses, namely, ligating the coronary sinus, produce equally good protection against infarction by arterial occlusion? They compared the effects of ligation of the anterior descending branch of the left coronary artery in dogs without previous ligation of the coronary sinus and in a group of dogs in whom the coronary sinus was first ligated. The former dogs all had evidence of infarction and the latter showed good evidence of a vasodilation by injection studies and almost none of infarction.

An earlier article by Blum and Gross appeared in 1936, entitled "Technique of Experimental Coronary Sinus Ligation." The early difficulties encountered and how they were overcome by the development of a good method of occluding the coronary sinus is the subject of this paper (Blum and Gross, 1936).

The third paper by Gross, co-authored with Gertrude Silverman and Arthur M. Master, dealt with electrocardiographic changes following coronary sinus occlusion in the dog's heart. Significant gross changes such as inversion of T waves, notching, and change in axis of QRS usually resulted from sudden complete or partial occlusion. Restoration of normal pattern usually evolved in the course of two to four weeks. The authors suggest that the changes could be due to temporary injury to myocardium related to oxygen insufficiency due to venous congestion (Gross, Master, Silverman, 1936).

Also, in 1936, an article appeared on haemodynamics following experimental coronary occlusion in dogs, co-authored with Milton Mendelowitz and Gerhard Schauer. The principal conclusion of this well-controlled study is that "following left anterior descending coronary branch ligation, in the open or closed chest there is an immediate appreciable fall in average cardiac output and also a delay in cyanide circulation time" (Gross, Mendelowitz, Schauer, 1936).

The fifth article was presented for publication in July 1936 and appeared in January 1937 entitled "Experimental Attempts to Increase the Blood Supply to the Dog's Heart by Means of Coronary Sinus Occlusion," co-authored with Lester Blum and Gertrude Silverman. This essay marshals evidence which casts much doubt on the value of pericardial adhesions for increasing the blood supply to the heart. "The well-known clinical observation that anginal pains not infrequently disappear during an attack of right-sided heart failure, led one of us to the thought that increased tension in the coronary sinus might accomplish the same result." This observation formed the principal basis for studying the effects of coronary sinus occlusion. The experiments reported in this article led to the conclusion that "it is desirable to produce a partial or a gradual occlusion in order to lower the mortality rate both of the initial procedure as well as of subsequent sudden arterial occlusion" (Gross, Blum, Silverman, 1937).

The next four publications, all in the *American Heart Journal*, appeared in June, July, and December 1937. They form a series devoted to various aspects of the haemodynamics of experimental coronary artery occlusion. The first three articles are co-authored with Mendelowitz and Schauer. The first publication deals with open chest experiments, the second with closed chest, and the third, with denervated heart experiments. The chief conclusion of this work is stated in the third article, "The ligation of the left anterior descending coronary branch in the dog is followed by cardiogenic hypokinetic circulatory failure and left ventricular congestive cardiac failure. The hypothesis that the decrease in minute volume is neurogenic is considered with some reservations, unsubstantiated."

The fourth in the series examines the effect of stellate ganglionectomy and concludes that this procedure does not affect the size of the infarct, but it tends to reduce immediate mortality and frequency of ventricular fibrillation.

The tenth article was published posthumously; co-authored with Bension Calef, it dealt with changes in the electrocardiogram following sudden occlusion of the left anterior descending coronary branch under various experimental conditions. Among their conclusions, they found no direct correlation between electrocardiographic abnormalities and size of infarct (Gross and Calef, 1937).

Louis Gross participated actively in the 1937 annual meeting of the Canadian Medical Association in Ottawa. An important feature of this event was the large number of scientific exhibits. His exhibit was entitled "Experimental Studies of the Blood Supply to the Heart in Relation to Coronary Occlusion." The exhibit consisted of charts, drawings, photographs, and roentgenograms which illustrated how the heart compensates for stenosis of coronary arteries. The physiological experiments in search of methods for increasing coronary arterial flow and myocardial blood were depicted. The volume of the *Canadian Medical Association Journal* for 1937, number 36, lists all the exhibits; Gross was awarded the first prize. The same volume also contains his obituary, on page 609. It is futile to speculate what he might have achieved if he had lived to continue working in this field, as he fully intended.

Mercier Fauteux began his experimental work in 1935, but his first publication in 1940 did not deal with his own experience. The article entitled "Positions Actuelles du Traitment Chirurgical de L'Angine de Poitrine" (*Un. Méd. Can.*, 1940: 69, 829-837), consists of a review of the literature and his opinions of the status quo. Concerning the physiological pathology, he states: "Mais quelles que soient les formes recontrées, un fait demeure constant et propre à chacune d'elles; un trouble de l'irrigation myocardique est à leur origine ou devient leur consequence immediate." (But whatever forms in which it [angina pectoris] is met one fact remains constant and unique in each case: a disturbance in myocardial irrigation is at their origin or becomes their immediate consequence." He regards the reports of surgical therapy by denervation, or by revascularization methods of Shaughnessy or Beck, as inconclusive but worthy of further exploration by well-designed protocols with adequate controls and in numbers sufficient to render statistically significant conclusions.

In October of 1940, he delivered an address before the Société

Médical de Montréal on "Les Conditions de la Recherche Scientific en Médecine" (The Conditions of the State of Scientific Research in Medicine). He deplored the polarization of the philosophers who attributed minor significance to experimental techniques and rational deductions, and the scientists who regarded these as paramount. He devotes much discussion to Claude Bernard as a role model. At one point he quotes him, "Nos idées ne sont que des instruments intellectuels qui nous servent à pénétrer dans les phénomènes; il faut les changer quande elles ont remplie leur rôle, comme on change un bistouri émoussé quand il a servi assez longtemps" ("Our ideas are only intellectual instruments which serve our penetration into phenomena; they must be changed when they have fulfilled their roles, as one changes a blunt scalpel which has been in use a long time").

The first report of experimental work, performed at McGill in Dr. Boris Babkin's Department of Experimental Physiology, appeared in 1940: "Experimental Study of Surgical Treatment of Coronary Disease" (*Surg. Gyn. Obst.*, 1940: 71, 151-155). Fauteux begins with quoting the work of Oppel (1913) and others who demonstrated the beneficial effect of ligating the accompanying vein when it is necessary to ligate an artery of a limb. He quotes Leriche who suggested that partial arteriectomy, which is so beneficial in the treatment of impaired arterial flow in the limbs, might also be effective in the coronary circulation. In a well-controlled study he demonstrated that ligation of the vena magna cordis before resection of a portion of the ramus descendens of the left coronary artery prevented death of the dogs, both in acute experiments and in dogs who had the vein ligated about a year before the arterial resection was performed. He also repeated the experiments reported by Gross in 1937. He reports a high mortality from coronary sinus ligation and concludes that ligation of the vena magna cordis is preferable. In the last paragraph he states that the results of these experiments suggest that in cases properly selected, coronary vein ligation may be expected to act as a preventive measure against a second attack of coronary thrombosis and also to improve the coronary circulation sufficiently to relieve the pain of angina of effort.

The report of the first patient he treated surgically at the Royal Victoria Hospital for angina pectoris is co-authored with J. H. Palmer (1941). The patient, a man of 54, who had had one infarct and experienced typical pain with very little exertion or by simply drinking cold water, benefited very greatly. Five months after the operation he could walk five miles without any discomfort. The operation was performed in April 1939. An addendum to the report states that during the year 1939-1940, five more cases had been treated with ligature of the vena magna cordis and the results would be reported at a later date.

Fauteux worked in Boston during the years 1942 to 1946. In 1943, he reported on experiments designed to test whether the nerve supply to the heart plays a role in initiating ventricular fibrillation and to search for the trigger mechanism that is involved. He concluded that myocardial ischaemia alone is not the cause of fibrillation. He found evidence which led him to state that the increase in intra-arterial pressure about the point of sudden occlusion initiated the neurogenic mechanism which produces ventricular fibrillation. The combination of pericoronary neurectomy plus ligature of the great coronary vein results in the maximum protection against death from ligature of coronary artery (Fauteux, 1943). This paper bore the title "Etudes expérimentales sur le traitement chirurgicale des coronaires (*Un. Méd. Can.*, 1943: 72, 1260-1262).

As one might expect it was followed in two years by "La Neurectomie Péricoronarienne Associé à la Ligature de la Grande Veine Coronaire dans le Traitment de Certaines Formes de la Maladie Coronarienne" (*Un. Méd. Can.*, 1945: 74, 425-431). He begins by reminding the reader that since 1935, he has had faith in the hypothesis that the three elements — mechanical impairment in blood flow, neurogenic vasoconstriction, and irritation of arterial sensory nerve fibres — are intimately connected so that they probably never function one at a time, but always in concert. He adduces arguments in favour of adding pericornary neurectomy to the surgical treatment of angina pectoris. The virtue of ligature of the great coronary vein is demonstrated in his report of the ten cases that had this operation between 1939 and 1944. The first patient, who had the operation in 1939, died two years later. The histological picture of the vasculature in the myocardium was exactly like the pattern demonstrated by Louis Gross in dogs after ligature of the sinus venosus. Seven patients were alive, all able to work and free from the pain they had before the operation. Some had relatively mild chest discomfort at times. At the end of this article, he reports in great detail the operation he performed in a man of 45, combining neurectomy and ligature of the great coronary vein in September 1944, about seven months before the publication of the article. The patient had become free of pain (Fauteux, 1945).

In November of 1945, he reported on experimental studies which confirmed the effectiveness of these surgical procedures and he describes a second case, a man who had angina pectoris, in whom the procedure was performed in June 1945.

The next publication summarizes the achievements up to 1945 and contains a detailed account of that first patient who had the operation in September 1944. As it appeared in the *American Heart Journal,* 1946: 31, 260-269, this article reached the specially interested audience more directly than the articles published in the *Union Médicale du Canada.* In the same year, again with Swenson, he published an article in *Archives of Surgery,* 1946: 53, 169-181, which contains essentially what he had previously written in French about pericoronary neurectomy for abolishing anginal pain in coronary disease. In the same year, he reported on an experimental study on the effectiveness of various procedures designed to prevent the occurrence of ventricular fibrillation during the cardiac surgery. He was able to demonstrate that the combined procedure, ligature of the great coronary vein and neurectomy, tends to eliminate reflex "irritation," and tends to prevent the initiation of ventricular fibrillation by elements which do produce it when this measure is not performed (Fauteux, 1946).

In April 1946, he delivered a paper on "Surgical Treatment of Angina Pectoris" at a meeting of the American Surgical Association. He marshalled the evidence in favour of the combined operation mentioned above and reported his experiences with 16 patients who had the operation since September 1939. Eleven who were alive in 1946, one six years after the operation, were all free from angina pectoris or the degree of pain was greatly diminished (Fauteux, 1947).

One month later he delivered a paper at the meeting of the American Association of Thoracic Surgery, on cardiac resuscitation. He reviewed the literature and cited his own experience with more than 200 experiments on dogs. He describes one human case of paroxysmal ventricular fibrillation of brief duration which was documented by electrocardiograms during cardiac surgery, a rare event in 1946. This essay describes the state of the art of cardiac resuscitation at the dawn of the current era. His paper elicited questions and comments by distinguished pioneers of cardiothoracic surgery, Evarts A. Graham, John H. Gibbon, Claude S. Beck, Clarence Crafoord. Otto Brantigan, of Baltimore, described a "rather unusual case of cardiac resuscitation in a 24-year-old white girl." At the end of the operation for removal of the right upper lobe of the right lung, cardiac arrest occurred. The intratracheal tube was in place and the lungs were kept well inflated. Ordinary cardiac massage produced only a few transient beats. It was decided to massage more vigorously. "One hand was placed posteriously under the heart and the other on the rather pliable sternum." Dr. Brantigan and his assistant took turns and after thirty-five minutes of vigorous massage, the heart began to beat normally and the blood pressure rose to normal. The patient recovered well, had no complications and had a normal convalescence. This unique experience belongs in the history of resuscitation as a precursor of the cardiac compression technique devised by Kouwenhoven, Jude and Knickerbocker, which has gained wide popularity known by the initials CPR, cardiopulmonary resuscitation (1960). Fauteux makes a strong plea for adequate preparation with the required instruments and drugs in the operating room for the contingency of cardiac arrest or ventricular fibrillation. He urged that "every operating room should be equipped with a good automatic respirator, an electrocardiograph, a defibrillator and the essential drugs." A pacemaker was on its way and would be added by Callaghan and Bigelow (1951) and by Paul Zoll (1952).

The last paper he wrote in this series reflects the methodical innovator. Its title is "Chirurgie Intracardiaque" (*Un. Méd. Can.*, 1947: 76, 1036-1048). The first paragraph tells what he had in mind.

> Il ne fait aucune doute que, s'il était possible d'entrer dans une cavité du coeur sous le contrôle de la vue et des doigts et d'y travailler le temps nécessaire sans risques sérieux, un pas considérable serait réalisé dans le dévéloppement de la chirurgie intracardiaque.
>
> [There is no doubt that if it were possible to enter a cavity of the heart under control of direct vision and of fingers, and to work there during a necessary period of time without serious risks, then a very considerable step would be realized in the development of intracardiac surgery.]

Of the eleven references in this paper, the tenth is on "Temporary Arrest of the Circulation to the Central Nervous System. Physiologic Effects," by L. W. Weinberger, M. H. Gibbon, and J. H. Gibbon (1940). These authors found that in cats, no animal survived after occlusion of the pulmonary artery for between 8 minutes, 45 seconds and ten minutes, 15 seconds. Fauteux carried out his study during 1945-1946 when he worked in the Harvard Laboratory of Experimental Surgery. He chose to work with dogs. He arrested circulation by obstruction of both venae cavae (including the azygos vein) or by obstruction of the pulmonary veins. He performed intracardiac procedures such as section of a valve. He resuscitated hearts after fibrillation or standstill set in. He measured the time between the beginning of obstruction and onset of cardiac arrest. He explored the problems and the methods of solving them. Was he aware of studies by Gibbon, by Lillehei, and others in search of a method of extracorporeal circulation? Nothing in this article would indicate a positive reply to this question.

Mercier Fauteux would have been one of the first, if not the first in Canada, to perform mitral commissureotomy and a little later, intracardiac surgery.

Dr. Fauteux's career ended at about the time when some of the new generation of thoracic surgeons were becoming cardiovascular surgeons, and within a few years, would be performing heart-lung preparations on their patients. The story of the spread of cardiovascular surgery into every region of Canada can be gleaned best by reading the minibiographies of the men who pioneered the new techniques. Their responses to the special questions contain the essential available facts and describe the mood of the times during that quarter of a century, about 1945 to 1970.

The minibiographies are presented in groups according to the provinces from east to west and in each group according to year of M.D. graduation.

Nova Scotia

Dr. Frederick Gerard Dolan, 19 February 1926, Dominion, Nova Scotia; St. Francis Xavier, B.Sc. 47; Dalhousie, M.D., C.M. 51; F.R.C.S.(C) 55.

The medical and surgical cardiologists in Halifax served the needs of all four Maritime provinces to a large extent. Some patients sought health care in Boston, or Montreal, or Toronto.

Dr. Dolan began his postgraduate training in surgery in Halifax at the Camp Hill and Victoria General Hospitals. In 1954, he decided to train in thoracic and cardiovascular surgery. This he accomplished at the Toronto General Hospital (1954-1955) and at the Hospital for Sick Children in Toronto (1955-1956). At the time that he completed the questionnaire in 1968, he was assistant Surgeon at the Victoria General and at the Children's Hospital in Halifax, and was also Assistant Professor of Surgery at Dalhousie University.

Dr. Dolan did not supply a bibliography; however, his name appears as co-author of three articles, one with Dr. Bigelow and two with Dr. Mustard. The first item is "The Effect of Hypothermia upon Risk of Surgery" (W. G. Bigelow, F. G. Dolan and F. W.

Campbell, *Bulletin de la Société International de Chirurgie,* 1955). The other two articles with Dr. Bigelow and colleagues deal with surgical treatment of constrictive pericarditis. The first article, written with Dr. Mustard, is "The Surgical Treatment of Total Anomalous Pulmonary Venous Drainage" (*Ann. Surg.*, 1957: 145, 379-387). The second article is on "Congenital Diverticulum of the Left Ventricle of the Heart" (W. T. Mustard, J. W. Duckworth, R. D. Rowe, and F. G. Dolan, *Can. J. Surg.*, 1958: 1, 149-153).

Dr. Dolan belongs to the generation of specialists in cardiovascular surgery who chose their careers when facilities for training had become available in Canada. He had all his postgraduate education for both adult and paediatric cardiovascular surgery in Toronto. As he served all the Maritime provinces in the general and in the children's hospital, he was well prepared for the work he was called on to do.

Quebec

Dr. Arthur Martin Vineberg, 24 May 1903, Westmount, Montreal; McGill, B.Sc. 24; M.Sc. (Biochemistry) 28; M.D., C.M. 28; Ph.D. (Experimental Physiology) 33; F.R.C.S.(C); F.A.C.S., F.A.C.C., F.A.H.A., F.A.C.C.P., C.P.S.Q. Thoracic Surg. 50.

In the course of premedical studies which began in 1920, Dr. Vineberg engaged in biochemistry research on amino acids; during the early years as a medical student, he continued this work and earned an M.Sc. During the last two years of the medical course he worked as "student assistant" with Dr. Edward Archibald who exercised a benevolent and inspiring influence on him. This led to his adoption of thoracic surgery as his specialty.

His postgraduate studies began with an internship in surgery at the Presbyterian Division at the Bellevue Hospital in New York (1928-1929). Supported by a Rockefeller Fellowship, he devoted the following year to experimental surgery at McGill, and the next year he served with Dr. J. C. Meakins in the Department of Medicine at the Royal Victoria Hospital. In the two years 1931-33 he had a residency in surgery with Dr. Edward Archibald as his chief. He followed a course of studies and experimental work during the years 1929-1933 which earned him the degree Ph.D. in physiology. In clinical surgery he treated pulmonary tuberculosis at the Mount Sinai Sanitorium and at the Grace Dart Hospital as well as at the Royal Victoria where he also did some general surgery and, emulating his chief, Dr. Archibald, he continued experimental research.

This program was interrupted during his service in the army but it was resumed when he re-entered civilian life.

In his minibiography Dr. Vineberg tells the story of how his studies of myocardial revascularization began.

> It was while I was a demonstrator in anatomy at McGill, 1935-42 that I became aware of the internal mammary arteries — how close they are to the heart. I was always wondering whether if they could be placed in the heart for myocardial revascularization. This idea apparently came to me in 1927, following a lecture in pathology given by the late Dr. H. Oertel. I had forgotten about this episode and was reminded of it by Dr. Eric McNaughton, surgeon at the Montreal General Hospital. Dr. McNaughton and I had just finished a wrestling match in the old gym. After a shower, I said to him: "You know, Dr. Horst Oertel said coronary artery disease involved the surface coronary arteries primarily, rarely their branches lying in the myocardium, except in patients with high blood pressure and severe diabetes." It was at this time that Dr. McNaughton reminded me that I had suggested: "Why can't we put the internal mammary artery into the heart muscles and bring the blood directly to the non-diseased myocardial arterioles?"

After discharge from the army medical corps in 1945, Dr. Vineberg resumed his career and among other things started to investigate myocardial revascularization in the McGill Department of Experimental Surgery. His interest in this subject was triggered by witnessing his father's fatal illness with angina pectoris and myocardial infarction in 1930-35. By 1950 the experimental evidence justified performing the operation of implanting a mammary artery in ventricular myocardium in a patient. By 1962 he added supplementary sources of blood with epicardiectomy and a free omental graft. In his minibiography he states, "Over 265 operations have been performed with excellent long-term results."

From the style in which he wrote his minibiography there emanates the image of an ever-enthusiastic person with a fertile imagination and a corresponding capacity for engaging in hard work, during long hours each day. In his late seventies the tempo had not changed from what it was in his forties. Nor had his conviction that the internal mammary artery implant is superior to any other presently available technique for myocardial revascularization, including the saphenous by-pass operation.

Dr. Vineberg submitted a detailed curriculum vitae together

with his bibliography. At McGill he rose to the position of Associate Professor of Surgery. There are longish lists of honours bestowed and special lectures he was invited to deliver in many cities of North America and some also in Europe. He was involved as founder or co-founder of four departments of cardiovascular surgery, namely at the Queen Mary Veterans Hospital, the Jewish General Hospital, the Montreal Institute of Cardiology and at the Royal Victoria Hospital where he was founder and director of the Sub-Department of Cardiac Surgery. In the last paragraph of his minibiography he states:

> I might add that during my time of activity I trained twenty-two young men a few of whom are full professors of surgery across the United States. Of the twenty-two, seventeen went through the Department of Experimental Surgery, sixteen received their M.Sc. and one a Ph.D. in experimental surgery.

Between 1930 and 1972 Dr. Vineberg's bibliography grew to 122 items. The first article related to the cardiovascular system, No. 21, is also the first on myocardial revascularization: "Development of anastamosis between the coronary vessels and transplanted internal mammary artery" (*C.M.A.J.*, 1946: 55, 117-119). The first clinical approach to this subject appears in an article co-authored with a pupil, Paul Niloff, "The value of surgical treatment of coronary artery occlusion by implantation of the internal mammary artery into ventricular myocardium" (*Surg. Gyn. Obst.*, 1950: 91, 551-561). In the 1950s, Dr. Vineberg performed the Smithwick operation for the surgical treatment of hypertension. He wrote about this subject in a chapter on cardiac surgery which he contributed to the book edited by H. F. Moseley (Mosby, 1952). Item No. 37 appears to be the first clinical report on the Vineberg operation, "Internal mammary artery implant in the treatment of angina pectoris: A three year follow-up" (*C.M.A.J.*, 1954: 70, 367-378). Interspersed among the articles on myocardial revascularization, there are such items as "Report of a case of successful operation for stenosis of common pulmonary vein (Cor Triatriatum)," co-authored with Osman Gialloreto (*C.M.A.J.*, 1956: 74, 719-723). The first report of open heart surgery is co-authored with A. R. C. Dobell and J. Guteluis, "Mitral Insufficiency, Report of an adult case treated with open heart surgery" (*C.M.A.J.*, 1958: 79, 273-275). His published book on myocardial revascularization by arterial/ventricular implants contains an extensive bibliography on this subject (Vineberg, 1982).

Dr. Georges Etienne Cartier, 27 November 1907, Montreal; Université de Montréal, M.D., 34; Certif. R.C.S.(C) 45; C.P.S.Q. 50.

Dr. Cartier did not mention details of his postgraduate training. At the Hôtel-Dieu of Montreal, he became the Chief of the Department of Cardiovascular Surgery. His bibliography reveals that he had a special interest in surgery related to the parathyroid glands and more especially to the peripheral vascular system and arterial pressure. An article on "Parathyroides et Chirurgie" appeared in 1941 in the *Journal de l'Hôtel-Dieu de Montréal.* In the *Union Médicale du Canada* of August 1953, he published an article on "Endarterectomie: Rapport sur Huit cas Opérées." Also in that year his article on "Indications Chirurgicales dans l'Hypertension" appeared in *Rapports du Congrés Français de Médicine,* XXIXe Session. Masson Cie éd., Paris.

In 1963, he wrote of his work on the surgery of the adrenal glands, "La Chirurgie des Adrenales" (*Un. Méd. Can.*, 92, 72). In several articles, Dr. Cartier reveals his concern about medical education in francophone Canada, e.g., "Reflexions sur l'Hôpital Canadien-Français en Fonction du Temps Present" (*Un. Méd. Can.*, 1958: 87, 467 and 581; also "Le Rôle Educateur de l'Hôpital" (*Un. Méd. Can.*, 1958: 87, 1176).

Dr. Joffre-André Gravel, 30 September 1915, Gravelbourg, Saskatchewan; University of Ottawa, B.A. 36; Laval, M.D. 41; F.R.C.S.(C) 48; Laval, Ms. 48; C.P.S.Q. Gen. Surg. 52; Thoracic Surg. 52; F.A.C.C.P. 53; F.A.C.S. 54; F.I.C.S. 62.

After serving one year as intern at the Hôtel-Dieu of Quebec, Dr. Gravel enlisted in the Royal Canadian Air Force and served as a medical officer in Canada and overseas. In response to the question as to how he chose cardiac surgery as his specialty, he wrote in 1965:

> As soon as the war was over, I did a postgraduate residency for three years at the Hôtel-Dieu of Quebec and obtained my F.R.C.S.(C) and M.S. in 1954. At this stage in 1948, the Dean of the Faculty of Medicine of Laval University, Dr. Charles Vezina, asked me if I would be interested in specializing in thoracic and cardiovascular surgery. This was in view of the future University Hospital (which, of course, we did not have yet).
>
> At that time, it was known that Professor C. Crafoord in Stockholm had a good service and I applied for a job as Foreign Assistant. It was too late in the year for me to get a good cardiac residency in the U.S.A. and besides, I liked the idea of some

European training. I knew that in the years to come, it would be easy to visit the U.S.

After Stockholm, I went to Hôpital Broussais in Paris for a few months and then in London, England where I took a job in the Thoracic Hospital. When I came back in 1951, I found very little of organized groups and joined the Canadian Heart Association.

Dr. Gravel received appointments as the Thoracic Surgeon in four Quebec hospitals and by 1963, his rank at the University was Professeur Agrégé.

In 1964, he was President of the Quebec Association of Thoracic Surgeons. His curriculum vitae contains a long list of societies which he joined and the many honours and awards he received.

Between 1948 and 1965, his bibliography grew to 57 items which include clinical and experimental studies mainly related to thoracic and cardiovascular surgery. In Quebec City, he pioneered this discipline. In 1951, he reported two cases of "Bronchogenic Cysts Associated with Anomalous Arteries Arising from the Thoracic Aorta" (*Thorax,* March 1951). Several publications appeared each year from 1951 to 1965.

In 1957, he wrote about "The Closure of Inter-Auricular Septal Defects Under Hypothermia" (*C.M.A.J.*, Jan. 1957). The following year he wrote "Le Traitement Chirurgical de la Tetralogie de Fallot" (*Laval Méd.*, mars 1958). With Dr. André McClish, he co-authored an article on "Circulation Extra-Corporelle et Cardioplegie: Rapport Préliminaire" (*Laval Méd.*, Feb. 1958). The bibliography indicates that together with his colleagues of the Quebec Institute of Cardiology, all types of cardiovascular surgical problems were dealt with as in any progressive, modern institution. The 57th item is "Communication Interauriculaire: Presentation de 46 Cas Opérés Sous Circulation Extracorporelle," co-authored with M. Beaulieu, J. A. Awad, J. P. Déspré̀s, J. P. Dechene, C. Hebert, and A. McClish (*Laval Méd.*, Feb. 1965).

Dr. Henry James Scott, 16 January 1918, Montreal; Bishop's University, B.A. 37; McGill, M.D., C.M. 41; Diploma in Surg. McGill, 46-51; F.R.C.S.(C); F.A.C.S.; Cert. Gen. Surg. 53; and Thoracic Surgery 55; C.P.S.Q.; F.A.C.C.P.

In 1968, when Dr. Scott filled in the questionnaire, he held the post of Senior Surgeon at the Montreal General Hospital and Associate Professor of Surgery at McGill. When Dr. Scott joined the surgical staff of the Montreal General Hospital in 1951, after returning from military service and after completing the McGill diploma course in surgery (1946-1951), he was specially trained for thoracic and cardiovascular surgery. In the early 1950s mitral commissureotomy was much in vogue. However, although the medical cardiologists favoured the operation in appropriate cases, Dr. Fitzgerald, Chief of the Department of Surgery, believed that re-stenosis would occur soon after commissureotomy, and caused a delay of several years before cardiac surgery took root at the Montreal General Hospital. Dr. Scott nevertheless actively exercised his special interest, working in the Department of Physiology in collaboration with Professor Hebbel Hoff and his colleagues until Dr. Rock Robertson became Chief of Surgery at the Montreal General Hospital.

The first item in his bibliography is an article co-authored with Dr. H. E. Hoff, "Medical Progress — Physiology" (*N. Eng. Med. J.*, 1948: 239, 89-95; 120-126; 176-181). The third item, co-authored with B. A. Levitan is on "Effect of Anti-Histaminics on Arrhythmias Following Coronary Artery Ligation" (*C.M.A.J.*, 1949: 61, 306-308).

The sixth item, co-authored with L. G. Hampton and F. N. Gurd, is entitled "Studies in Therapy of Haemorrhagic Shock and Associated Myocardial Damage" (*Surg. Forum,* 1954: 490). The eighth item reflects his clinical cardiovascular surgical experiences: "Aortic Stenosis in Adults. Evaluation of Diagnostic Criteria of Patients for Surgical Treatment," co-authored with P. A. Gorman, J. B. Calotayud, R. F. P. Cronin, and E. A. S. Reid (*Am. Ht. J.*, 1962: 64, 625-630). The ninth item is "Surgical Closure of Interventricular Septal Perforation Complicating Myocardial Infarction," co-authored with A. R. C. Dobell, R. F. P. Cronin, and E. A. S. Reid (*J. Thorac. & Cardiovasc. Surg.*, 1962: 43, 802-809). The twelfth item, co-authored with his surgical colleague, A. R. C. Dobell, is "Hypertrophic Subaortic Stenosis: Evolution of a Surgical Technique" (*J. Thorac. & Cardiovasc. Surg.*, 1964: 47, 26). The nineteenth item, co-authored with his pupil, W. J. Keon, entitled "Effect of Closed Left Heart Bypass on Acute Myocardial Infarction with Shock," was in course of preparation in 1968. This also was, in part, incorporated in Dr. Keon's thesis for the degree M.Sc.

Dr. Edouard D. Gagnon, 2 December 1915, Montreal, Université de Montréal, B.A. 36; M.D. (*summa cum laude*) 42; F.R.C.S.(C) 47; Cert. in Gen. Surg. R.C.P.&S.(C) 47; Cert. in Gen. Surg. S.P.S.Q. 50; Cert. in Thor. Surg. C.P.S.Q. 52; Cert. in Thoracic Surg. R.C.S.&S.(C) 55; F.C.C.P. 53.

Dr. Gagnon's father, Dr. O. A. Gagnon, and his mother whose maiden name was Kathleen Hull, endowed their son with both

English and French languages and cultures. This endowment probably had some influence in his selection of educational institutions. Thus, after premedical education in French schools and graduation in medicine from the Université de Montréal in 1942, he went, not to Paris, but to Toronto where he joined the Gallie course, serving internships, residencies, and working on research projects until 1948. In that year, he joined the surgical staff of the Notre Dame Hospital and of the Université de Montréal Medical School. He was the first of his generation of graduates of this school who chose to go to Toronto for his postgraduate studies. He will be remembered best as the Canadian pioneer of mitral valve surgery. The story of this aspect of his career is well told by his medical colleague, Dr. Paul David, in relating his own minibiography. They chose a patient, a boy of seventeen, who suffered from haemoptisis and symptoms of congestive cardiac failure related to severe mitral stenosis. They decided to treat him surgically. They went to Philadelphia to learn the technique from Dr. Charles Bailey and his staff. On their return, Edouard Gagnon performed the operation on lower animals and completed his own preparation while Paul David administered medical care to their patient, Normand Fleury, who lived in the hospital until the day of the operation, 27 February, 1950. They had invited me to function as consultant. I firmly approved of surgical therapy for this boy and attended the operation. Gagnon and David reported the case in their article "Le Traitement Chirurgical de la Sténose Mitrale: Commissureotomie" (*Un. Méd. Can.*, 1950: 79, 1142). The same report also appeared in English in the *C.M.A.J.*, 1950: 63, 537. In Toronto, Dr. Wilfrid Bigelow performed his first mitral commissureotomy at about the same time; his first article on this subject appeared in *C.M.A.J.*, 1953: 69, 588, co-authored with colleagues and was a review of a group of cases.

In 1972, responding to my request for follow-up information about Normand Fleury, Gagnon wrote:

> This patient died at the Institute of Cardiology in Montreal, Mar. 5, 1963 when he was operated upon for Starr valve replacement having recurrence of approximately three years duration. He, therefore, had marked improvement for approximately ten years at which time he showed signs of progressive re-stenosis leading to further surgery.

In 1972, when Dr. Gagnon updated his curriculum vitae he held the following posts: Hôpital Notre Dame, Chief of the Division of Cardiovascular and Thoracic Surgery; Senior Surgeon. At the

Queen Mary Veterans Hospital, Consultant in Thoracic and Cardiac Surgery and Chief of Thoracic Surgical Service. At the Institut de Cardiologie de Montréal, he served as Senior Consultant in Surgery from 1954 to 1959. Clinical Professor of Surgery at the Université de Montréal was his final academic title.

Dr. Gagnon's bibliography grew to 39 items between 1948 and 1968. The first item, "Bronochogenic Carcinoma, 12-Year Survey of Operative Results" (*C.M.A.J.*, 1948: 61, 12) indicates his special interest in thoracic surgery. On a number of occasions he published the same article in both languages in the medical journals, as he did with the first report on mitral commissureotomy.

In 1958, he published an article on the theme of the indications for surgical treatment of heart disease (*Un. Méd. Can.*, Nov. 1958: 87).

In 1963, he wrote two chapters in the book on accident surgery edited by H. S. Moseley, namely "Injuries to the Tracheobronchial Tree," and "Injuries to the Heart and Great Vessels."

Dr. David Ross Murphy, 26 March 1917, Montreal; McGill, B.Sc. 39; M.D., C.M. 42; M.Sc. Exper. Surg. 49; Diploma in Surg. McGill 50; F.R.C.S.(C) 52; C.P.S.Q. 54; F.A.C.S. 57.

In 1968, Dr. Murphy's status was Professor of Surgery at McGill, Surgeon-in-Chief at the Montreal Children's Hospital, and Director of Cardiovascular Surgery and Paediatric Surgery. He was also Consultant in Surgery at the Royal Victoria and the Alexandra Hospitals.

Dr. David Murphy graduated in Medicine in 1942, about four years after Dr. Robert Gross had taken the epoch-making step in surgery of ligating the patent ductus arteriosus in a child. About three years after he graduated, the first Blalock-Taussig operation was performed. His career began at the inception of the modern era of cardiovascular surgery. Moreover, he enjoyed a close relationship with one of his teachers in surgery, the late Dr. Fraser B. Gurd who had performed the first ligation of a ductus arteriosus for the treatment of sub-acute bacterial endocarditis at the Montreal General Hospital in 1943. Unfortunately, the ductus was too fragile to permit successful ligation and the patient died. Dr. Gurd had good vision of the near future for he encouraged David Murphy to take a special interest in cardiovascular surgery. Thus, in 1943, Dr. Gurd tried to arrange for his intern, Dr. David Murphy, to attend a surgical meeting in Cleveland because some interesting cardiac surgery was to be discussed by Dr. Claude Beck. Although Murphy was not able to attend the meeting (he was then in the Armed Forces) this incident initiated a special interest in cardiovascular surgery which became firmly established during his service as a resident in the Montreal Children's Hospital. He rounded out his postgraduate training by visiting various centres of cardiovascular surgery in the United States during a six-month period.

As a member of the Canadian Cardiovascular Society, he has given liberally of his talents and time in serving on committees and in various offices, including that of the Presidency and as Chairman of the Medical Advisory Committee of the Canadian Heart Foundation.

Between 1951 and 1965, his bibliography grew to 20 items. Quite appropriately, the first article reflects his state of mind as he began his career at the Montreal Children's Hospital; it is "Congenital Cardiovascular Anomalies Amenable to Surgery" (*McGill Med. J.*, 1951).

In 1953, he wrote on "The Present Status of Extracorporeal Circulation" (*Can. J. Surg.*). In 1959, he wrote the chapter on "Cardiac Surgery" in the *Textbook on Surgery,* edited by H. F. Moseley, published by Lippincott. In 1965, he published a paper on "Biologic Evaluation of Blood After Prolonged Recirculation Through Film and Membrane Oxygenators" (*Ann. Surg.*, 1965).

Dr. Gordon M. Karn, 12 March 1920, Toronto; McGill, B.Sc. 42; M.D., C.M. 43; M.Sc. 49; McGill Dipl. in Surg. 51; F.R.C.S.(C) 52; C.S.P.Q. (Gen. Surg.) 52.

Dr. Karn's postgraduate studies lasted eight years, ending in 1951 with the Diploma in Surgery from McGill University.

During the year 1947-1948 at McGill, his experimental work was on the lymphatic drainage of bone, and in 1949-1950, he worked at the Harrison Department of Experimental Surgery at the University of Pennsylvania on liver regeneration. After returning to Montreal, he was appointed Lecturer in Surgery at McGill and Associate Surgeon at the Montreal Children's Hospital. He resumed his research and in 1952-1953, he studied problems related to arterial grafts. He did not supply any comments on the special questions nor his bibliography.

Dr. Maurice Beaulieu, 19 February 1920, Rivière-du-Loup, Quebec; Collège Ste-Anne de la Pocatière, B.A. 41; Laval, M.D. 45; C.S.P.Q. 54; F.R.C.P.(C).

Between 1949 and 1953, Dr. Beaulieu served as Resident in Thoracic Surgery in Quebec City and in New York at the Sea View Hospital;

in 1953, he had a residency in Cardiovascular Surgery in Newark, New Jersey at St. Michael's Hospital.

In 1953, he was appointed to the Department of Surgery at the Hôpital Laval and to the staff of the Quebec Institute of Cardiology. When he filled in the questionnaire in 1972, he was Professeur Agrégé in Surgery of Laval University and Consultant to the Laval University Hospital Centre.

He wrote the following comments on the special questions:

> I decided to specialize in cardiovascular and thoracic surgery when I was studying thoracic surgery in New York (1951-1952). I had no difficult obstacles to overcome in obtaining special training. I did apply for and received a provincial bursary to support me during my stay in New York. The Laval Hospital, where I began to work on my return to Quebec, was at that time the only institution in this region where tuberculosis was treated both medically and surgically. Later I was able to participate actively in the creation of a section in which it was possible to treat cardiac patients surgically. This section is now the Institute of Cardiology of Quebec City.

Dr. Beaulieu's bibliography is of considerable interest. The first twenty-one items appeared between March 1950 and April 1961 and were by him alone. The first article in which he was the senior author with Dr. J. A. Gravel was published in April 1961, "Cardiotomie Pour Ablation d'un Cathéter Intra-Veineux" (*Laval Méd.*, 1961: 31; 458-461). During those first ten years, the major part of his work concerned pulmonary surgery. In 1956, however, he published a monograph on "Malformation Cardio-Vasculaires" (143 pages, Presses Université Laval, Québec). In more recent years, his bibliography reflects his involvement in experimental and clinical cardiovascular surgery with several colleagues on his team.

Dr. Lloyd Douglas MacLean, 15 June 1925, Calgary, Alta.; University of Alberta, B.Sc. 46; M.D. 49; University of Minnesota, Ph.D. 57; F.R.C.S.(C) 64; Cert. Amer. Board of Surg.; Cert. Board of Thoracic Surg.; F.R.S.(C) 71.

Dr. MacLean's postgraduate studies lasted from 1949 to 1956. They began with one year of rotating internship at the University of Alberta Hospital, followed by a year of surgical internship and then five years of surgical residency at the University of Minnesota Hospitals. He then joined the staff of this University and rose to Associate Professor of Surgery while serving as Surgeon-in-Chief of Ancker Hospital in St. Paul, Minnesota.

In 1962, he came to Montreal to occupy the post of Surgeon-in-Chief at the Royal Victoria Hospital and Professor of Surgery at McGill.

Dr. MacLean did not offer any comments on the special questions, but in 1965 he did supply his bibliography of 110 items which reflect the nature of his work between 1952 and 1965. In 1971, he reported that the number of publications had increased to 170. Of the first 110 items, the cardiovascular system is the subject of 50 items. The first of these deals with shock, a subject which engaged Dr. MacLean's interest for many years. In the year 1955-1956 he co-authored six articles on shock; the sixth is "Studies on the Circulatory Changes in Dog Produced by Endotoxin from Gram-Negative Micro-Organisms" co-authored with M. H. Weil, M. D. Vischer, and W. W. Spink (*J. Clin. Invest.* 1956: 35, 1191-1198). An early paper related to coronary artery surgery is "A Comparison of Toxicity of Various Agents Used in Coronary Angiography" co-authored with R. S. Flom and F. J. Lewis (*Lancet,* 1957: 431-433). His interest in vascular surgery is reflected in "Atherosclerotic Changes in Grafts of the Thoracic Aorta" with R. S. Flom, C. E. Turbak, and F. J. Lewis (*Surg.*, 1958: 44, 356-360). An important contribution to the study of the physiology of ventricular fibrillation appears in "The Influence of Temperature and Coronary Occlusion on the Ventricular Fibrillation Threshold" with C. M. Phibbs and L. M. Levy (*Surg. Gyn. Obst.*, 1959: 109, 216-222). In the same year he wrote an article on "Some Aspects of the Surgery of Congenital Heart Disease" (*Lancet,* 1959: 79, 382-384). He reported a case of inominate arteriovenus fistula with a review of the literature, with W. F. Mazzitelo (*J. Thor. & Cardiovasc. Surg.*, 1960: 39, 770-778). Dr. MacLean was an early investigator of defibrillation, as is noted in the 57th item of his bibliography, "Ventricular Defibrillation — An Experimental Investigation of Voltage Requirements and the Effect of Electrode Size" with R. A. Vantym (*J.A.M.A.*, 1961; 175, 471-474). To approach the end of this random selection of publications which reflect Dr. MacLean's substantial contributions to cardiovascular surgery, there is the 67th item entitled "Cardiovascular Surgery in Marfan's Syndrome," with R. J. Blanchard, A. Davitt, and J. A. Culligan (*Ann. Surg.*, 1963: 158, 990).

Before the dramatic report of a cardiac transplantation by Barnard in 1967, Dr. MacLean was studying problems related to organ transplantation. Soon after his arrival in Montreal, he worked in this field as reflected in the 82nd item, "An In Vitro Test to Detect the Degree of Antigenic Difference Between Individuals," with B. Bain, J. Lowenstein and S. Briers (*Surg. Forum,* 1964: 15, 151). This interest was very likely inspired by his work on kidney transplantation about which there are several articles co-authored with nephrologists of the Royal Victoria Hospital.

Dr. Emile Marie Bertho, 20 July 1922, St. Connec-Côtes-du-Nord, Bretagne, France; Baccalauréat Mathématiques, Rennes, France, 43; Faculté de Méd. Paris, M.D. 50; C.P.S.Q. General Surgery 57; Thoracic Surgery 60; F.R.C.S.(C) 58; F.I.C.S. 58; F.A.C.G. 59; F.A.C.S. 59; F.A.C.C.P. 60; F.A.C.A.S. 61; F.I.C.A. 62; F.A.C.C. 67.

Dr. Bertho's postgraduate studies began with two years in Nantes. He then spent 1950 to 1951 in Canadian and American hospitals, which led to specialization in thoracic and cardiovascular surgery.

In 1958, he was Associate in Research at the Cleveland Clinic, and later that year, he returned to Chicoutimi to become the Chief of Thoracic and Cardiovascular Surgery at the Hôtel-Dieu, St. Vallier, Chicoutimi, Quebec, Hôpital de Chicoutimi Inc.

In commenting on the special questions, he wrote that he had always been interested in cardiovascular surgery and began special training after residencies in general surgery. There were difficult obstacles to overcome in finding the most suitable place to settle. He convinced the authorities in Chicoutimi that their hospital needed a Department of Thoracic and Cardiovascular Surgery. In this he was eminently successful, as his accomplishments demonstrate.

He performed his first experimental heart operation with closed chest in Chicoutimi in 1958, and the first operation with extracorporeal circulation in 1959. The first closure of a patent ductus arteriosus in a patient was performed by him in March 1959 and the first open-heart operation for an interventricular septal defect took place in November 1959; the patient was a six-year-old child who made an uneventful recovery. In 1962 he performed a replacement of an aortic valve by a prosthesis in a patient. Cardiac transplantation was performed in laboratory animals. The first was on 3 January 1963, about five years before Barnard's operation in a human, and by 1971, 130 had been performed. The experimental laboratory had a facility for the care of 500 animals which included 150 dogs. Its museum, in 1971, exhibited over 3000 anatomical specimens. In that year, a number of surviving dogs with valve prosthesis had been observed for over 12 years. By 1971, the clinical experience included cardiovascular or thoracic operations on 900 patients . . . and during this period, over 150 students, externs, interns, residents, and teaching Fellows were associated with the department, led and administered by Dr. Bertho. A remarkable record indeed for a surgeon working outside a university centre.

Between 1953 and 1968, his bibliography grew to 56 items of which 40 dealt with experimental and clinical subjects related to cardiovascular surgery. In 1971, he wrote that the list had grown to over a hundred. The first of the 40 items bears the title "Stenose Valvulaire Aortique; Maladie Chirurgical" ["Aortic Valve Stenosis; A Surgical Disease"] (*Un. Méd. Can.*, 1956: 85, 671-675). He was an early pioneer of open-heart surgery. His first publication related to this field is entitled "Résultats des 30 Premières Circulations Extra-corporelles Totalles pratiqués dans le Laboratoire" ["Results of the First 30 Extra-Corporeal Circulations Performed in the Laboratory"] (*Un. Méd. Can.* 1960: 89, 809-822). An item which reflects his versatility is "Resection d'un Aneurysme Cérébral à l'aide de l'Hypothermie Profonde, de l'Arrêt Circulatoire Total et l'Exanguinnation" ["Resection of a Cerebral Aneurysm with the Aid of Deep Hypothermia, Total Arrest of Circulation, and Exsanguination"] (*Laval Méd.*, 1962: 31, 414-418).

His exploration of the surgical treatment of coronary artery disease appears in several articles, one of which is titled "Anatomie Comparée Normale des Artères et des Veines Coronaires du Coeur de Différentes Espéces Animales" ["The Comparative Anatomy of the Coronary Arteries, and Veins of the Heart in Different Animal Species"] (*Arch. d'Anat., d'Histol. et Embryol. Normales et Experimentales,* 1964: 47, 283-309). It is interesting to anyone associated with a university centre to note that in Chicoutimi, a non-university hospital provided patients which made possible the following item "Co-arctation de l'Aorte (à propos de 20 cas)" ["Coarctation of Aorta (Concerning 20 cases)"] (*Saguenay Méd.*, 1967; 14, 151-173).

In 1968, the following article was in press "Coquetol Revascularisant du Myocarde: Etude Experimentale et Clinique sur 45 Chiens et 30 Humains" ["Revascularizing Cocktail of the Myocardium: An Experimental and Clinical Study of 45 Dogs and 30 Humans."]

Dr. Bertho has won many awards including the Grand Prix de L'Union Médicale du Canada; these and the list of exhibits he has made and lectures he has delivered are among the documents in the archives of the Canadian Cardiovascular Society.

Dr. Anthony Richard Curzon Dobell, 13 May 1927; McGill, B.Sc. 49; M.D., C.M. 51; F.R.C.P.&S.(C) 57; Dip. Amer. Bd. of Surg. 57; C.P.S.Q. General Surg. 57; Thoracic Surg. 59; F.A.C.S. 60; Cert. Amer. Bd. of Thor. Surg. 62; F.A.H.A.

Postgraduate education for Dr. Dobell began with internship at the Montreal General Hospital (1951-1952), followed by four years at Jefferson Medical College under Dr. John H. Gibbon. This experience establishes Dr. Dobell as the earliest Canadian pioneer in the field of devising and applying artificial extracorporeal circulation in research on animals, and in clinical surgery of congenital and acquired cardiovascular disease. He has described the problems he encountered in introducing this precious new technique in the three McGill teaching hospitals in his comments on the special questions. He was working with the pioneer of artificial extracorporeal circulation when Dr. Morley Cohen of Winnipeg was working with Dr. C. Walton Lillehei, the pioneer of open heart surgery. Lillehei was using a human source of extracorporeal circulation by the heart lung preparation method invented for physiology in 1881 by H. Newell Martin, the Professor of Biology at Johns Hopkins University, a new university whose Medical School was opened in 1889.

In 1971, Dr. Dobell was Professor of Surgery at McGill, Surgeon in Charge of Cardiovascular Surgery at the Royal Victoria Hospital, Director of Cardiovascular Surgery at the Montreal Children's Hospital, Assistant Surgeon at the Montreal General Hospital, and Consultant in Cardiovascular Surgery at the Santa Cabrini Hospital.

In 1965, Dr. Dobell wrote the following:

> I never really decided to specialize in cardiac surgery but my interests always took me in that direction. I found myself trained in thoracic and general surgery and was particularly attracted to cardiovascular surgery as the most dynamic area of surgery at that time. I had the opportunity to work with the pioneer of extracorporeal circulation, Dr. John H. Gibbon of Philadelphia, and participated in some of the first open-heart operations.
>
> I returned to Montreal in 1956, and found little interest in open-heart surgery except at the Montreal Children's Hospital. Here, I was given support by Dr. D. R. Murphy and experiments were performed on animals in the Donner Building of McGill University. This led to open-heart operations being performed at the Montreal Children's Hospital in 1957.
>
> The major obstacle was simply the general apathy of responsible surgeons in Montreal, particularly at the Montreal General

Hospital, the institution at which I interned and with which I corresponded while in Philadelphia. It was Dr. D. R. Webster, Surgeon-in-Chief of the Royal Victoria Hospital, who encouraged me to return to Montreal and gave me a position as a Teaching Fellow at the Royal Victoria Hospital. He suggested I contact Dr. David Murphy and I remember we met for lunch at a prominent local restaurant. Things have proceeded steadily since then. Once the technique was proven at the Montreal Children's Hospital, it was brought into the Royal Victoria Hospital and then in 1960, in association with Dr. Henry Scott, open-heart surgery finally arrived at the Montreal General Hospital, the surgical department of which had undergone a complete change since the arrival of Dr. H. R. Robertson as Chief of Surgery.

I might add that I returned to Montreal as an exciting cosmopolitan city and not to friends or relatives that we have here. I think, too I have always been interested in helping McGill University.

The first item in Dr. Dobell's bibliography represents extracurricular work he did as an undergraduate, "Potassium Metabolism and Physiology" (*McGill Med. J.*, 1951: 20, 169-175). The next one deals with pioneer work on open heart surgery, "The Closure of Interventricular Septal Defects in Dogs During Open Cardiotomy with the Maintenance of Cardiorespiratory Functions by a Pump Oxygenator" by John H. Gibbon, Bernard J. Miller, Anthony R. C. Dobell, Hans C. Engell, and George B. Voigt (*J. Thor. Surg.*, 1954: 28, 235). At the beginning of his career in Montreal, he wrote the third item, "Open-Heart Surgery" (*McGill Med. J.*, 1958: 27, 94-99) and in the same year, for a wider audience, "The Present Status of Extracorporeal Circulation," with John R. Gutelius, Gordon M. Karn, and David R. Murphy (*Can. J. Surg.*, 1958: 2, 78). There follow several articles every year, co-authored with surgical and medical colleagues of all three McGill teaching hospitals, the Montreal Children's, the Royal Victoria, and the Montreal General.

By 1971, the bibliography had grown to 51 items.

Dr. Pierre Grondin, 18 August 1925, Quebec; Laval, B.A. (*magna cum laude*) 45; M.D. (*magna cum laude*) 51; California Bd. of Med. Exam. 56; C.S.P.Q. 59; F.R.C.S.(C) 59; C.P.S.Q. Thoracic Surg. 65.

Whether by design or through necessity, Dr. Grondin began his postgraduate career with three years in general practice in his native city, Trois Rivières, an excellent foundation for the practice of any specialty. Then he embarked on a program of education in surgery.

In 1954, the year in which open-heart surgery with extracorporeal circulation was announced, he chose to specialize in cardiovascular surgery. He began with a year at the University of Pennsylvania Postgraduate School in basic science related to surgery, then four years of residencies in general surgery, a year of practice as a general surgeon in Trois Rivières (1960-1961) and finally, two years in Houston, Texas in cardiovascular surgery at Baylor University and the hospitals associated with it. In 1964, he was invited to become Chief Surgeon of the Montreal Heart Institute. Accepting this post, he also was appointed to the Faculty of Medicine of the Université de Montréal in 1971 — his title was Associate Clinical Professor. His curriculum vitae lists many honours and awards, and both active and honorary membership in many societies.

As a medical student, in 1947, Dr. Grondin published an article on Michel Sarazin. This reflects an interest in the achievements of Canadian pioneers in the domain of science and education. There follow three items on surgery of the abdomen, and beginning in 1959 with a prize-winning essay on "Thromboendarterectomie Aorto-iliaque" (*Laval Méd.*, 1959: 30, No.2), his publications are related almost entirely to the cardiovascular system.

Dr. Grondin contributed very greatly to the rapid progress of the Montreal Institute of Cardiology. During the beginning of the current era of great achievements in cardiovascular surgery, he met the challenges with the necessary technical skills, scientific knowledge, and effective personal leadership as Surgeon-in-Chief. Soon after the announcement of the first heart transplant by Barnard, Dr. Grondin performed his first and by February 1969, he and his team had performed nine such procedures. Realizing that because of tissue incompatability all the patients died, he and Dr. Paul David decided to postpone any further heart transplanting until the problems related to immunity would be solved.

Dr. Gilles Lepage, 20 November 1926; Université de Montréal M.D. (*cum laude*) 51; C.S.P.Q. (Thor. Surg) 58; F.R.C.S.(C) (Thor. and Cardiovasc. Surg.) 62.

Dr. Lepage began postgraduate studies with a surgical internship at the Hôtel-Dieu de Montréal (1951-1952) followed by surgical residencies in Tennessee (1952-1954), North Carolina (1955), and in England (February 1956-March 1958). The details are fully documented in his curriculum vitae. His comments on the special questions tell the story of his training for cardiothoracic surgery.

> Quite early in my student days, I decided that I wanted to become a surgeon. It appeared to me then that surgery was the best way of helping sick people in a maximum fashion. At that time, in 1948, medical therapy seemed to be purely symptomatic and accomplished very little by way of altering the fundamental aspects of any given disease. Tuberculosis was still a major cause of illness and death, and I selected thoracic surgery as a specialty because this discipline promised to achieve important progress in the treatment of disease. Moreover, it was quite easy to obtain financial assistance for studies related to tuberculosis. I needed that kind of backing because I could not obtain it from my family who were in financial straits at the time. Cardiac surgery was not in the picture in 1951-1952. In that year, cardiac surgery was only beginning to learn to speak. Thus, I had a training in general surgery to begin with, which lasted three years. Then I had two years of training in thoracic surgery. During the latter part of the training in England, I heard the beginning of discussions about open-heart surgery with hypothermia. At that time, extracorporeal circulation was still in the stage of animal experimentation. My chief at the Southampton Thoracic Surgery Unit, where I was Senior Registrar, sent me to the National Heart Hospital in London to learn cardiac catheterization from Dr. Paul Wood. I learned the art in the course of about two weeks. During that time, my chief was visiting Guy's, Brompton, and the Middlesex Hospitals where they were performing open-heart surgery with hypothermia and cardiac arrest. After these few weeks of study, we returned to Southampton, where I organized the haemodynamic and angiographic laboratory, the first in the southwest of England; and my chief, Mr. Paul Chin, initiated the first open-heart surgical unit in the region. These are the circumstances under which I began my experience in cardiac surgery. On my return to Montreal in 1959, I found that there was an opening for a cardiac surgeon at the Institute of Cardiology. I seized this opportunity and have continued to work only as a cardiovascular surgeon since then. One may say that I grew along with the growth of cardiac surgery and of extracorporeal circulation and I have had the immense privilege of having had a front seat in the course of my life as a cardiovascular surgeon in the application of the new techniques which have revolutionized the treatment of heart diseases.

As I mentioned above, I did not choose cardiac surgery, but rather thoracic surgery. It was in the course of my training that cardiac surgery was born and quite naturally it grew out of thoracic surgery. When my training finished, I had had the experience of cardiac surgery related to the few conditions which lent themselves to surgical therapy at that time, namely, several congenital heart conditions like interatrial septal defect, patent ductus arteriosus, coarctation of the aorta, closed heart surgery for mitral stenosis and occasionally for aortic stenosis.

As mentioned earlier, on my return to Montreal in 1959, after an absence of seven years, the Institute of Cardiology already had an excellent reputation and I offered it my services. I was finally accepted at the Institute, mainly because Dr. Paul Stanley, one of my confrères who remained in close contact with the Montreal institution had decided to develop his career at the Hôtel-Dieu. My appointment was also influenced by the fact that Paul could not devote any time to the Institute, and it needed a young surgeon to assist the chief who required someone with knowledge and skill for the management of the techniques related to open-heart surgery with extracorporeal circulation or hypothermia. During the first years, the results of cardiac surgery were somewhat depressing but thanks to the support and the sympathetic understanding of Dr. Paul David, the Director of the Montreal Institute of Cardiology, I persevered in this career. I should mention that on many occasions, I was tempted to return to pulmonary surgery and to give less attention to cardiac surgery. In 1962, however, an important change occurred at the Institute. Dr. Jean-Luis Lamy, the Chief of Surgery, resigned to develop a department at the Maisonneuve Hospital, apart from the Institute, which was due to move from this hospital to a separate building. His departure promoted me to the role of Senior Surgeon, and I certainly do not regret having followed Dr. David's advice, to persevere.

In 1972, when Dr. Lepage submitted his curriculum vitae, he was Professeur Adjoint de Clinique at the Université de Montréal and in addition to his principal hospital appointment of Surgeon at the Montreal Institute of Cardiology, he was Consultant in Cardio-Thoracic Surgery to the Jean Talon, the Fleury, and the Notre Dame Hospitals.

Dr. Lepage's bibliography begins with an article which he co-authored in 1959 on "Open-Heart Surgery" (*Un. Méd. Can.*, 1959: 88, 1360-1377). By 1973, his bibliography had reached number

40; most of the items are written with co-authors. The article on "Evaluation of Surgically Treated Cardiac Abnormalities — A Study of 1,650 Cases" (*Un. Méd. Can.*, October 1972: 101) reflects the extensive experience he has accumulated in a relatively short period of time. The remaining 38 items deal with the cardiac surgery that has evolved during this little more than a decade. Dr. Lepage was among the first to insert cardiac pacemakers and also to replace the diseased valves with prostheses. He was an important member of Dr. Pierre Grondin's team which performed nine cardiac transplants and, shortly after this, initiated a long series of cases of coronary artery disease treated by the coronary by-pass operation. Dr. Lepage has been and is a loyal stalwart of the Montreal Institute of Cardiology.

Dr. Peter Ernest Blundell, 21 August 1923, Toronto; University of Toronto, M.D. 54; F.R.C.S.(C); F.A.C.S.; C.S.P.Q.; F.A.C.C.P.

After one year of internship at the Toronto General Hospital, Dr. Blundell went west for a one-year internship at the Shaughnessy Military Hospital, Vancouver. He returned to the Toronto General Hospital for the years 1958 to 1962. He spent part of the next year at the Frenchay Hospital, Bristol, England and part of the time at the Mayo Clinic. He returned to University of Toronto with the status of Lecturer in 1964. However, in 1965, he began his career at the Montreal General Hospital and McGill University. By 1968, he had been promoted to Assistant Professor of Surgery. He did not write any comments on the special questions. Between 1964 and 1967 he co-authored 11 articles, all but one related to cardiovascular surgery, both clinical and experimental. The first item, co-authored with Dwight C. McGoon of the Mayo Clinic, is "Fate of Starr-Edwards Valve in the Aortic Area of Calves" (*Jr. Thor. & Cardiovasc. Surg.*, 1964: 48, 704). The first paper on work done at the Montreal General Hospital, co-authored with J. K. MacFarlane, N. G. Sutherland, and Sean Moore, is "Histology of Aortic Valve Heterografts and Homografts in Calves" (*C.M.A.J.*, Abstract, 1967: 98, 112).

Dr. Jean-Paul Déspres, 6 February 1929, Ste-Perpetue, L'Islet, Quebec; Laval, B.A. 49; M.D. 54; F.A.C.S.(C) General Surgery 59; F.A.C.S. Thoracic Surgery, 66.

Dr. Déspres began postgraduate training at Hôtel-Dieu de Québec (1955-1959), continued at the Hôpital Laval (1959-1960). Then he spent a year at the University Hospital in Edmonton and finally the year 1961-1962 at Hôpital Laval.

In 1968, when he filled in the questionnaire, he was Professor of Surgery at Laval University and on the surgical staff of Hôpital Laval and the Quebec Institute of Cardiology. Dr. Déspres did not comment on the special questions and did not provide his bibliography.

Dr. Jacob Rosensweig, 1 December 1930, Montreal; McGill, B.Sc. 51; M.D., C.M. 55; Ph.D. (Experimental Surgery) 70; A.O.A. Cert. Thoracic Surg. C.P.S.Q.; Amer. Bd. Thoracic Surg. F.R.C.S.(C); F.A.C.S.; F.A.C.A.

Dr. Rosensweig's postgraduate studies continued from 1955 to 1962. He returned to Montreal in 1962 to occupy posts of increasing responsibility in the Department of Cardiothoracic Surgery at the Royal Victoria and the Jewish General Hospitals.

In 1971, he moved to the U.S.A. to occupy the post of Professor of Surgery at the University of Connecticut and Chief of Surgery and Director of the Division of Thoracic and Cardiovascular Surgery at the Mount Sinai Hospital, Hartford, Conn.

In 1971, he wrote about the special questions as follows.

> My interest in thoracic and cardiovascular surgery developed during the first year of surgical training at the George Washington University Hospital. I was attracted by the work of Doctors Brian Blades, Owen Gwathney and Paul C. Adkins. The nature of the problems challenged my imagination and influenced my decision to pursue this aspect of surgical endeavour. My subsequent training qualified me in both general and thoracic surgery. Through an affiliation with the University of Pittsburgh I was privileged to work in the laboratory of Dr. Don Fisher where I gained an understanding of cardiac haemodynamics, became proficient in cardiac catheterization, and trained in cardiac surgery under Drs. Edward Kent and George McGovern.
>
> I returned to Canada in July 1961 to assume a position in Cardio-Thoracic Surgery at the Jewish General Hospital in Montreal. My subsequent activities have been both clinical and investigative. In 1962, an experimental research program was initiated, which gradually expanded to encompass several projects. Primary interests related to cardiac pacing, assisted circulation, the artificial membrane lung and cardiac transplantation. The Quebec Heart Foundation and the Medical Research Council greatly facilitated these efforts, and the Canadian Cardiovascular Society served as a stimulus. The latter provided an important opportunity to report our findings and to learn about

the work of others across Canada. The social benefits of the Society have also been very meaningful.

I feel very privileged to have been part of "Cardiology in Canada" during a period (1961-1971) in which great strides were made and cardiology and cardiac surgery reached the current level of sophistication and excellence. Two specific personal achievements have been most gratifying — (1) The demonstration of a positive clinical role for assisted circulation (counterpulsation) in treating acute coronary disease, now extended to provide open-heart surgery circulatory support of patients with low output syndrome. (2) The demonstration that hyperacute or accelerated rejection of allografts involved two distinct phases, the initial being exclusively platelet-related and aborted by the use of platelet aggregation inhibitors. Recently, I established the University of Connecticut School of Medicine Pacemaker Clinic for monitoring patients throughout the state by transtelephone transmission of their electrocardiograms. It has proved to be an effective and convenient way of following such patients — well received by both patient and referring physician.

Dr. Rosensweig's bibliography begins with an article he wrote as an undergraduate, "Systemic Diseases of Connective Tissue" (*McGill Med. J.*, 1954: 23, 91). There follow three articles concerning surgery of the gastrointestinal tract, then the first related to thoracic surgery, "Modern Surgical Management of Pulmonary Tuberculosis; Proceedings, Scientific Sessions," twenty-fifth anniversary of the Jewish General Hospital, September 21, 1959. With S. Chatterjee, he studied coronary circulation and co-authored "Haemodynamic Validity of the Ameroid Ischaemic Heart Preparation" (*J. Surg. Res.*, 1968: 8, 471). He became interested in counter pulsation, and co-authored with S. Chatterjee and F. Merino, "Treatment of Acute Myocardial Infarction by Counter Pulsation" (*J. Thor. & Cardiovasc. Surg.*, 1970: 59, 243). Dr. Rosensweig presented a chronological list of papers he delivered and articles he published that numbers 46 between 1954 and 1972.

Dr. Claude Labrosse, 20 April 1930, Buckingham, Quebec; University of Ottawa, B.A. 52; Laval, M.D. 56; C.S.P.Q.; F.R.C.S.(C).

After several years in general practice, Dr. Labrosse began training for cardiothoracic surgery. He spent the years 1961-1964 at the Toronto General Hospital, 1965-1967 at the Hôpital Laennec, Paris, France and the Frenchay Hospital in Bristol, England. Finally, he devoted the years 1968 and 1969 to work at the Toronto General and the Sick Children's hospitals. He joined the staff at Laval University in 1969 as Assistant Professor of Surgery but in 1970, he established himself as Professor and Head of Cardiovascular and Thoracic Surgery at the Sherbrooke University Medical Centre.

Dr. Labrosse made brief and very informative comments about the special questions.

> In the first year of medicine, after anatomy dissecting sessions, I decided I wanted to be a surgeon. In the second year of medicine, I studied the physiology of the heart and became most interested in it. I therefore decided that I had to go into cardiac surgery to please both my head and my hands.
>
> Money was the main obstacle. I, therefore, went into general practice in order to pay my debts and earn money for specialized studies. I was simply offered the job that I now hold in Sherbrooke and decided to accept it after consulting with senior advisors.

Dr. Labrosse's bibliography grew to 17 items between 1962 and 1970. All but two are co-authored and many with colleagues of the Toronto General Hospital. Most are related to cardiovascular surgery.

In 1965, with J. J. Galley, J. Langlois, J. Maurel, E. Hazan, and J. Mathey, he published an article on "Deux Cas de Rupture de la Trachée Opérés Avec Succés dans les Premières Heures l'Une Trachés-bronchique, l'Autre Oesotrachiale" (*Mem. Acad. Chir.*, 1965: 19, 626).

Dr. Yves Castonguay, 23 September 1929, Montreal; Université de Montréal, M.D. 55; C.P.S.Q. Gen. Surg. 59; Cv. & Thor. Surg. 65.

Dr. Castonguay's postgraduate training lasted until 1965, when he was certified in Thoracic and Cardiovascular Surgery. By 1972, when he filled in the questionnaire, he had reached the status of Professeur Adjoint Clinique at the Université de Montréal and was on the Active Surgical Staff of the Montreal Institute of Cardiology and the Maisonneuve-Rosemont Hospital. Dr. Castonguay did not write any comments about the special questions. His bibliography begins as co-author with Y. Windart and L. Pesant on "Les Porphyries et Leurs Manifestations Pseudo-chirurgicales" (*Un. Méd. Can.*, 1960: 89, No. 12). The next item, co-authored with P. Grondin and G. Lepage is an early article related to open heart surgery at the Montreal Institute of Cardiology, "Remplacement Simultané des Valvules Mitrale et Aortique" (*Un. Méd. Can.*, 1964: 93, 1043-1049).

By 1979, his bibliography had grown to 27 items, all co-authored. He was on the surgical team which initiated the coronary bypass procedure and total cardiac transplants at the Montreal Institute of Cardiology.

Dr. Luc Bruneau, 1 May 1933, Montreal; Université de Montréal, B.A. 52; M.D. 58; C.S.P.Q. 62.

Dr. Bruneau did not list details of postgraduate training; his bibliography offers a clue in the following item: co-authored with Aratolio B. Cruz, Robert L. Master, Robert L. Simmons and C. Walton Lillehei, "A New Caged Meniscus Prosthetic Heart Value" (*Surg.*, 1965: 58, 995). The previous data indicates he worked at the University of Minnesota. During his tenure of a staff appointment at the Hôtel-Dieu de Montreal, he wrote an article on "Rupture Traumatique de l'Aorta Thoracique: A Propos de Trois Cas Opérés" (*Un. Méd. Can.*, 1972: 101, 1055).

In brief comments on the special questions, Dr. Bruneau informed us that he came under the influence of Dr. Georges Etienne Cartier and Dr. Paul Stanley during his first year of surgical internship. He was thus involved in much cardiovascular surgery and decided to continue training in this field. As he was married he had numerous financial responsibilities. He overcame his financial problems with loans and frugal living. He returned to Montreal to continue his association with the two men who played such an important role in the development of his career.

Dr. Claude M. Grondin, 23 November 1934, St. Casimir, Portneuf, Que.; Laval, B.A. 56; M.D. 61; F.R.C.S.(C) Thor. & Vasc. Surg; F.A.C.S. 69; Amer. Bd. of Thor. Surg. 70; F.A.C.C.

Dr. Grondin emulated his brother Pierre to the extent that he chose to train for cardiothoracic surgery. To this end, he spent the years 1962 to 1969 at the University of Minnesota. He qualified in General Surgery and Thoracic and Cardiovascular Surgery. He returned to Montreal to join the surgical staff of the Institute of Cardiology. He did not make any comments on the special questions. When he filled in the questionnaire in 1972, he was Professeur Adjoint (Chirurgie) at the Université de Montréal.

Dr. Claude Grondin's bibliography begins with seven items which he co-authored with colleagues at the University of Minnesota. The remaining fourteen, published after 1969, are co-authored with colleagues of the Montreal Institute of Cardiology.

All deal with cardiovascular subjects, clinical and experimental. An interesting item, co-authored with R. S. Elliot and J. E. Edwards, is "Dissecting Aneurysm in a Mother and Son with Marfan's Syndrome" (*Am. Ht. J.*, 1969: 77, 301). The first item related to work at the Institute of Cardiology, co-authored with G. Lepage, G. Castonguay, Y. Meere, and P. Grondin is "Aorto-Coronary Venous Bypass Grafts: Initial Blood Flow Through the Graft and Early Postoperative Patency" (*Circulation,* 1970: 43, 111, 106).

He was a member of the team that performed nine total cardiac transplants.

Dr. Jean Edouard Morin, 28 June 1936, Quebec; Laval, B.A. 56; M.D. 61; F.R.C.S.(C); F.A.C.S.; C.P.S.Q. Cardiothoracic Surg. 68.

Dr. Morin served internships at St. Sacrement Hospital (1960-1961) followed by a year at Hôpital de l'Enfant Jésus. Then he spent the years 1962-1967 at Yale University. On his return to Quebec, he had a teaching Fellowship in Surgery at Laval University for one year after which he moved to Montreal. In 1972, when he filled in the questionnaire, he was Assistant Professor of Surgery at McGill and Assistant Surgeon at the Royal Victoria Hospital. He did not make any comments on the special questions.

Dr. Morin's bibliography begins in 1965 with several articles related to cancer. In 1970, he co-authored an article with Anthony R. C. Dobell on "A Safe Technique for Cordis Pacemaker Battery Change" (*Jr. Thor. & Cardiovasc. Surg.*, 1970: 59, 721-722).

Ontario

Dr. Gordon Murray, 29 May 1894, Oxford County, Ontario; University of Toronto, M.B. 21; A.O.A.; F.R.C.S. (Eng.) 26; F.R.C.S.(C) 31; F.A.S.A.; F.A.C.C.; I.S.A.; F.I.C.A.; Hon. F.C.S. (Brazil); Hunterian Professor, R.C.S.

The Canadian Cardiovascular Society initiated the Annual Lecture program in 1961. With an invitation to deliver this lecture the Society seeks to honour the lecturer for scientific achievement. Until 1967, when the Keith lecture became an important function of the annual meeting, the Annual Lecture was the only such honour in the gift of the Society. All the lecturers have been members of the Society. Dr. Gordon Murray, a charter member, delivered the 1963 lecture. One aspect of this event, which I now recall vividly, is my astonishment of how little I then knew of his very important pioneering accomplishments. As Dr. William Bigelow spoke in introducing him, I became acutely aware of this ignorance. About a year later, I visited Dr. Murray, interrupting his office schedule for about a half hour, and came away with the two books Murray had written in which he tells of his work, especially of the innovations. Historians have recognized his achievements. Richard H. Mead, in his book on the *History of Thoracic Surgery* (1961) starts the chapter on Atrial and Ventricular Septal Defects with this sentence, "The first surgical attack on atrial septal defects was made by Gordon Murray of Canada, who in 1948 reported on his experiments in dogs." Among Bigelow's reminiscences of the period immediately after World War II, when he resumed his career in Toronto, he has written,

> Clinically, there was not enough heart surgery for two surgeons and Gordon Murray was perfectly capable of handling what was available, so that I interested myself, the first three or four years on the staff, in the peripheral vascular field and carried out research.

Reading the first forty pages of his book, *Medicine in the Making* (Murray, 1960), in which he tells of his very happy childhood on a farm and his experiences in the small primary school, he clearly and eloquently credits his mother (née Elizabeth Conway) with inspiring him to learn about natural phenomena in the human environment. He relates how his mother organized a successful demonstration of procreation by showing the difference in appearance of a fertilized and a non-fertilized egg in the course of a number of days during which her six children observed the growth of a chick embryo. His father, John, a successful building entrepreneur, hoped Gordon would follow his older brother's example and become an engineer. But he chose to be influenced by what his mother taught him in her amateur way and he elected to study medicine. His medical studies were interrupted in 1915, early in his sophomore year, when he enlisted in the 26th Field Artillery as a gunner, and so found himself on active duty in France. Of this experience he wrote:

> The first signs of active warfare aside from wet clothing, tired horses, 'cooties' in blankets and clothing, and restless sleep, was the appearance of many puffs of pretty white smoke. These anti-aircraft puffs followed a very definite line across the sky and at a ridiculous distance from them was a beautiful white Taube German airplane. Compared with the dive bombers, the jet planes and the atomic bombs of the present time, this was child's play with toys. But, however it might be in the air, on the

> earth's surface there was grim reality with the big guns firing tremendous crumps both ways. The poor horses flinched under the saddles, and with erect ears, dilated snorting nostrils, and staring eyes, beheld in horror the results of the latest lethal inventions of man.

Fortunately, Murray himself was spared for a brilliant career in the vanguard of twentieth-century surgery.

He disposes of the medical undergraduate years, 1918-1922, by mentioning that he was "elected with a few others to the Honour Medical Society of the University, the Alpha Omega Alpha." He began his postgraduate career by devoting a year to general practice in his home town, Stratford, Ontario, as assistant to Dr. Lorne Robertson. Writing of this period in his 1960 autobiography, he gave high praise to the education of the doctor that is provided by general practice. He emphasized the fact that it affords the opportunity of meeting challenges which tax one's ingenuity in solving unexpected technical as well as social human problems. The appearance of these problems reveals also the lacunae in knowledge which call for research. The next step, postgraduate training away from home, posed a choice between a centre in North America and the possibility of going to the other side of the Atlantic. He visited the Mayo Clinic and recognized its virtues, but allowed himself to be influenced by his parents and by those friends who advised the other option. During the next five years, 1923-1928, he worked mainly in London, England. Among the going-away presents which his friends gave him, he received a biography of Louis Pasteur. He refers to this as one of the books which influenced his future course. He greatly admired Pasteur's inventiveness and hard work and greatly deplored the fierce opposition Pasteur encountered from his "establishment" colleagues. And in this connection, he writes of Lister and his similar experience in Edinburgh and Glasgow. In London the opposition to Lister was less active. These historical events prepared Murray for the opposition he encountered when he proposed innovations which initiated controversy.

Needless to say, a fixed goal of his five years in England was achieved when he passed the necessary examinations to become a Fellow of the Royal College of Surgeons. His postgraduate studies largely designed to prepare him for clearing these hurdles afforded him broad clinical experience. Soon after arriving in London he was appointed Senior Resident Medical Officer of the Westend Hospital. During the 18 months that he served in this post he was associated with a research project on the treatment of tertiary syphilis with hyperthermia. This association brought him in contact with the leading neurologists of London and also with prominent general surgeons, the pioneers of brain surgery. He studied anatomy at St. Mary's Hospital Medical School in preparation for the fellowship exams. His teacher, Professor Ernest Fraser, liked him very much and appointed him to the staff as a demonstrator with a salary of £400 per year. He served for three years in this capacity and benefited greatly from the experience. Following the end of his stay at the Westend Hospital he worked at St. John's Hospital in Leicester Square in dermatology and orthopaedics. This period was followed by a residency in general surgery at the Hampstead General Hospital, then similar residencies at University College Hospital, and at the All Saints Hospital where he dealt with genito-urinary problems. Next, he had an appointment in general surgery at St. Bartholomew's Hospital where he took notice of the pioneer work in thoracic surgery by Mr. Fred Roberts. Here, he also learnt about new developments in the treatment of peripheral vascular disease, notably lumbar sympathectomy for Buerger's disease.

When the time came for returning homeward he took cognizance of the fact that "there were more great journals and medical periodicals published in America than in Europe and Asia combined," and chose to visit New York before settling in Toronto. He secured a residency in the New York Hospital to work with Dr. Eugene Pool. Of this period he later wrote: "It was in the field of operative surgery and surgical technique that I profited most by experience in the United States." During his stay in New York he also worked with Dr. Royal Whitman in orthopaedics and with Dr. W. B. Coley in general surgery. Toward the end of Murray's stay in New York, Dr. Coley offered him a staff appointment in the hospital and a partnership in his office but he chose to return to Toronto where he was to have a residency in surgery at the Toronto General Hospital. And of this he later wrote: "Thus was made the decision to stay in Toronto, regretted on many occasions in later years." An enthusiastic innovator, he was destined to experience frustration and to breed controversy. Eventually he did reap some well-earned rewards and awards. His bibliography of seventy-seven items from 1930-1962, the list of important lectures delivered and the rewards and honours he received, appear in his two books (Murray, 1960 and 1963).

The first article related to the cardiovascular system is "Embolism in Peripheral Arteries," (*C.M.A.J.*, 1936). In the course of the next twenty-six years there followed forty-two publications in this field, which include experimental and clinical work on cardiac valves, septal defects, tetralogy of Fallot, blood transfusion, thrombosis and embolism, anticoagulants (notably heparin), and kidney transplantation. In 1936, together with L. B. Jaques, T. S. Perret, and C. H. Best, he pioneered the treatment and prevention of peripheral thrombosis by intravenous heparin. In 1938, with F. R. Wilkinson and Ross Mackenzie, he co-authored an article on "Reconstruction of the Valves of the Heart." This reported study, in progress since 1932, that resulted in an effective method of treating significant mitral insufficiency. As a prosthesis he used an inverted vein which he reinforced by inserting a piece of tendon into its lumen. He attached this in the path of the mitral valve so that it reduced the degree of regurgitation. He demonstrated the experimental animals at the hospital's seminars and meetings but received little if any encouragement from his confrères. He performed the operation on a number of patients who were referred to him by physicians who were not on the staff of the hospital. In writing of this in 1960 he declared: "It never got a break and was not countenanced in medical circles in Canada." In 1940 he wrote an article related to war surgery, "Heparin in Surgical Treatment of Bloodvessels." Very soon after the Blalock-Taussig operation was described, he went to Baltimore, observed and learned the technique so that on his return he began collecting a series of cases in which he performed the operation. He was the "first in the British Commonwealth to carry out this procedure," and published a paper on the "Tetralogy of Fallot" and its surgical treatment in the *British Medical Journal* of 1947. He began experimental work on transplantation of kidneys in animals in 1932 and pioneered this procedure in humans. A good case can be made for the conclusion that Gordon Murray was the first pioneer in cardiac surgery, as William Stairs Morrow was the first physiologist-cardiologist in Canada.

Young surgeons who completed their training in general surgery before entering military service returned from the war in 1946, ripe for research and specialization. Two such young men, who chose to settle in Toronto, were destined to play important roles in creating centres of cardiovascular surgery in Canada, W. G. Bigelow and W. T. Mustard.

Dr. William Thornton Mustard, 8 August 1914, Clinton, Ontario; University of Toronto, M.D. 37; M.S. 47; F.R.C.S.(C) 47; F.A.C.S. 48; A.A.P.; A.S.T. & Cv. S.; F.A.H.A.

"Bill" Mustard, about a year younger than Bill Bigelow, after completing secondary school education entered the University of Toronto Medical School, graduating M.D. in 1937. Postgraduate training began with the year 1937-1938 at the Toronto General Hospital, followed by a year at the Hospital for Sick Children. Then he went to New York for the year 1939 at the New York Orthopaedic Hospital. Finally, he entered the Gallie postgraduate course in surgery in July 1940. This training was interrupted in September 1941 when he enlisted in the Canadian Army Medical Corps. He rose to the rank of Officer Commanding No. 7 Field Surgical Unit. He was decorated M.B.E. Demobilized in June 1947, he resumed his civilian career beginning with two residencies in surgery: the first at the Hospital for Sick Children in Toronto, July 1945 to January 1946, then at the New York Orthopaedic Hospital, January 1946 to December 1946. At about this time Dr. John Keith became chief of cardiology at the Sick Children's Hospital. Presently, the need for a surgeon who would specialize, full-time, in paediatric cardiovascular surgery made itself felt. Dr. Mustard accepted this new challenge.

Lacking the kind of personal reminiscences provided by John Keith and by Bill Bigelow, we must look at Mustard's bibliography to glean an impression of his contributions. Between 1945 and 1965, he authored or co-authored sixty-four articles. First on the list is "The Problem of the Damaged Artery in Forward Surgery" (*C.M.A.J.*, 1945: 53, 128-130). In this article he revealed his early interest in vascular surgery. The second item is also related to his war experience: "The Technique of Immediate Restoration of Vascular Continuity After Arterial Wounds. Indications and Results" (*Ann. Surg.*, 1946: 134, 1). Four years later, as his contribution to the Festschrift in honour of Dr. W. E. Gallie, he chose to write on "Traumatic Arterial Thrombosis, Based on Cases Treated at the Battlefront." In the first paragraph on the treatment of arterial contusion and thrombosis, after having discussed the problems of differential diagnosis, he declares:

> In the treatment of these interesting cases one cannot do too much too soon. The dictum of watchful expectancy is to be condemned; frequently too little is done too soon and too much too late. It is the opinion of the author that if the diagnosis is

doubtful it is better to prove or disprove this at open operation than to wait until death of the limb demonstrates the lesion.

This reminds one of the famous lines spoken by Brutus in Shakespeare's *Julius Caesar*: "There is a tide in the affairs of men which taken at the flood leads on to fortune, omitted, all the voyage of their life is bound in shallows and miseries." Bill Mustard took the tide in flood. The third item in the bibliography marks the beginning of his career as a paediatric cardiovascular surgeon; it is "The Operation for Closure of the Patent Ductus Arteriosus" (*C.M.A.J.*, 1947: 57, 340-341). The eighth item marks him as one of the early pioneers in exploring the possibility of open-heart surgery with the use of a heart-lung preparation: "Experimental Intracardiac Surgery with Extracorporeal Circulation" (*Surg.*, 1951: 30, 684-688).

The fifteenth, a breakthrough event, deals with "A Surgical Approach to Transposition of the Great Vessels with Extracorporeal Circuit" co-authored with A. L. Chute, J. D. Keith, A. Sirek, and R. D. Rowe. This new procedure has come to be known as the Mustard Operation. In the same year, his work with Bill Bigelow and J. G. Evans on "Some Physiologic Concepts of Hypothermia and Their Applications" was published (*J. Thor. Surg.*, 1954: 28, 463-480). Ten of his sixty-four publications deal with subjects which called for his skills in orthopaedic surgery, the remainder reveal a wide range of clinical, surgical subjects, and experimental projects all related to paediatric cardiovascular disease. Forty-one colleagues, medical and surgical, associates and pupils, appear as co-authors in forty items. He was the sole author of twenty-four. He served on a panel of five editors of a two-volume textbook of paediatric surgery which appeared in 1962. W. T. Mustard in paediatric surgery and John D. Keith in paediatric medicine gave leadership in the creation of the training centre for paediatric cardiology at the Hospital for Sick Children which has been, and remains, second to none in the world. They and their associates established at Sick Children's a service for the diagnosis and treatment of cardiovascular disease whose reputation for excellence became and remains world-wide.

Dr. Wilfred Gordon Bigelow, 18 June 1913, Brandon, Manitoba; University of Toronto, B.A. 35; M.D. 38; M. S. 38; F.R.C.S.(C); A.S.A.; S.T.S.; Great Britain and Ireland (Hon); A.A.T.S.; F.A.H.A.; LL.D. (Brandon University).

Wilfred G. (Bill) Bigelow was twenty-eight years old when he enlisted in the Canadian Army Medical Corps. After completing his secondary education in Brandon, Manitoba, he had earned the B.A. degree in 1935, the M.D. and M.S. degree in 1938 at the University of Toronto and experienced surgical internship and residencies for three years. He served overseas from 1941-1946. Bill Bigelow's 1965 letter to the archivist in response to the special questions greatly merits being quoted here.

> I would think that vascular surgery entered my mind during the second great war. I was a surgeon in the Sixth Casualty Clearing Station and preparing myself for a Normandy invasion by reading traumatic and surgical war papers. I commenced to feel that the one area that appeared to demand attention was the vascular area. Before going to Normandy, I was able to obtain a private supply of heparin in London, and as well as arterial sutures, I obtained some Blakemore-Lord tubes. For a variety of reasons my attempts at vascular surgery in the Casualty Clearing Station in Normandy were not very successful, but I was disturbed to see amputations carried out in otherwise good limbs because of arterial insufficiency.
>
> On returning to Toronto I did some reseach in the laboratory, interesting myself in local hypothermia, and when I was invited to come on the staff of Toronto General Hospital I requested special training in vascular surgery. I was sent to Johns Hopkins to study peripheral surgery but there was a change in staff and I landed up in the laboratory supervised by Richard Bing and had the good fortune to be present when the first cardiac catheterizations were carried out for congenital heart disease with estimations based on the Fick principle. Here I watched the blue-baby operations and heard about the work of Gibbon. The idea of general hypothermia with interruption of the circulation occurred to me at this time and although there was very little evidence that surgery would progress much beyond the shunting procedure for tetralogy of Fallot, nevertheless the hypothermia concept was the first stimulus to consider cardiac surgery as an eventual goal.
>
> I early on became interested in the micro-circulation so that the research attacked both ends of the vascular system.
>
> On returning to Toronto after the war the department was not geared for fundamental research involving team work with basic disciplines. Finally space was found. There was the usual difficulty of obtaining financial support from granting bodies for an idea before it has been worked upon. I founded our laboratory at

the end of the first year's research with five thousand dollars worth of borrowed equipment. With reports of successful experiments research grants were obtained and these borrowed bits of equipment were eventually paid for.

Clinically, there was not enough heart surgery for two surgeons and Gordon Murray was perfectly capable of handling what was available so that I interested myself, the first three or four years on staff, in the peripheral vascular tree, and carried out research. With the beginnings of surgery of acquired heart disease I went to Philadelphia and watched Charles Bailey do what I believe was his fourth or fifth case of mitral stenosis and enticed Bill Greenwood to come along so that I would have some support on returning. As in most fields, this area of surgery was slow in developing, and most of the early cases were referred by general practitioners; but with close cooperation with the cardiologists we soon had a team approach to the surgery of both congenital and acquired heart disease. I believe the Toronto General Hospital had one of the early combined medical-surgical cardiovascular investigative units and we did have the first established surgical division for cardiovascular surgery with a staff of three in 1957, all limiting our practice to cardiovascular surgery. All junior appointments to our staff have been full-time, Dr. Raymond Heimbecker being the first true geographical full-time appointment at the General Hospital in surgery apart from the department head.

Regarding the choice of location I have never planned my life to any degree. My father, a surgeon in Brandon, Manitoba, and a graduate of Manitoba, sent me unquestioningly to Toronto for my medical degree with the advice that he thought Toronto offered the best medical training in Canada, but I was further advised that I should leave Toronto once I had my degree and obtain postgraduate training elsewhere. The reason for this latter advice was, in my father's opinion, that in those days Toronto was far too provincial to be able to offer a first class postgraduate training (1931)! He thinks they have improved a good deal since but I might say this opinion was not an uncommon one on the prairies. I dutifully applied for surgical training at the Mayo Clinic when it was recommended that I apply for the Gallie course of postgraduate surgical training [in Toronto]. This application was accepted and after the war, once again with plans to go out and set up practice in Vancouver, I was asked to come on the Toronto General Hospital staff.

The invitation to be a charter member of the Canadian Heart Association (now the Canadian Cardiovascular Society) arrived in an unauspicious envelope in a rather hectic postwar household with a full quota of children running about. This important invitation was fortunately picked out of the fireplace and I was proud indeed to be able to reply to it and associate my name with the great Canadian names in cardiology at the time. At some of the very early meetings our early experience with mitral stenosis proved an interesting sounding board for opinions from our associates. Some years ago I spoke to Dr. Paul David requesting that there be larger surgical representation in the Society and his response was enthusiastic and effective.

In 1968 Bill Bigelow wrote a six-page introduction to a precious book of 115 pages entitled *Forceps, Fin and Feather,* memoirs which his father composed at the age of eighty-five, two years before his death. Wilfred Abraham Bigelow, a native of Nova Scotia, a direct descendant of Isaac Bigelow who founded Kingsport, Nova Scotia in 1761, became a surgeon and organized the first private clinic in Canada in Brandon, Manitoba. Bill's mother, Grace Gordon, the daughter of a Scottish family who emigrated to Western Canada, had completed her training as a nurse in London, England, and practised in Minneapolis before her marriage to Dr. Bigelow in 1905. Bill, the third of four children, the only one to choose a career in medicine, elected to pioneer on the new frontier of cardiovascular surgery. By 1965 his bibliography contained 66 items, all related to some aspect, physiological or surgical, of the heart, blood vessels, or blood. The first two reveal his early interest in hypothermia, "The Modern Conception and Treatment of Frostbite" (*C.M.A.J.*, 1942: 47, 529) and "Some Uses of Dry Cold Therapy and a Proposed Cooling Cabinet" co-authored with E. C. G. Lanyon (*Br. Med. J.*, 1944: 1, 215). These items were followed by a whole series of articles on experimental and clinical work in the study and application of hypothermia which established him as a world authority on the subject. In 1951, he co-authored with J. C. Callaghan the article on "An Electrical Artificial Pacemaker for Standstill of the Heart" (*Ann. Surg.*, 1951: 134, 8), a milestone in the history of pacemakers as we know them now. Soon after Charles Bailey began to perform valvoplasty on cases of mitral stenosis, Bill Bigelow performed the operation in Toronto at about the same time as Edouard Gagnon did his first commissureotomy in Montreal. The bibliography contains items on cardiac resuscitation, pericardiectomy for constrictive pericarditis, ruptured aneurysm of sinus of Valsalva, direct vision surgery for mitral insufficiency, ventricular myotomy in hypertrophic sub-aortic stenosis, internal mammary artery implantation for coronary artery disease, and thromboendoarterectomy for peripheral arterial disease. This partial list offers an impression of the wide range of subjects Bigelow studied and dealt with in clinical surgery. Moreover, his co-authors, medical colleagues and surgical associates and assistants, are among those who contributed to the development of cardiology in Canada; fifty-six different names appear in the titles of the sixty-six articles, offering some measure of the contribution Bigelow has made as the chief of a training centre for cardiovascular surgery.

By 1957, about a decade after Bigelow resumed his life work following war service, his achievements and those of his medical colleagues came to be recognized as requiring the creation of a special cardiovascular unit. Another five years elapsed after the creation of the unit on paper until the opening of the greatly expanded and modernized physical facilities for its work at the Toronto General Hospital. At the opening ceremonies on 19 January 1962, Edouard Gagnon brought greetings and good wishes from the Université de Montréal and the Notre Dame Hospital. He alluded to the fact that a Fellowship for the specialty of Cardiovascular and Thoracic Surgery was being initiated by the Royal College of Physicians and Surgeons of Canada in 1962. The other guest of honour, Dr. Henry Swan, spoke of the great potentialities for progress on behalf of the patient, inherent in the cardiovascular unit. Henry Swan had performed the first operation under direct vision for closure of an interatrial septal defect using hypothermia. Bill Bigelow, in an eloquent address, paid tribute to Gordon Murray, the pioneer of cardiovascular surgery in our part of the world and to the dedication of those who formed the personnel of the unit. His vision of the future appears in the following sentences:

> I think the Toronto General Hospital should take on a major responsibility as a postgraduate training centre for Canada with a strong representation of their staff active in international societies and returning to interpret world surgery to Canadian trainees.
>
> It is not enough to teach a postgraduate student how to diagnose and treat disease skilfully. Postgraduate training is not complete unless he comes in contact with research: this will: 1) stimulate him, 2) teach him research methods, and 3) prepare him for changes which will occur in the future.

> Finally, what of those who strive for excellence? It is not seeking after an easy cheerful existence but excellence does have its rewards. It must surely be motivated by some deep-seated instinct, akin to sex. When one considers the trials, tribulations, and frustrations encountered on the road to excellence, the analogy can be reasonably extended.

In the course of his career, Dr. Bigelow received many awards and honours, notably the degree LL.D. from Brandon University, Professor Emeritus, Department of Surgery, Toronto University, Honorary Fellow, the Royal College of Surgeons, England, Lister Prize and Peters Prize, University of Toronto, the Gairdner Prize, Award of Merit of the Canadian Heart Foundation, and the Award of Merit of the City of Toronto. He served as president or member of the council of several surgical organizations, both national and international. He was President of the Canadian Cardiovascular Society during the two years 1971 and 1972. Cardiovascular physiology and surgery benefited very greatly from his achievements in Canada.

Dr. James Alistair Key, 31 May 1915, Scotland; University of Edinburgh, M.B., B.Ch. 39; F.R.C.S. (Eng.); A.A.T.S.; F.A.H.A.

Dr. Key had all his education in Edinburgh. He attended the famous Watson's College (1929-1934) and Edinburgh University where he obtained his medical degree in 1939. He served in the British military forces during World War II. His return to civilian life began with a surgical appointment at Guy's Hospital (1946-1948), then on the staff of the Royal Victoria Hospital in Newcastle-on-Tyne (1948-1952). During the year 1950-1951 as a Rockefeller Research Fellow, he worked at the Toronto General Hospital with Dr. Bigelow. He tells of this period and its significance:

> My decision to specialize in cardiovascular surgery was largely fortuitous. I became interested during the war in vascular surgery and continued this interest when the war was over and when I really started to do my postgraduate training in earnest. I was fortunate enough to gain a Rockefeller Research Scholarship, and worked at one of the centres where the necessary laboratory facilities were available for micro-circulation technique, namely, in Toronto where I spent a very pleasant year and during this time I was exposed to the work of such people as Dr. Bigelow who was then doing his studies on hypothermia and Dr. Mustard at the Sick Children's Hospital and Dr. Gordon Murray. I think this was

the real beginning of my interest in cardiac as opposed to pure vascular surgery.

I was then invited to return to Toronto and become a member of the staff at the Toronto General Hospital which I did and again encouraged mainly by Dr. Bigelow, my interest in both vascular and cardiac surgery increased. Subsequently, I was appointed as one of the staff of the Cardiovascular Surgical Service when this was formed as a special surgical division and since then my interest has been pretty well exclusively in this field.

I think my answer to the first question has covered certain of the points asked in your second question as to the experiences I had in planning and carrying out my special training and again I think they were to some extent fortuitous and I think I was lucky especially in getting my research fellowship and in happening to pick on Toronto as the place to come to. I was also not a little influenced by the fact that I could not think of a nicer society of surgeons to grow up amongst than those at the Toronto General and on my part the wisdom of my choice has been amply borne out in my life and work here. I think membership of the Canadian Cardiovascular Society has had its most rewarding effect in meeting other cardiovascular surgeons and cardiologists because, in a highly specialized field such as ours, we tend to be cut off a little bit from the general society of other surgeons and colleagues and the main pleasure I have derived has been to meet other people who are working in the field, who talk the same language, and who face the same problems, make the same mistakes but always, like me, seem to find enough success in our work to bolster up the enthusiasm and dedication which is necessary in the field of high risk surgery.

In conclusion, I think one of the most rewarding aspects of my career has been that of taking part in opening up cardiovascular surgery, and in some small measure, helping to provide the signposts towards surgical treatment which simply did not exist prior to the 1950s. It is rather wonderful to be able to look back on the early days when we operated on patients with mitral disease who very often were in severe failure with bilateral pleural effusions, when our operative mortality in certain groups was in the region of 20-30%, and to think that now we are rather upset if we have one to two cases in 100 who die as a result of surgery. I can't help feeling, however, that had the fates ordained it otherwise I could well have embraced some other field of surgery and been perfectly happy in it but I'm certainly continually grateful to these same fates that my interests and opportunities led me into this field.

Between 1950 and 1965, Dr. Key was author and co-author of eleven articles, almost all related to cardiovascular surgery; for example, the first item is "Bloodvessels of a Gastric Ulcer" (*Br. Med. J.*, 1950: 2, 1464), and the eleventh, "The Recognition and Management of Peripheral Arterial Injuries" (*C.M.A.J.*, 1965: 92, 1154). It is interesting to note that in common with Dr. Bigelow and Dr. Mustard, his interest in cardiovascular surgery began with experience in military service during World War II. His comments reveal that he is keenly aware of the fact that he was a pioneer in cardiovascular surgery. He has articulated what others also have felt.

Dr. Donald Richard Wilson, 15 July 1917, Saskatoon, Saskatchewan; University of Saskatchewan, B.A. 39; University of Toronto, M.D. 42; F.R.C.S.(C) 50; F.A.H.A.

Dr. Donald Wilson, a contemporary of Keith, Bigelow, and Mustard, provided only the bare skeleton of a minibiography. He took the Gallie course in 1948-1951. When he filled in the questionnaire in 1965 he was Chairman of the Department of Surgery at the University of Toronto, and Chief of Cardiovascular Surgery at the Toronto Western Hospital. In Dr. Bigelow's bibliography his name appears as co-author on "Surgical Treatment of Chronic Constrictive Pericarditis" (*C.M.A.J.*, 1956: 75, 814), and again in an article on "Subtotal Pericardectomy for Constrictive Pericarditis" (*Surg.*, 1957: 41, 102), and a third item on "Chronic Aorto-iliac Obstruction" (*C.M.A.J.*, 1957: 77, 747).

Dr. Eric Charles Grundy, 24 March 1918, Toronto; University of Toronto, M.D. 43; F.R.C.S.(C); F.A.C.S.; F.C.C.P.

The rather meagre documentation of his career that he provided indicates that Dr. Grundy obtained the degree M.D. at the University of Toronto in 1943 and devoted the years 1946-1951 to the course in surgery in the teaching hospitals of the University of Toronto. Then he spent a year in England at the Northern Regional Thoracic Surgery Centre at Newcastle-on-Tyne. He has pursued his surgical career in Toronto at St. Joseph's Hospital, Queensway General Hospital, and the Mississauga Hospital.

Dr. Clare Brenton Baker, 20 September 1922, Biggar, Saskatchewan; University of Saskatchewan, B.A. 43; University of Toronto, M.D. 47; F.R.C.S.(C).

Postgraduate education began with internship at the Toronto General Hospital (1947) followed by three years at the Hague and one at Utrecht in Holland. Next, he spent a year at St. Michael's Hospital, Toronto, and one at Johns Hopkins Hospital. In 1968, when he sent his curriculum vitae, he was Chief of the Division of Cardiovascular Surgery at St. Michael's Hospital, Consultant in this specialty at the Scarborough General Hospital, and Assistant Professor of Surgery at the University of Toronto. He offered no comments on the special questions, nor his bibliography. He and his associate, Dr. J. Yas, accomplished a notable achievement, the performance of three cardiac transplants in 1968; one of those patients lived for four years.

Dr. Raymond O. Heimbecker, 29 November 1922, Calgary, Alberta; University of Saskatchewan, B.A.; University of Toronto, M.A. 49, M.D. 47; M.S.; F.R.C.S.(C); F.A.C.S.; A.A.T.S.; F.A.H.A.; F.A.C.C.

It appears that Bill Bigelow and Bill Mustard created the two earliest principal centres of postgraduate training in cardiovascular surgery in Ontario. By 1965, Bigelow's bibliography reveals fifty-four co-authors, namely, trainees who, with few exceptions, became pioneering cardiovascular surgeons in other Canadian hospitals, or abroad. A few became members of Dr. Bigelow's own staff. Dr. Raymond O. Heimbecker was the first of these latter. In 1965, he wrote:

> My initial interest in cardiovascular surgery was during my undergraduate days at the Toronto General Hospital in 1946-1947 when Dr. Gordon Murray was doing some of the pioneer work in the Blalock anastamosis for tetralogy of Fallot and some of the closures of septal defects. Cardiovascular surgery was certainly an unknown entity at that time, but Dr. Murray's keen and inquiring mind ... was a great stimulus to me. Even in 1949 it appeared that cardiovascular surgery should only be a hobby to be undertaken by interested surgeons.... Robert Janes, Wilfred Bigelow, and further contact with Gordon Murray paved the way for my entry into this specialty. Contact with Sir Russell Brock and Dr. Paul Wood in England broadened my interest and knowledge of the field.... The Canadian Cardiovascular Society has been a wonderful platform upon which to exchange information with fellow Canadians and above all to build up a fellowship.

After two years of internship and residency at the Toronto General Hospital Dr. Heimbecker spent a year (1949-1950) with Dr. Alfred Blalock at Johns Hopkins. Then, after another four years of work in Toronto, he received a Travelling Fellowship in 1955 and went to England, where he came under the influence of Sir Russell Brock and Dr. Paul Wood. On returning home he began his career in the newly created post as geographical full-time Cardiovascular Surgeon on Dr. Bigelow's staff. This position provided him the opportunities to serve in the care of patients, to teach undergraduates and postgraduate trainees, and to continue his interests in research. Between 1950 and 1965, his bibliography grew to fifty-two items. The subjects include physiological experimental studies, clinical experiences, inventions of instruments and new techniques, editorials, and reviews. The majority are co-authored with medical and surgical associates and trainees. Because of the training he had experienced in Canada, Dr. Heimbecker was better prepared to benefit from his studies in the United States and in England than those of the previous generation who began their special training in cardiovascular surgery abroad. He was among the first Canadian cardiovascular surgeons to enjoy these privileges. Many emulated him in subsequent years. Until 1974 he worked in Toronto; in that year he became the first Professor and Chief of Cardiovascular Surgery at the University of Western Ontario in London.

Dr. John C. Coles, University of Western Ontario, M.D. 48; F.R.C.S.(C); General Surgery, Thoracic Surg. and Cardiovascular and Thoracic Surg.; F.A.C.S.; F.A.C.C.

Dr. Coles did not respond to the questionnaire. He is mentioned as a senior teacher in the minibiography of Dr. Samuel C. Carroll and as a co-author of nine items in Dr. Carroll's bibliography. In 1971, he was Assistant Professor of Surgery at the University of Western Ontario and on the staffs of the Victoria and the St. Joseph's Hospitals.

Dr. George Aubrey Trusler, 17 November 1926, Toronto; University of Toronto, M.D. 49; B.Sc. (Med.); F.R.C.S.(C); F.A.C.S., Ms. (Tor.); F.A.H.A.; A.A.P.

Between 1949 and 1955 Dr. Trusler served internships and residencies in medicine and pathology in Toronto, and spent 1952-1953 in research at the Banting Institute. In January 1955 he started training for surgery. His comments on the special questions succinctly and very effectively describe how he chose to become a cardiovascular surgeon.

While I was training in general surgery under Professor R. M. Janes at the Toronto General Hospital, I spent a year in basic research with Dr. W. G. Bigelow. Subsequently, I received my general surgical training on Dr. Bigelow's ward (Ward c at the Toronto General Hospital). At this time Dr. Bigelow was gradually changing this ward from a mixed service to a cardiovascular service. The post of Resident in Cardiovascular Surgery was created and at Dr. Bigelow's request, I became the first man to occupy this position. At that time I had no firm design to specialize in cardiovascular surgery because I could not see any promise in finding a position and an area in which to practise. Six months later when I had just completed my general surgical training, Dr. W. T. Mustard at the Hospital for Sick Children, Toronto requested that I join him on the staff of that hospital to do cardiovascular surgery. For this purpose I spent six months on a McLaughlin Travelling Fellowship in the United States and then twelve months as Resident in both Paediatric General and Paediatric Cardiovascular Surgery at the Hospital for Sick Children.

In June 1965, Dr. Trusler was Assistant Surgeon at the hospital, Honorary Research Associate of the Research Institute of the Hospital for Sick Children and Clinical Teacher in the Department of Surgery at the University of Toronto. When Dr. Mustard retired, Dr. Trusler was appointed Chief of Cardiovascular Surgery at the hospital. He attained the rank of Assistant Professor at the University. Between 1949 and 1965, his bibliography contains twenty-five items. The first item, written when he was an undergraduate, is on "Headache." The second, co-authored with J. C. McBernie, F. G. Pearson, A. G. Gornall, and W. G. Bigelow, is on a "Study of Hibernation in Relation to the Technique of Hypothermia for Intracardiac Surgery" (*Surg. Forum,* 1953: 4, 72-77). The majority of the articles deal with cardiovascular subjects; in the early years he co-authored a few articles on paediatric surgery related to the gastrointestinal tract.

Dr. George David Hooper, 21 October 1926, Ottawa, Ontario; McGill, M.D., C.M. 50; Diploma Surgery 56; F.R.C.S.(C) General Surgery and Thoracic Surgery; F.A.C.C.P. 58.

In the course of his training, Dr. Hooper held appointments at the Montreal General and the Montreal Children's hospitals, Guy's Hospital, London, England, Royal Victoria Hospital, Montreal, and Royal Edward Laurentian Hospital, Ste. Agathe, Quebec.

In 1965, he was Assistant Professor, Cardiothoracic Surgery at the University of Ottawa and Consultant in Cardiac Surgery at Ottawa Civic and Riverside Hospitals as well as at the National Defence Medical Centre. In addition, he was Consultant in Thoracic Surgery at the Royal Ottawa Sanitarium. Dr. Hooper appears to have been the first specially trained cardiothoracic surgeon who practised in Ottawa. He did not submit any comments on the special questions, nor his bibliography.

Dr. Samuel Edwin Carroll, 20 December 1928; University of Western Ontario, B.A. 56; M.D. 53; F.R.C.S.(C) General Surgery 58; F.R.C.S.(C); Cardiovascular and Thoracic Surgery 64; C.S.C.I.; F.A.C.C.

After junior internship at the Victoria Hospital, Dr. Carroll began his training in general surgery, a four-year course (1954-1958) with Professor Angus D. McLachin, Chief of Surgery at the University of Western Ontario. From July to December 1958 he was resident in Pathology, working with J. C. Paterson at the Westminster Hospital in London, Ontario. He then spent a year as Registrar in Surgery at Edgware General Hospital and as Research Assistant at St. Mark's Hospital in London, England. On returning home he worked as part-time assistant to Dr. J. C. Coles, in thoracic and cardiovascular surgery (1960-1963).

During the first six months of 1961, he worked in the Surgical Laboratory of the Children's Hospital Medical Centre in Boston, with Dr. R. B. Gross, studying hypothermia. In January, 1961 he was appointed Research Fellow of the Ontario Heart Foundation and in January, 1963, he became Cardiovascular Surgeon at the Westminster Hospital and at St. Joseph's Hospital in London, Ontario.

In 1964, his appointment with the Ontario Heart Foundation changed to Part-Time Associate.

Dr. Carroll did not write any comments about the special questions but did include his bibliography of twenty-four items published between 1954 and 1965. The first item is on "Lobotomy," published in *University of Western Ontario Medical Journal* (1954: 24, 131), probably written when he was an undergraduate. The earliest article on a cardiovascular subject is co-authored with Drs. J. C. Coles, G. A. Sears, and G. W. Manning entitled "Intracardiac Phonocardiographic Studies of the Aortic Valve" (*Proceedings of the Canadian Society for Clinical Investigation,* 1961). The twelfth publication is on a method of providing adequate cerebral blood flow during carotid artery thromboendarterectomy, co-authored with Drs. J. C. Coles and N. Gergely (*C.M.A.J.*, 1962: 86, 835).

Dr. Ronald James Baird, 3 May 1930, Toronto; University of Toronto, M.D. 54; B.Sc. (Med.) 56; F.R.C.S.(C); Gen. Surg. 59; Thor. and C. V. Surg. 64; F.A.C.S. 64; F.A.H.A.; C.S.C.I.

As a medical undergraduate student, Dr. Baird "believed he would become an internist with special interest in cardiovascular disease." During his junior internship he became fascinated with surgery and influenced by Dr. Gordon Murray, Dr. Wilfred Bigelow, Dr. Donald Wilson, Dr. James Key, and Dr. Raymond Heimbecker, he chose to specialize in cardiovascular surgery. During the year 1954-1955 he worked at research on hypothermia with Dr. Bigelow. The next five years were devoted to training in general surgery and cardiovascular surgery at the Toronto General, Sunnybrook, and Sick Children's hospitals. Then followed a year of travel in Europe and in the United States. On returning home he joined the staff of the University of Toronto and of the Toronto General Hospital, and became Research Associate of the Ontario Heart Foundation. Thus began his distinguished career. By 1972 he had become Chief of Cardiovascular Surgery at the Toronto Western Hospital and Professor of Surgery at the university. Among his many responsibilities and honours were chairman of the medical committee of the Ontario Heart Foundation in 1970, and in the same year secretary-treasurer of the Canadian Cardiovascular Society.

The first item in his bibliography was written as an undergraduate student: "The Etiology and Pathology of the Nephrotic Syndrome" (*U. of T. Med. J.*, 1953: 31, 101-106). The second item, his thesis for the degree of B.Sc., is "A Study in Hypothermia with Special Reference to Brown Fat" (*U. of T. Med. J.*, May 1956: 47). In 1965 there were twenty-four items in his bibliography. The majority deal with subjects related to the cardiovascular system and are co-authored. The twenty-fourth item is his thesis for the degree of Master of Surgery, "The Mechanism of Vasodilatation Which Follows Arterial Gas Embolism" (*U. of T. Med. J.*, May 1964: 70).

Dr. Trusler and Dr. Baird exemplify the maturity of cardiovascular surgery in Toronto. They belong to the first generation of specialists in cardiovascular surgery who obtained their training in Toronto and engaged in research which produced significant innovations, mainly, the application of hypothermia to the technique of intracardiac surgery.

Dr. Paul Field, 12 January 1931, Swansea, South Wales; University of London, King's College and Medical School, M.B., B.S. 54; L.L.M.C. 54; F.R.C.S. (Edin.) 61; F.R.C.S.(C) 62; F.A.C.S. 65; F.R.C.S.(C) Cardiovascular and Thoracic Surgery 65; F.A.H.A.

Dr. Field's postgraduate training began with an internship in Surgery at Chelmsford in England in 1953-1954 and there followed internships, residencies, and registrarships on both sides of the Atlantic during the years 1954 to 1962. The year 1961-1962 found him as assistant resident in Cardiovascular Surgery at the Massachusetts General Hospital. He served as clinical assistant to Dr. W. A. G. Bigelow in the Cardiovascular Unit at the Toronto General Hospital during the year 1965-1966.

Dr. Field's response to the questionnaire provides a very good description of pioneering cardiovascular surgery in a medical centre which does not have a medical school.

> Having always been interested in thoracic surgery and having worked in this field with Dr. George R. Walker who is a general and thoracic surgeon in Sudbury from 1955 to 1957, my training was planned in order to take me to a thoracic unit in Great Britain in 1959. There I spent two years working with Mr. R. H. Belsey, F.R.C.S. who was at that time becoming involved in his first cases of open-heart surgery. Assisting with these stimulated my interest in the cardiac side of surgery, in addition to my well-established interest in surgery of the lungs and oesophagus. While in Boston, I was assistant resident at the Massachusetts General Hospital. 1961-1962, I worked with Dr. R. R. Linton whose life is almost entirely devoted to peripheral arterial reconstruction. This training interested and equipped me for a future involving this part of cardiovascular and thoracic surgery. My final decision to confine myself to this specialty was not made until my arrival back in practice in Sudbury in 1962, when it was apparent that no one in the community was providing a service in the field of cardiovascular surgery and it has therefore since then been my endeavour to get established in this field and to set up a unit for treatment of cardiovascular and thoracic investigation and treatment.
>
> My training was primarily planned to fulfil the requirements of the Royal College for the Fellowship in General Surgery. However, during the training, I obtained as much experience in thoracic surgery as I possibly could. Following my decision to specialize in cardiovascular surgery, the Royal College de-

manded a further four months of training. After consultation with Dr. W. G. Bigelow, I was welcomed to an appointment at the Toronto General Hospital as clinical assistant for a period of six months in order to fulfil the requirements of the College. There do not appear to have been any major difficulties that would have prevented my qualification in the specialty of cardiovascular surgery. My establishment in Sudbury has developed from the need for a cardiovascular unit in this area and the promise that my wishes to develop such a unit seem to be gradually becoming realized.

The Canadian Cardiovascular Society did play a part in the development of my career, mainly in introducing me to men of common interest throughout Canada. I was introduced to the Society through the group of Toronto surgeons who are already known to me but most people outside of Toronto in this field were entirely strangers to me. Through the two meetings of the Society which I have attended since my being made a member, I have met a very large number of people who I feel I now know as friends. I think that this aspect of the role of the Society is a very important one to a person whose primary training has not been undertaken at a Canadian medical centre.

I have inaugurated in Sudbury, a Journal Club which is attended by various sectors of the medical and nursing profession. This club meets twice monthly and all attending members are responsible for presentation of papers from journals that they have recently read and we are endeavouring to build up an index system of all papers presented.

In 1965, Dr. Field was in the process of establishing the Cardiothoracic Unit at the Sudbury Memorial Hospital which serves the population of the region known as Northern Ontario. His appointment as Research Associate in the Faculty of Science at Laurentian University provided him with facilities for research.

Dr. Field's bibliography for the years 1959 to 1962 includes a thesis on "An Experimental Approach to Portal Hypertension Using Parenchymatous Splenic Anastamosis." This essay was submitted to the Royal College of Physicians and Surgeons in fulfilment of the requirements for the Medal in Surgery in June 1959. In the same year he published an article on "Establishment of Parenchymatous Spleno-Pulmonary Venous Anastomosis" (*Nature,* 1959: 184, 703). He has also published an article on "Cholelithiasis Associated with Congenital Malformation of the Cystic Duct in a Young Child" (*Br. J. Surg.*, 1960: 48, 78).

Dr. John Lloyd Provan, 9 August 1931, Newport, England: University College, London, B.Sc. 53; M.B.,B.S. 56; M.S. (London) 68; F.R.C.S. (Eng.) 61; F.T.S.; F.A.S. (Great Britain & Ireland).

The story of Dr. Provan's education and eventual emigration to Toronto is well told in his own words.

> As a student I was always interested in physiology of the cardiovascular system and had no explanation why this should be the case. But I found it easy to understand and rather more enjoyable than other aspects of physiology. I maintained this interest at University College Hospital working as a clerk for Dr. Kenneth Harris (Chief of Medical Cardiology) with whom I subsequently fell out because at that stage of my career I preferred rowing to spending long hours in the outpatient clinic, a situation which did not entirely meet with his approval! After graduation in medicine at University College Hospital I decided to specialize in surgery and for part of my training spent two years working at University College with Professor Sir Roy Cameron and Professor R. S. Pilcher. The latter was Professor of Surgery at University College Hospital at that time and his main interest was in thoracic surgery. He had just started doing peripheral vascular surgery which was relatively new in 1956 and he was also interested in the Vineberg operation, having been stimulated by Arthur Vineberg when he visited him in Montreal in 1955. I started to study with Professor Pilcher, and published a paper on "The Histological Features of Internal Mammary Implants," and largely guided by Professor Pilcher's interest in the field I also spent some time working on the development of a bubble oxygenator for cardio-pulmonary bypass. Also at this time, we were doing experiments using veno-venous cooling for hypothermia and we started putting this into practice while I was still a Research Fellow. After I got the English F.R.C.S. I went to work with Professor Pilcher as a Resident in Surgery and continued my interest in the field of cardiovascular surgery.
>
> In England at that time there was very little formal training in cardiology or cardiovascular surgery and training was very largely a hit or miss experience, depending upon what jobs were available at the moment when an intern or resident was facing the end of a one-or-two-year appointment in a given hospital. I was lucky to be kept on at University College Hospital and even more lucky when Professor Pilcher suggested, through his association with Dr. R. Shaw at the Massachusetts General Hospital, that I

should go and work there for a year. This I did in 1964-1965, coming under the tutelage of Dr. W. G. Austen, now Chief of Surgery at that hospital. Dr. Shaw had retired due to ill health after the arrangements had been made for my attendance over there. Upon returning to University College Hospital in 1965, I became more heavily committed to cardiac surgery but was eventually forced to leave the English system by the lack of posts which were available for cardiac surgeons at that time. I think the main obstacle to my progress was the fact that a training scheme for cardiovascular surgeons had gradually started in Britain by which time I was rather too senior to have entered it. As no post was available at University College Hospital, where I was happily practising, and as Professor Pilcher had retired, I felt that it was time to seek fields elsewhere and when my post at Wellesley Hospital was offered I was very pleased to come.

Dr. Provan came to Toronto in 1969 to occupy the post of Staff Surgeon which was his status in 1972 when he wrote the above lines.

During the years 1961-1972 Dr. Provan's bibliography grew to twenty-four items. There are five articles related to cardiovascular surgery which he co-authored with Dr. Austen and several of his colleagues. The remaining nineteen include several concerning thoracic surgery which involved the lungs and the esophagus, and several which deal with peripheral vascular surgery.

Dr. Provan's experience during the years of training suggests that Dr. Bigelow and Dr. Mustard initiated their training centres somewhat earlier than such centres were formed in Great Britain.

Dr. Alan Stephen Trimble, 11 June 1932, Toronto; University of Toronto, M.D. 56; B.Sc. (Med.) 58; F.R.C.S.(C) 64; F.A.C.S.

Dr. Alan Stephen Trimble, an early recruit of the 'Bigelow School,' wrote as follows in 1968.

I decided to go into cardiovascular surgery during a basic research year (1957) spent with Dr. W. G. Bigelow after my junior internship. I had initially intended to go into neurosurgery, however, interest in the project — we were working on hypothermia at the time — and the influence of this man led me to go into cardiovascular surgery.

My training was organized through the Gallie Course at the University of Toronto under the direction of Dr. W. G. Bigelow. No obstacles were encountered and I decided to practise in Toronto because it had been my home.

He supplemented the Torontonian postgraduate studies with sojourns in San Francisco at the Presbyterian Medical Center and in Jackson at the Mississippi Medical School. In 1968 his official status was Clinical Teacher, Department of Surgery, University of Toronto, and Surgeon, Division of Cardiovascular Surgery, Toronto General Hospital, and Research Associate, Ontario Heart Foundation. The first item of his bibliography is an article on "Fibrosis of the Ampulla of Vater" (*Arch. Surg.*, 1961: Vol. 83, 458), which he co-authored with four colleagues. By 1968, the list grew to twenty-six items, mainly related to cardiovascular surgery; there are a few relating to other problems of thoracic surgery. Nearly all are co-authored with forty different medical and surgical colleagues. This number reflects the great influence exercised by the 'Bigelow School' in the training of generations of cardiovascular specialists.

Dr. Edward Joseph Peter Charette, 10 January 1935, Troy, New York; St. Patrick's College, Ottawa, B.Sc. 55; Ottawa University, M.D. 59; McGill, M.Sc. (Surgery) 62; F.R.C.S.(C); F.A.C.S.; F.C.C.P.; F.A.C.A.; C.P.S.Q., F.A.H.A.

Dr. Charette went to McGill for his postgraduate training in surgery from 1959 to 1967; this included a year of experimental surgery (1961 to 1962), residency in Cardiovascular Surgery and earning the degree M.Sc. with his thesis on "The Lymphocyte and Shock Resistance" (1962). In 1968, he joined the surgical attending staffs of the Kingston General and Hôtel-Dieu hospitals and Queen's University Medical School. In 1972, his status was Assistant Professor of Surgery and also Consultant to the Canadian Armed Forces, Ongwanada, and the Kingston Psychiatric hospitals. The McGill special training program in Cardiovascular Thoracic Surgery started in 1964. He had not had any special interest in this field until, in 1964, he worked as Resident in Cardiovascular Surgery at the Montreal Children's Hospital for some weeks as substitute for the Resident who was on holiday. This experience led him to become the first to enter the new special course.

The first item in his bibliography is the thesis for his B.Sc. degree, "Evolution and Man." The thesis for the M.Sc. degree mentioned above is the next item. There follow four articles co-authored with Drs. Jegier and Dobell, on work achieved during training. The final five are subjects related to thoracic surgery and to cardiovascular surgery co-authored with colleagues of Queen's University Medical School and Kingston Hospitals. Dr. Charette's experience exemplifies the long period of formal training required in preparation for a career in cardiovascular and thoracic surgery. He had this training at McGill and its associated hospitals, and enriched the Queen's University Medical School, where his career is evolving.

Dr. Wilbert Joseph Keon, 17 May 1935, Sheenboro, Quebec; St. Patrick's College, Ottawa, B.Sc. 57; University of Ottawa, M.D. 61; F.R.C.S.(C) Gen. Surg. 66; Cv. and Thor. Surg. 68; F.A.C.C.; F.A.H.A.

After a junior internship at the Ottawa Civic Hospital (1961-1962), Dr. Keon entered his training for cardiothoracic surgery. The years 1962-1966 were devoted to general surgery at the Montreal General Hospital and also to research which formed the subject of his thesis for the degree M.Sc. on "The Investigation of Closed Left Heart By-pass" (McGill University, 1964). During the year 1965-1966 he was Chief Surgical Resident at the Montreal General Hospital; the following year he was Senior Cardiovascular Resident on Dr. Bigelow's staff and during the year 1967-1968, he served as Senior Resident in Cardiovascular Surgery on Dr. Mustard's staff. After these two years in Toronto, he spent approximately eight months at the Peter Bent Brigham Hospital and Harvard Medical Center as Research Associate. When Dr. Keon filled in the questionnaire in 1971, his academic status was Associate Professor of Surgery and Head of the Sub-Department of Cardiothoracic Surgery, the University of Ottawa. His clinical appointment was Director of the Cardiac Unit of the University of Ottawa and Head of the Department of Cardiothoracic Surgery, Ottawa Civic Hospital. Dr. Keon did not include any comments on the special questions but did provide his bibliography. The nine articles published between 1967 and 1970 reflect his work with colleagues during his years of training. The eleventh is entitled "Emergency Aorto-Coronary Venous Bypass Graft in Cardiogenic Shock" and is co-authored with S. Z. Abbas, K. R. Shankar, and A. F. Nuno (*C.M.A.J.*, 1971: 105, 1293-96). This first publication after he began his career in Ottawa reflects the skilful, confident surgeon, a good omen for great achievements in the course of a successful career. He belongs to the generation of cardiothoracic surgeons whose principal training took place in Canadian centres and who proceeded to bring fresh stimulus for the growth and maturation of an additional Canadian centre of cardiology.

Dr. Bernard Sidney Goldman, 23 February 1936, Toronto; University of Toronto, M.D. 60; B.Sc. (Med.) 62; F.R.C.S.(C);F.A.C.S.; F.A.C.C.; F.A.H.A.

Dr. Goldman had all his education in Toronto, including the University of Toronto postgraduate training course (1961-1966). He supplemented this education with studies abroad as Registrar in Thoracic Surgery at Frenchay Hospital, Bristol, England (1967), and as Research Fellow, Cardiovascular Surgery, Harvard Medical School, Massachusetts General Hospital, Boston (1968). His official status in 1972 was Assistant Professor of Surgery, University of Toronto, Staff Surgeon, Division of Cardiovascular Surgery, Toronto General Hospital, and Consultant (Cardiovascular Surgery) at the New Mt. Sinai Hospital, Toronto. In response to the question as to how he chose to specialize in cardiovascular surgery he wrote in 1972 the following:

> The decision to specialize in cardiovascular surgery was prompted by an interest in cardiopulmonary physiology and the specific desire to perform surgery, and to care for the acutely ill patient. The decision to study cardiology was made at the end of the third undergraduate year at medical school while working as an extern and in the same year, the decision to combine cardiovascular physiology and surgery was made after a session on the surgical service. There were no special plans or people to rely on until one was actually in the special training program. Most obstacles were overcome by perseverence rather than by any actual mentor or patron other than the friendship that a particular senior surgeon provided me during difficult times. Later, during difficult times in training, Drs. Mustard and Bigelow who were my respective chiefs in my senior residency years encouraged and assisted me.

Between 1962 and 1972 Dr. Goldman's bibliography grew to thirty items. The first, his thesis for the B.Sc. degree is "Studies in Hypothermia with Special Reference to Natural Hibernation" (University of Toronto, 1962). The thirtieth item bears the intriguing title "Pacemaker Panic" and like all the remainder except the thesis, is co-authored with colleagues.

Dr. Goldman contributes an interesting story concerning when and how he became interested in becoming a cardiovascular surgeon, namely, as a third year undergraduate medical student. It appears that the subject itself, rather than inspiration derived from a teacher, stimulated him. In this respect his experience appears to be similar to that of Dr. Provan. His story also reflects the fact that he belongs to the generation which began to take for granted the specially organized training program for cardiovascular surgery. To become aware of how the current opportunities for training, including financial support, came into existence, physicians and surgeons of this generation would have to read about the trials and tribulations of their pioneering teachers, such as Gordon Murray, Wilfred Bigelow, William Mustard, and their contemporaries at home and abroad.

Manitoba

Four men pioneered cardiovascular and thoracic surgery in Manitoba. All graduated in medicine at the University of Manitoba and began postgraduate training with internships and residencies in Winnipeg area hospitals, went to four different centres to acquire expertise in the specialty, and returned to work at clinical care of patients, research, and teaching in Winnipeg and St. Boniface.

Dr. Colin Campbell Ferguson, 30 October 1921; University of Manitoba, M.D. 45; F.A.C.S.; F.R.C.P.(C); F.A.A.P.

Dr. Ferguson devoted the years 1946-1947 to work in Pathology at McGill, 1947-1948 to Surgery at McGill, 1948-1949 to Surgical Research at the University of Pennsylvania, 1949-1950 again to Surgery at McGill, and the years 1950-1953 to Cardiovascular Surgery at Harvard.

In the course of these years, he became a Fellow of the Royal College of Surgeons (Canada), earned the Diploma in Surgery at McGill and of the American Board of Surgeons, and became a Fellow of the American Academy of Paediatrics.

In 1965, his official status was Professor and Head of the Department of Surgery, the University of Manitoba, and Surgeon in Chief, The Children's Hospital, Winnipeg.

At first glance, his bibliography is unique; it begins with a list of seven motion picture films. He made the first film in 1953 on "The Surgical Treatment of Pectus Excavatum." The third film, made in association with Dr. G. Cumming, deals with "Pulmonary Atresia in a Two Week Old Infant." The next film, entitled "Open-Heart Surgery" was made in 1962. The seventh, also made with Dr. Cumming, is about "Tumour of the Pulmonary Valve."

The list of forty publications begins with an article he co-authored with C. Collins-Williams on "Infectious Mononucleosis" (*C.M.A.J.*, 1946). The fourth item "Abdominal Incisions in Infants and Children," co-authored with R. E. Gross (*Ann. Surg.*, 1953: 137, 349) marks the beginning of his writings on paediatric surgery.

In 1954, he wrote a review entitled "The Surgery of Congenital Heart Disease" (*Man. Med. Rev.*, 1954: 34, 13). The twentieth item is "Patent Ductus Arteriosus, A Review of 36 Cases Treated by Surgery," co-authored with H. W. Chestnut (*Can. J. Surg.*, 1958: 2, 55) and in the same year there appeared the "Surgical Treatment of Transposition of the Great Vessels" (*C.M.A.J.*, 1958: 79, 551). The forty-three publications during the years 1946 to 1965 include a wide variety of subjects related to paediatric general surgery, some editorials, medical history, and number 43, which was due to be published in the *Manitoba Medical Review* in 1965, entitled "Report of a Surgical Tour of the United Kingdom as James IV Surgical Traveller."

Dr. Morley Cohen, 18 November 1923, Winnipeg; University of Manitoba, M.D. 48; University of Minnesota, Ph.D. 54; Diploma Amer. Board Surgery F.R.C.S.(C) 55; F.A.C.S. 57; Diplomate Amer. Board Thoracic Surgery 58; F.A.C.C.P.

Dr. Morley Cohen had all his basic education in his native city. He graduated from the Manitoba University Medical School in 1948, and served as Assistant Resident in Surgery at the St. Boniface Hospital and Teaching Fellow in Surgery, University of Manitoba during the year 1948-1949. From June 1949 to June 1950, he was Resident in Pathology at the Deer Lodge Veterans Hospital and Demonstrator in Pathology at the University. During six months from June to December 1950, he was Senior Resident in Surgery, as well as Teaching Fellow in Surgery for the University. Then, as good judgement and good luck would have it, he became a Fellow in Surgery at the University of Minnesota for the years 1950-1954. Thus, he had the opportunity to contribute to the beginning of open-heart surgery with the technique of a heart-lung preparation, and contribute he did — very significantly.

Dr. Owen Harding Wagenstein was appointed Professor of Surgery at the University of Minnesota in 1930, twenty years before Morley Cohen had the good fortune to be accepted into the special academic training program which Dr. Wagenstein had organized soon after his appointment. The training included clinical surgery in the hospital, experimental surgery in the laboratory, and fulfilment of requirements for the degree Ph.D. in surgery. Four years were devoted to this course. His young but senior co-worker, Dr. C. Walton Lillehei, had joined the course on returning from World War II; he graduated in 1950.

In that year, Lillehei was found to have a rare type of malignant tumour in the neck. The illness related to the surgical operation, radiation therapy, and convalescence lasted many months, until the spring of 1951, when he resumed his normal way of life, namely, assiduous work from early morning to late at night in general surgery, with a special interest in the cardiovascular system. Thus, it happened that Dr. Wagenstein invited him to fill the vacancy created when Dr. Clarence Dennis accepted a Professorship of Surgery at New York Downstate College of Medicine. Dr. Dennis had been one of a small coterie of men in all the world, working on the creation of an artificial heart-lung machine. His progress had reached the stage at which he had used the machine, unsuccessfully, in two operations. One of the conditions of his moving to New York was that the college should buy his apparatus from the University of Minnesota, so that he could continue his research in his new laboratory. Dr. Wagenstein arranged for this money to be assigned to pursuing the same type of goal in his department; Dr. Lillehei undertook to do the work. The events described so far form the background for appreciating how it came about that the title of Dr. Morley Cohen's doctoral thesis is "Studies on Experimental Methods for Intracardiac Surgery — The Development and Physiologic Basis" (1954).

Dr. Lillehei, well-informed about the literature on the subject, chose to search for a new approach. He began by selecting an effective pump and when Cohen joined him in the work, he had chosen the double Signamotor pump: one motor drove two pumps, one for receiving, the other for delivering precisely the same amount of blood. They sought to answer the question of how long the circulation could be stopped without damaging the heart. Their experiments revealed that, if drainage from the azygos vein was retained, the small amount of blood which circulated significantly prolonged the duration of life of the animal. This fact strongly suggested the circulation rate to be achieved by an artificial heart-lung machine need be only a fraction of the normal amount, especially if hypothermia would also be used. Various ideas were explored which proved useless; these are described in the thesis. A fertile idea emerged out of conversation between Cohen and Herbert E. Warden, who had entered the special course some time after Cohen. They became close friends. One day in September 1953, Warden said to Cohen, "Wouldn't it be nice if we could plug a patient into an oxygen supply the way a fetus is plugged into its mother?" According to Leonard Engel, who relates this story in considerable detail, the two men had on their minds the fact that Morley's wife Joan was experiencing her first pregnancy and this may have led Warden to make the remark (Engel, 1959). The next morning (Sunday), when they met in the lab, Cohen greeted Warden with "Why not? Why not plug the patient into a donor to breathe for him?" Out of this exchange there developed the plan for a human heart-lung technique (cross-circulation). The breakthrough event occurred on the 26th of March, 1954. The first patient, a one-year-old boy with an interventricular septal defect, had his father as donor. Warden and Cohen monitored the father during the operation by Dr. Lillehei, who was assisted by Dr. Richard L. Varco, a senior member of the surgical staff. The infant was making good post-operative progress when on the eleventh day he suddenly died of pneumonia. Three and a half weeks later the second case was done and this child survived. Between the spring of 1954 and that of 1955, forty-five such operations were performed. Radical correction of tetralogy of Fallot was accomplished for the first time with this technique. The work was announced at a session of the World Congress of Cardiology in September 1954. In 1955, Drs. Lillehei, Cohen, Warden, and Varco received the Lasker Award for Medical Research, each a gold statuette and a $1,000 cheque.

Between 1949 and 1964, Dr. Cohen's bibliography grew to thirty-six items, the majority related to cardiovascular surgery. The first article, co-authored with four colleagues including Dr. Lillehei is on "Tolerance of the Canine Heart for Temporary Complete Venacaval Occlusion" appeared in 1952. The following year, with Dr. Lillehei, he co-authored an article on "Autogenous Lung Oxygenator with Total Cardiac By-Pass for Intracardiac Surgery." These studies represent the work done in the experimental laboratory, preliminary to intracardiac surgery in humans. Item fourteen crystallizes both the experimental and clinical work, "The Direct Vision Intracardiac Correction of Congenital Anomalies by Controlled Cross Circulation. Results in 32 Patients with Ventricular Septal Defects, Tetralogy of Fallot and Atroventricularis Communis Defects" (*Surg.*, 1956: 38, 11-30). The four physicians who received the Lasker awards — Lillehei, Cohen, Warden, and Varco — co-authored this article. Soon after he returned to Winnipeg to begin his career as a pioneering cardiovascular surgeon, Dr. Cohen published an article in the *Manitoba Medical Review* (1955: 35, 489-494) entitled "Recent Advances in the Surgery of Congenital Heart Disease." Item number 25 is on "Mitral Valvulotomy — Results in a Preliminary Survey of 104 Cases" (*C.M.A.J.*, 1956: 74, 788-792). At the 1963 meeting of the Canadian Cardiovascular Society he and Dr. Mymin presented a paper on "Prosthetic Valve Replacement in Management of Aortic Valve Diseases."

In 1965 when Dr. Cohen submitted his curriculum vitae, he held the following posts: Member of the Active Staff, Department of

Surgery, Director of the Surgical Research Laboratory, and Director of the Cardiopulmonary Surgical Unit of the St. Boniface Hospital. At the University of Manitoba, he was Professor of Surgery.

Dr. Janoslaw Barwinsky, 15 October 1926, Ukraine; University of Manitoba, M.D. 55; Diploma in Surgery 59; Diplomate Amer. Board Surg. 62; Thoracic Surg. 63; Cert. R.C.S. General Surg. 61; Thoracic Surg. 61; F.R.C.S.(C) 64; F.A.C.S. 64; F.A.C.C.

During the first three years after graduation, Dr. Barwinsky worked in the surgical training program of the University of Manitoba teaching hospitals; then he spent three years as Resident in Training in Thoracic and Cardiovascular Surgery at Cleveland Metropolitan General Hospital associated with Western Reserve University School of Medicine. He stated that he "decided to take the training in Thoracic and Cardiovascular Surgery at the end of his third undergraduate year" and that he had no special experience which he could identify as the stimulus for making this choice. His principal concern was to make a good choice in selecting the "right place for postgraduate training." He has been very happy with his choice.

By 1965, when he completed the questionnaire, he was in charge of the Cardiovascular Research Laboratory at the St. Boniface General Hospital, a member of the Active Surgical Staff of this hospital, on the Courtesy Staff of the Winnipeg General Hospital, the Children's Hospital and the Misericordia Hospital. His status at the University of Manitoba Surgical Faculty was Demonstrator and Half-Time Tutor.

His bibliography begins with an article on "The Cardiac Output in Response to Surgical Trauma," which he co-authored with Dr. Clowes (*Arch. Surg.*, 1960: 81, 212). The last paper in his bibliography of four items published between 1960 and 1964 is on "Surgical Management of Complete Heart Block" (*Man. Med. Rev.*, 1964: 43, 187).

During these four years, he presented papers at five meetings of Societies.

Dr. Allan Rae Downs, 14 October 1930, Preeceville, Saskatchewan; University of Manitoba, M.D. 54; F.R.C.S.(C).

Dr. Downs had his primary and secondary schooling in Preeceville. He entered the University of Manitoba in 1947 and graduated M.D. in 1954. During the first four years after graduation, he served internships and residencies at the Winnipeg General Hospital. In 1958-

1960, he enjoyed the advantage of a McLaughlin Fellowship which made possible postgraduate studies in England, at St. Mary's Hospital in London and at the Southampton Chest Hospital. He returned to Winnipeg in 1960.

In 1968, when he completed the questionnaire, he was Associate Surgeon and Associate Director of the Intensive Care Unit at the Winnipeg General Hospital, and Associate Professor of Surgery in the Faculty of Medicine of the University of Manitoba. Dr. Downs did not supply his bibliography.

Saskatchewan

Dr. Eric Musard Nanson, 4 January 1915, Geraldine, South Canterbury, New Zealand; Otago University, B. Med., B. Surg. 39; F.R.C.S. (Eng) 47; F.R.C.S.(C) 54; F.A.C.S. 56; F.R.A.C.S.(N.Z.) 70.

From 1939-1941, Dr. Nanson served internships at Christ Church Hospital and in 1940, he was a Demonstrator in Anatomy at Otago University. He served in World War II as Captain in the New Zealand Medical Corps (1941-1945). After the war, he resumed postgraduate training first in New Zealand (1945-1947), then in England (1947-1950). He obtained a Rockefeller Fellowship in 1950, and spent a year at Johns Hopkins Hospital. He returned to England where he became Assistant Consultant in Surgery at the Bristol Royal Infirmary (1951-1952).

During the next two years, he worked on the surgical staff of Johns Hopkins Hospital. From 1954 to 1969, he pioneered thoracic and cardiovascular surgery in Saskatchewan as Surgeon-in-Chief, University Hospital, Consultant Surgeon in City Hospital, St. Paul Hospital, and Saskatoon Sanitarium. In 1969, he returned to New Zealand to occupy the post of Professor of Surgery, School of Medicine, Aukland University.

> As regards specialization in cardiology, I got into the matter of cardiovascular surgery by chance more than by design. I was working at Johns Hopkins Hospital in the Cardiopulmonary Laboratory under a Rockefeller Fellowship because I wished to work under Dr. Blalock. Then came the Korean War and a shortage of house staff suddenly developed in Johns Hopkins. I was offered the residency in cardiovascular surgery for six months out of the year I had my fellowship. This enabled me to get training under Dr. Blalock. I then went back to Bristol University on the teaching staff and the staff of the Bristol Royal

Infirmary in 1950 and began doing the first cardiac surgery in the southwest area of England. I introduced mitral valvulotomy to this area and also the surgery of congenital heart disease. Thereafter, I came back to Hopkins and I continued on doing some of this work and when I came up to Saskatoon, I developed cardiovascular surgery in the province of Saskatchewan. Consequently, with the advent of open-heart surgery, I brought in a young fully-trained cardiovascular surgeon and I retreated out of routine cardiovascular and cardiac surgery, except for certain special areas like portal hypertension and certain aspects of peripheral vascular disease.

Dr. Nanson's bibliography from 1941-1971 contains 83 items. The first is "Aspiration of Massive Pleural Effusions" (*N.Z.M.J.*, 1941). The fifth is on "Treatment of Cardiac Arrest." (*B.M.J.*, 1949). The fourteenth is on "Present Status of Cardiac Surgery" (*N.A.M.J.*, 1951). The fifteenth is "A Case of Thrombus in the Left Auricle Simulating Mitral Stenosis" (*Thorax*, 1952). Thirty-two articles are directly related to the cardiovascular system, a few deal with thoracic surgery and the remainder are on a wide variety of subjects in general surgery. Dr. Nanson had adopted the practice of writing an overview article such as the fourteenth, every few years. Very appropriately, his inaugural address to the University of Auckland in 1971 bears the title "Whither Surgery."

Dr. Whitner Bennett Firor, 6 January 1932, Baltimore, Maryland; John Hopkins University, M.D. 53; F.R.C.S.(C) 66; F.A.H.A.; F.A.C.S.; F.A.C.C.

After a year of internship at Johns Hopkins, Dr. Firor served as assistant resident in General Surgery at the Hospital for Sick Children in Toronto (1958-1959), then in a similar post at the Toronto General Hospital in 1959. After this, he had an assistant residency in Neurosurgery at the Toronto General.

In 1960-1961, he was a Fellow in Cardiovascular Surgery at the Hospital for Sick Children. During the next two years, he served as assistant resident and as resident in this department. He worked in pathology at the Toronto General Hospital as assistant resident in 1962 and in the same hospital, was resident in Cardiovascular Surgery in 1963-1964. His formal postgraduate education was concluded with a year as McLaughlin Fellow in Uppsala, Sweden, studying thoracic surgery.

When he updated his curriculum vitae in 1971, he was Associate Professor of Surgery at the University of Saskatchewan since 1966.

> I am actually a cardiovascular surgeon rather than a cardiologist. I first became interested in this specialty during my junior internship while on a tour of duty on the cardiac surgery team. I did not make the final decision to enter cardiovascular surgery as a specialty until about two years later, however. I had no particular difficulty in arranging for training in this specialty as the University of Toronto, where I received most of my postgraduate surgical training, already had a well organized program for training surgeons in this specialty.

Dr. Firor's bibliography between 1960 and 1967 grew to ten items, all related to cardiovascular surgery. In 1967, he reported on "Massive Systemic Tumour Embolism During Pneumonectomy; Successful Removal by Means of Balloon Catheter" (*Can. J. Surg.*, 1967: 10, 200).

Alberta

Dr. Will Carleton Whiteside, 16 August 1900, Lamont, Alberta — 19 January 1967, Ottawa; University of Alberta, M.D. 28; F.R.C.S.(C); F.I.C.S.; Dipl. Amer. Bd. Thoracic Surg.

Dr. Whiteside belongs to Alberta by virtue of his having been born in Lamont, and because he began his career as a surgeon with a special interest in thoracic surgery in Edmonton. He first performed pulmonary lobectomy in 1938, mitral commissureotomy in 1952, and closure of an interatrial septal defect in 1954. He was the first pioneer of thoracic and cardiovascular surgery in Alberta. In 1956, he moved to Victoria, British Columbia, where he sought to contribute to the creation of a modern department of cardiovascular surgery and also to the Medical School at Victoria University. Thus, he also belongs to British Columbia. He died prematurely on 19 January 1967 of acute myocardial infarction. The onset of the illness occurred dramatically as he was attending a session on cardiovascular disease at the meeting of the Royal College of Physicians and Surgeons in Ottawa.

Dr. Whiteside responded generously in 1965 to the archivist's request for information. In addition to answering all the formal questions, he wrote an interesting letter and provided an autobiography, a book of 89 pages which was privately printed in 1950 about his primary and secondary education. He wrote "Public schooling was an ever-changing process because the life of a minister of the Methodist Church at that period was not stable; rather like the sands of the desert." The schools attended were: Star School, Alberta and the Academy in Inverness, Quebec; Upper Arthurette (The Red School House) in New Brunswick; Linton Corner School, Bayfield School, and South Devon School (New Brunswick) across from Fredericton; and Mount Allison Academy, Sackville, N.B. "Here, one worked the four year schedule into two years in an effort to make up for time lost prior to this period." Matriculating from this fine academy, he graduated in 1921.

In an essay on *The Little Red School House,* he reveals that the eldest of his four siblings, a sister aged 15, took the place of their deceased mother in the parsonage. She did all the cooking and baking, and nearly all the cleaning. She also walked the two miles to the Little Red School leading the others who were old enough to attend. He writes of very limited resources; butter or jam was beyond their means. Lunch brought to school was home-baked bread and molasses spread over each slice. Sometimes he succeeded in trading a slice for bread and jam, which his companions had.

In Chapter I, he lists the ways in which he earned the money he needed during his high school and university years. He did receive one hundred dollars from his father for his education which "was repaid early to help him carry on." To earn money he sold newspapers, *The Gleaner* and *The Canadian Pictorial Magazine* in Fredericton; he also worked in a fish factory on Saturdays, as well as working during the haying and fruit seasons in New Brunswick. He clerked in a jewelry store (Birks) at Christmas, was a Fuller Brush agent, became a steward and slung hash on the CPR Alaskan run (Victoria-Skagway) during four summers and also sold shoes in Edmonton, etc.

He graduated M.D. at the University of Alberta in 1928. During the next two years, he served internship and residency in surgery at the Moses Taylor Hospital in Scranton, Pennsylvania and affiliated hospitals in New York. During 1930-1931, he studied in Edinburgh (six months), London (two months), and Vienna (four months). Dr. Whiteside devoted half a page in his autobiographical memoir to a thumb-nail sketch of the famous Professor Jakob Erdheim, the most popular and probably the best teacher of pathological anatomy in Vienna from 1913 to the end of his life in 1937. The "sketch" is dated 8 a.m., 10-3-30 (presumably 10 March, 1930). Dr. Erdheim is the only teacher he mentions in his notes about this period in Europe. He alludes to his keen powers of observation, and states:

> Professor Erdheim works 18 hours per day. . . . During the morning, he did ten complete autopsies himself from start to finish

and followed each by an exacting report dictated to his assistant ... he has done over 66,000 autopsies during his time of service.... He lectured in the afternoon on diverticulitis and its pathology.

Chapter VI consists of a diary covering 17 July to 13 August 1930, which records the daily events of a rare experience. Apparently, Dr. Whiteside applied for the post of medical officer for Sir Thomas Lipton's *Shamrock V* expedition, accompanied by the yacht *Erin* from Josport, England to Newport, U.S.A. There were eleven applicants; he was selected for the job. He met with beautifully calm seas and also with a severe storm. He developed "a beastly nasal abscess near the inner canthus of the right eye" which caused him some anxiety. He had the experience of transferring a member of the crew from the *Shamrock* to the *Erin* during a storm. The man had acute appendicitis. He performed the operation. The "anaesthetist was a lawyer and the Captain was the assistant." He ends the story with his arrival in Newport, R.I., followed by a brief stay in New York; then he travelled to Philadelphia, Scranton, Boston, St. John, Fredericton ... Sherbrooke, Montreal, Winnipeg, Edmonton, Vancouver, and finally Victoria, after one of "Life's Grandest Experiences." He does not mention the yacht race for the America's Cup, which Sir Thomas Lipton, a very good sport, failed to win for the fifth time.

In 1931, he received an appointment on the teaching staff of the University of Alberta, and became associated with the University Hospital, the Royal Alexandra, the General, and Misericordia hospitals in Edmonton. He obtained training in thoracic surgery by spending some months in leading centres, e.g. in Sweden with Drs. Crafoord and Bjork, with similar men in the U.S.A., and in England with Sir Russell Brock.

Dr. Whiteside did not provide a formal bibliography. He listed four books that he had written, namely: *Principles of Surgery, A Book for Nurses; Toward the Diagnosis of Congenital Heart Disease; Nomadic Life of a Surgeon* (the autobiographical memoir); and *Surgical Manual for Interns*. In addition, he had published 42 papers in various journals. Dr. Whiteside did not give details about his books.

During World War II, he served overseas with the rank of Major. The book contains a picture of Dr. Whiteside, with Queen Elizabeth at the bedside of a patient in No. 11 Canadian General Hospital.

Dr. Cecil Melville Couves, 22 December 1919, Lang, Saskatchewan; University of Saskatchewan, B.A. 40; University of Manitoba, M.D. 45; F.R.C.S. (Edinburgh) 52; F.A.C.S. 56; F.R.C.S.(C); F.C.C.P. 62; Certification Thoracic Surgery 63; F.A.C.C. 72.

For Dr. Couves, postgraduate education began with pathology at the Winnipeg General Hospital (January to July, 1945). Then he started training in surgery at the University of Edinburgh, Royal Infirmary (July 1951 to October 1952), followed by two years (October 1952 to October 1954) at the University of Sheffield Royal Infirmary. For specialized training in cardiovascular and thoracic surgery, he worked with Dr. Michael DeBakey at Baylor University for two years (1954-1956). He began his career in Alberta as Research Fellow in Cardiovascular and Thoracic Surgery at the University of Alberta, (1957-1958).

In 1972, when Dr. Couves completed the questionnaire, he was Professor of Surgery and Acting Chairman of the Department of Surgery at the University of Alberta. His hospital appointments to five hospitals in Edmonton were all as Consultant in Thoracic and Cardiovascular Surgery. The list of special appointments to committees related to administration, to postgraduate as well as undergraduate teaching, and to several extracurricular interests, such as the Edmonton Symphony Orchestra, membership in Alpine Climbing expeditions, and a choral group, numbers twenty-two.

In 1972 his current research was on three projects, namely: 1) immunologic enhancement of the allografted canine lung; 2) the artificial heart. The heart-assist devices, and 3) membrane oxygenation in respiratory distress.

The list of medical organizations and societies of which he is a member is longer than that of most cardiologists who mentioned this item, namely, twenty-five; this list does not include his fellowships in the Royal Colleges of Surgeons of Edinburgh and of Canada.

Dr. Couves' bibliography of 61 items in 16 years begins with an article on "Haematologic Changes in Hypothermic Dogs" (*Surg. Forum,* 1956: 6) co-authored with Robert C. Overton and Wayne L. Eaton. Judging by the identity of his co-authors it appears that the first fifteen items, all related to cardiovascular and thoracic surgery, represent work done in 1954-1956, the two years which he was with Dr. Michael DeBakey. The fourteenth title is "Penetrating Injuries of the Chest: Clinical Results in the Management of 769 Patients," co-authored with A. Richard Gray, William H. Harrison, and John M. Howard (*Am. J. Surg.,* 1960: 100, 709) and the fifteenth is

"Severe Non-Penetrating Injuries of the Chest: Clinical Results in the Management of 216 Patients," co-authored with the same colleagues (*Amer. J. Surg.*, 1960: 100, 715).

The sixteenth item, co-authored with Dr. J. C. Callaghan, represents the first publication after Dr. Couves began his career at the University of Alberta. Its title is "Acute Peripheral Arterial Occlusion" (*Surgical Clinics of North America,* 1960: 40, 1275). The twenty-sixth item is of special interest, "Acute Pulmonary Embolism: Successful Embolectomy Using Cardiopulmonary By-Pass," co-authored with Brian J. Sprance and Robert S. Fraser, his medical cardiological colleagues. Couves' special interest in organ transplantation is reflected in item 42, "Perfusion of Isolated Organs for Prolonged Functional Preservation," co-authored with R. L. Fish, D. R. Brown, D. F. McFarland, D. Budney, K. G. Dristas, and K. Rowaleski in *Organ Perfusion and Preservation,* John C. Norman (ed.) Appleton-Century-Crofts, New York, 1968: 217-227. The sixtieth article is on "Experiences with a Sac-Type Artificial Heart," co-authored with D. T. Morris (*C.M.A.J.,* 1971: 105, 483-487). These few selected titles reflect his wide range of interest in clinical and experimental surgery. Thirty-five co-authors took part in the work, a good measure of the very significant influence exerted by Dr. Couves as a teacher and as a leader in research.

Dr. John Carter Callaghan, 1 October, 1923, Wentworth, Ontario; University of Toronto, M.D. 46; A.O.A., B.Sc., M.S.; F.R.C.S.(C); F.A.C.S.; F.A.H.A.; F.A.C.C.

Dr. Callaghan devoted nine years to postgraduate education before beginning his career in cardiovascular and thoracic surgery at the University of Alberta in 1955. Some understanding of the unique features of Dr. Callaghan's course of training may be gleaned from his comments in 1965 on the special questions.

> My decision to enter cardiac surgery occurred first of all through anatomy in which I was fascinated. At the age of 15, I dissected sheep and cow hearts which I obtained from the local butcher store. I used to enjoy dissecting the vessels. I had a cousin who was in first year Biology at McMaster University and prior to his joining the army in 1939, was at Bold, Muskoka, my summer home and he used to tell me about his biology and loaned me one of his biology books. I probably dissected three hearts and was fascinated by the texture of the muscle, by the arteries, and the valves with the strings dangling from them, etc. etc.

After completion of a junior internship at the Toronto General Hospital (1946-1947), he worked as a demonstrator in the Department of Anatomy and also as a part-time Medical Officer at the Lyndhurst Paraplegic Centre, Lyndhurst, Ontario (1947-948). Then, the appetite for adventure, as well as the opportunity to earn some money, took him to Aklavik in the Northwest Territories, as Medical Officer, Indian and Eskimo Affairs, Department of National Health and Welfare. When he resumed his training he responded to a stimulus he experienced during the internship.

> During my rotating internship, I was with Gordon Murray, who impressed me very much (a fascinating individual) and I helped him with some of the early Blalock [Blalock-Taussig] operations that he did. After my junior internship, I worked with Grant in Anatomy, and he gave me the job of dissecting lungs for the broncho-pulmonary segments. Of course, to carefully dissect off the lungs from a specimen meant that the heart had to be utilized and I used to enjoy dissecting the heart and blood vessels, etc. At that stage, when I came back from Aklavik to continue my postgraduate education, I had the good fortune to work with Dr. Bill Bigelow in the Banting Institute at the University of Toronto.

His official status for the year 1949-1950 was Research Fellow, Department of Surgery, University of Toronto.

> We began working on hypothermia, or deep freeze techniques to partially suspend metabolism and permit intracardiac surgery. During this period, I became fascinated by heart action under low temperature. I noticed that flicking or tweaking the heart would create a heart beat. Beginning with a simple physiological electrical stimulator, I finally developed techniques of intravenous electrodes and direct electrodes on the heart to stimulate it as body temperatures fell. Dr. Bigelow suggested I should invite Mr. Hopps of the National Research Council to work with us on a circuitry which was to provide us with our own simple machine to deliver a set current to the heart to fire it. This was the beginning of the pacemaker. We could find only one reference in the literature, namely, that of Dr. Albert S. Hyman in 1930, who stuck needles into guinea pigs and got a heart beat.

This precious paragraph crystallizes one very early event in the story of the evolution of the cardiac pacemaker, which has become an effective prolonger of the duration of life for very many human beings.

During the year 1950, Callaghan also served as senior intern, Department of Medicine at the Sunnybrook Hospital. He began training to become a surgeon with the appointment as assistant resident in Surgery at the Hospital for Sick Children and a similar status at the Toronto General Hospital (1951) and continued in the latter post in 1952. The following year, he became senior resident at the Wellesley Division and Fellow in Cardiac Surgery at the Toronto General Hospital.

During the years 1953-1955, he enjoyed the advantages of a McLaughlin Travelling Fellowship. Thus, he worked with Sir Russell Brock at Guy's Hospital in 1954 and with Dr. Frank Gerbode at Stanford University, San Francisco, in 1955.

In common with most comments on the special questions, those by Dr. Callaghan ignore the question of "the influences which led you to choose the place where you practise Cardiology." He did choose the city of Edmonton and began with the University appointment as Lecturer in Surgery in 1955. Three years later, he was promoted to Assistant Clinical Professor and in 1960 to Professor of Surgery and Head of the Division of Thoracic and Cardiovascular Surgery.

In 1965, when he composed his curriculum vitae, he was a member of the Specialty Committee in Cardiovascular and Thoracic Surgery of the Royal College of Surgeons and also an examiner. He held a post as Consultant in Thoracic and Cardiovascular Surgery in the Department of Veterans Affairs.

In 1965, he mentioned the projects for which he received financial support from the National Research Council, the Defence Research Board, the Department of National Health and Welfare, the Alberta Heart Foundation, and the Department of Public Health. The projects included studies on extracorporeal circulation, congenital heart disease, assisted circulation in acute coronary heart disease, valvular replacements, and artificial placenta. These projects contributed to the training of residents and interns and made for the accumulation of a significant bibliography which Dr. Callaghan did not submit.

Dr. Lawrence Perrin Sterns, 13 May 1930, Ottawa; Queen's University, M.D., C.M. 55; M.Sc. (Surg.) University of Minnesota, 68; F.R.C.S.(C); F.A.C.C.; F.C.C.P.

Dr. Lawrence Perrin Sterns attended Rothesay Collegiate in New Brunswick before beginning his medical education at Queen's University. Following graduation, Dr. Sterns had a junior rotating internship (1955-1956) and junior assistant residency in Surgery at the Montreal General Hospital (1956-1957). The next two years were devoted to special training in thoracic and cardiovascular surgery at the University of Minnesota, 1957-1958 as junior assistant resident and 1958-1959 in cardiovascular research. During the next two years, he again worked at the Montreal General Hospital (1959-1960) as senior assistant resident in Surgery. In 1960-1961, he was senior assistant resident in Surgery at the Queen Mary Veterans Hospital. He then returned to the University of Minnesota to engage in cardiovascular research during the next four years; this included one year (1963) devoted to the study of pathology of the cardiovascular system.

In 1965, a decade of postgraduate studies was marked by his obtaining the degree Ph.D. His thesis, the twentieth item in his bibliography, bears the title "Selective Cardiac Hypothermia" (University of Minnesota Press, 1966).

Dr. Sterns made brief but substantial comments on the special questions. With respect to his choice of specialty, he wrote in 1968:

> Decision was made to specialize in cardiovascular surgery during my penultimate year in medical school. The field was new and extrapolation of the advances made in the early 1950s indicated that much more was to be done.

About the question concerning obstacles related to carrying out the plan of training and the choice of place in which to settle, he wrote:

> I would not have been able to complete my training in cardiovascular surgery had it not been for the financial generosity of the U.S. Public Health Service and the professional encouragement of C. W. Lillehei. The main obstacle in my career came upon completing of my training when I wished to return to Canada and found that most doors were closed to me. Unfortunately, I was not allowed to return to Montreal, and through a stroke of good luck was invited to join the staff of the University of Alberta.

It seems likely that he might have remained in the United States, but for that "stroke of good luck," for during the year July 1965 to August 1966, he was in private practice and also continued research in Minneapolis. In August 1966, he went to Edmonton and began his career as Lecturer, Division of Cardiovascular Surgery, at the University of Alberta.

Dr. Sterns' bibliography grew to 35 items between 1960 and 1968. All except his thesis for the doctorate mentioned above are co-authored and all but two items are from his work in Minneapolis as a member of the group associated with Dr. C. W. Lillehei. The thirty-three articles deal with the wide variety of subjects, both experimental and clinical, which required study during the pioneering of extracorporeal circulation for intracardiac surgery. There are some items of non-cardiac, thoracic surgery, such as "Traumatic Rupture of the Right Diaphragm," co-authored with N. K. Jensen and W. R. Schmidt (*Dis. Chest,* 1967: 51, 205-207). Sterns is one of four men associated with Dr. J. C. Callaghan as the authors of two papers presented at the annual meeting in January 1967, of the Western Regional Group of the Medical Research Council. The first is on "Experimental Studies on Effective Blood Volume During Extracorporeal Circulation Using Non-Blood Prime" and the second is on "Experimental Revival of Cardiac Function After Cardiac Arrest."

Dr. Sterns worked with the early pioneers and prepared himself well for a fruitful career in cardiothoracic surgery.

British Columbia

Dr. Ross Robertson, 24 January 1902, London, Ontario; University of Toronto, M.D. 26; F.R.C.S.(C) General Surgery, Orthopaedic Surgery and Thoracic Surgery.

Dr. Robertson's curriculum vitae does not mention an internship, but states that from 1927-1935, he was in general practice in Wellington, Ontario, a small town on the shore of Lake Ontario about fifty miles southwest of Kingston. In response to the question, how he arrived at the decision to specialize in cardiothoracic surgery, he stated:

> My best friend, who was practising medicine in New York, developed tuberculosis and was treated in Muskoka Hospital. While visiting him, I realized that many patients required surgery.
>
> In 1936, I took postgraduate work at Brompton Hospital in London, England under Mr. Tudor Edwards and in 1937, at Toronto Western, under Dr. Robert Janes. While at Brompton, I watched Tudor Edwards operate on a patient with constrictive pericarditis. This, along with the fact that the twin sister of my first wife, Mary Newburn, had severe mitral stenosis, led me to wonder why there was no operation for this and aroused my interest in cardiac surgery.

He qualified for three specialties, earning the F.R.C.S.(C) for Orthopaedics, Thoracic, and Cardiovascular Surgery. During the years 1937-1941, he served as Thoracic Surgeon at the Muskoka Hospital and the Toronto Hospital for Tuberculosis. From 1941 to 1945 war service in the Royal Canadian Air Force intervened. On returning to civilian life he settled in Vancouver. In 1972, his status in the Vancouver General Hospital was Associate in Thoracic Surgery, 1945 to 1962, Honorary Attending Staff, 1963; and Consulting Thoracic Surgeon, 1963-1968 at Shaughnessy Veterans Hospital. At the University of British Columbia, he was Clinical Assistant Professor of Surgery until 1962, when he retired from teaching. He retired from practice in 1972. During the twenty-seven years of his career in Vancouver, he gave vigorous leadership in establishing excellent thoracic and cardiovascular surgical services.

In 1947, he performed his first Blalock-Taussig operation on 11 March, pericardectomy on the 12th, and ligature of a patent ductus arteriosus on the 14th. He first performed mitral commissureotomy in January 1951, only a few months later than Gagnon in Montreal and Bigelow in Toronto. In January 1956, he removed an atrial myxoma, performing intracardiac surgery with the aid of hypothermia. In March 1955, he began inserting the Hufnagel aortic valve prosthesis and in 1957, he started performing the Vineberg procedure in the treatment of coronary artery disease.

Comparing Dr. Ross Robertson's training with that of his peers, he remains a unique example of a general practitioner who, inspired by clinical problems which he confronted in close friends, obtained good training and pioneered thoracic and cardiovascular surgery in British Columbia. The first item in his bibliography of twenty articles belongs to the general practitioner period, "A Case of Parkinsonian Rigidity" (*C.M.A.J.*, 1929: 21, 204-205). The second item marks the beginning of his career as a specialist, "Indications for Surgery in Pulmonary Tuberculosis" (*C.M.A.J.*, 1941: 44, 107-113). In the same year he published "Extrapleural Pneumothorax" (*J. Thor. Surg.*, 1941: 10, 697-700). There follow two articles related to war surgery. Soon after he settled in Vancouver, he wrote on surgical conditions of the heart and great vessels (*Vancouver Medical Journal,* March 1947). The tenth item, co-authored with S. T. R. Sargeant is on "Reconstruction of the Oesophagus" (*J. Thor. Surg.*, 1950: 20, 689-701). This was also the subject of a film made for the American College of Surgery Film Library in 1951. The remaining fifteen articles reflect the wide range of subjects he dealt with in thoracic and cardiovascular surgery. He is the sole author of eleven of the first sixteen articles; the remainder are co-authored with one, occasionally two, colleagues and only once with three.

On 1 June 1972, his colleagues tendered a dinner in his honour to mark his retirement. The following excerpts from the address by Dr. D. S. Munroe are appropriate to this minibiography of Dr. Ross Robertson.

> I cannot claim that Ross did the first heart operation in Western Canada because in 1935 the late Dr. Schinbein assisted, I believe, by W. Elliott Harrison, did a pericardectomy on one Teddy Bennett — a boy in his twenties. Teddy was temporarily improved but the operation was incomplete and there were no antibiotics for tuberculosis and furthermore, the diuretics available at that time were very much less potent than those available today. More than one intern learned to do paracentesis abdominis and paracentesis thoracic on poor Teddy, who lasted many months.

After recounting Dr. Robertson's early surgical experiences, notably those three in one week of March 1947, and his first mitral commissureotomy in 1951, Dr. Munroe continued:

> It is important to realize that all this surgery was done without any investigation beyond history, the examination, minimal laboratory work, the electrocardiogram, and the X-ray. This was before right heart catheterization was done in Vancouver, long before the left side of the heart could be haemodynamically investigated, excepting for the measurement of the gradient across the aortic valve, and a very long time before coronary angiography was developed. Confidence and courage based on rapidly developing knowledge and experience were the order of the day. Meanwhile, internists, cardiologists, and paediatric cardiologists kept coming to Vancouver. One date is important — John Osborne arrived in October 1953, and this date marks the beginning of the development of the sophisticated investigation that can now be done here. . . . But to get back to our honoured guest . . . Dr. Millas defined science as knowing and art as doing. In the past, art has nearly always preceded science and this has often been so in the practice of medicine. Our predecessors, for example, knew how to use the foxglove long before the pharmaceutical actions of digitalis were worked out. . . . This is part of the art of medicine; very many other things enter into it including honesty, motivation, compassion, the ability to explain, and the ability to persuade. Finally, there is that ill-defined

and difficult-to-describe, but nonetheless very definite entity, whereby a man inspires confidence in a patient immediately or after some time, or occasionally never. I am sure our guest possesses all of these qualities in good measure and it has never ceased to astound me that he is able to set the patient at ease and gain his full confidence even after a short interview—and often the risk of the recommended procedure is not inconsiderable.

Dr. Robertson's secretary, Miss M. Russell, who assembled the minibiographical documents, added this comment:

> For many years, the Robertsons hosted a Cardiac Picnic at their waterfront home in West Vancouver for cardiologists, nurses, resident surgeons and their wives and families, barbecue ... swimming ... boating ... and water skiing and skin diving; about 60 turned up each year.
>
> Camellias and roses are Dr. Robertson's specialties and each year his patients enjoyed the beauty of these flowers at their bedside tables.

Dr. Robert Humphrys Gourlay, 13 February 1917, Vancouver, B.C.; McGill, M.D., C.M. 42; M.Sc. (Exper. Surg.) 49; Diploma in Surgery, 51; R.C.S.(C) Cert. Gen. Surg. 50; Thoracic Surg. 52.

In his first postgraduate year, Dr. Gourlay was a Fellow in Pathology at McGill. From 1946 to 1950, he took the Diploma Course in Surgery at McGill. In 1965, his status was Clinical Associate Professor of Surgery at the University of British Columbia, Chief of Surgery at St. Paul's Hospital, Consultant in Thoracic Surgery at Shaughnessy Hospital, and Consultant in the same specialty at the Children's Hospital in Vancouver.

He worked with Dr. Ross Robertson and in 1950 co-authored an article with him, "Carcinoma of the Lung. A Review of 252 Cases" (George Fekovitch, Ross Robertson, and Robert H. Gourlay, *C.M.A.J.*, 1956: 75, 207-209). The last item in the bibliography received in 1965 was an article on "Combined Replacement of Aortic and Mitral Valves with a Caged Ball Prosthesis" (*C.M.A.J.*, 1964: 90, 1363-1366).

Dr. Robert Toshio Miyagishima, 14 April 1934, Vancouver, B.C.; University of British Columbia, B.A. 56; M.D. 60; F.R.C.S.(C) 50; F.R.C.S.(C) Gen. Surg. 66; Cardiovascular and Thoracic Surg. 67; F.A.C.S. Thoracic Surg.

During his undergraduate period, Dr. Miyagishima won the Sandoz Haematology Prize in 1957 and enjoyed the privileges of the Nemetz

Scholarship in this same year, and a Research Scholarship in 1960. Postgraduate training, before returning to settle in Vancouver, consisted of the following:

1960 - 1961
Intern, Toronto General Hospital

1 July 1961 - 30 June 1962
Assistant Resident (General Surgery) Vancouver General Hospital

1 July 1962 - 30 June 1963
Research Fellow Ontario Heart Foundation, Banting Institute

1 July 1963 - 30 June 1964
Associate Resident (General Surgery) Vancouver General Hospital

1 July 1964 - 30 June 1965
Resident (General Surgery) Vancouver General Hospital

1 July 1965 - 30 June 1966
Resident, Cardiovascular Surgery, Toronto Western Hospital

1 July 1966 - 1 January 1967
Resident, Cardiovascular Surgery, Hospital for Sick Children, Toronto

1 January 1967 - July 1967
Registrar (Thoracic Surgery), Frenchay Hospital, Bristol, U.K. (Mr. Belsey)

Dr. Miyagishima made no comments about the special questions. His bibliography begins with the thesis for the degree M.D. which bears the title "Effect of Extracorporeal Circulation on the Respiratory Distress Syndrome" (May 1960). By 1972, it grew to eighteen items, fourteen co-authored with Dr. Ronald J. Baird and in some cases with other additional colleagues. Early in the history of coronary by-pass surgery, he co-authored an abstract of a paper published in the *Annals of the Royal College of Physicians and Surgeons of Canada,* January 1971, entitled "Autogenous Saphenous Vein Aortico-Coronary By-pass Graft." His co-authors were A. M. Gerein, D. I. Peretz, Dr. Kavanagh-Gray, R. G. Pitman, J. Boone, and M. Twohig. The remaining sixteen items deal mainly with cardiovascular surgery.

In 1972, Dr. Miyagishima's status at the University of British Columbia was Clinical Associate Professor of Surgery and at the St. Paul's Hospital, he was a member of the Active Surgical Staff and Director of Surgical Research.

Dr. Philip Godfrey Ashmore, 13 February 1926, Vancouver; University of British Columbia, 42-44; University of Toronto, M.D. 48; F.R.C.S.(C) 55; Cert. Gen. Surg. 55; Cert. Thoracic Surg. 62.

Dr. Ashmore began his training for surgery in traditional manner as Demonstrator in Anatomy, University of Toronto, 1950-1951. The following year he served as senior intern in Surgery at the Hospital for Sick Children. This period was followed by part of the year 1952 as senior intern in Surgical Pathology and also as senior intern in Surgery at the Toronto General Hospital. The year 1954-1955, as a University of Toronto Fellow in Surgery, he held a residency in Surgery at Sick Children's Hospital. His training was capped by a year in England at Guy's Hospital as Hon. Registrar to Sir Russell Brock. A McLaughlin Travelling Fellowship financed this experience.

Dr. Ashmore made brief but very informative comments on the special questions.

> I arrived at my decision to specialize in paediatric cardiac surgery after spending approximately two years in the Hospital for Sick Children in Toronto working in general and cardiothoracic surgery. My association with the problems of congenital heart surgery at that time (1953-1955) brought to my attention the challenge and reward associated with surgery in children suffering from congenital heart disease. My general interest in paediatric surgery has continued, however, and I continue to practise general and thoracic surgery in children as well as cardiac surgery in this age group.
>
> My plan for special training was almost coincidental rather than an organized campaign to become a cardiac surgeon. Once I was working in the field of paediatric surgery, I recognized the emergence of paediatric cardiac surgery as a special area of interest and my only additional training at that time was obtained by spending a year in Great Britain on a McLaughlin Fellowship working with Sir Russell Brock at Guy's Hospital and also spending a considerable amount of time with the cardiac group at the Hospital for Sick Children at Great Ormond Street. I chose to practise cardiac surgery in Vancouver simply because given the choice, why would anyone want to practise anywhere else?

The first item in Dr. Ashmore's bibliography is "Papilloma of the Bronchus" (*J. Thor. Surg.*, 1954: 27(3), 293). By 1968, sixteen items had accumulated which reflect his wide interests in thoracic surgery. A noteworthy article is on "Cardiopulmonary By-pass in the Infant" (*Surg.*, 1963: 54(2): 361).

In 1968, when Dr. Ashmore submitted his curriculum vitae, he held the following hospital posts: Member of the Attending Staff at the Vancouver General Hospital and of the British Columbia Cancer Institute, and of the Visiting Staff of the Children's Hospital. In that year he was Clinical Associate Professor of Surgery at the University of British Columbia.

CHAPTER THIRTEEN

Pacemakers, Monitors, Coronary Care Units and Resuscitation Teams

> In order to do this in man one electrode should be applied in front over the area of the cardiac impulse, and the other over the region of the fourth dorsal vertebra behind, so that the induction shocks may traverse the organ. The electrodes should be of considerable extent (for example, large sponge electrodes) and they and the skin should be well moistened with salt solution. The shocks employed should be strong, sufficient to excite powerful contraction in the voluntary muscles. Such a method, it seems to me, is the only rational and effective one for stimulating by direct means, the action of a heart which has been suddenly infeebled or arrested in diastole by causes of a temporary and transient character.

These sentences are from an article on "Cardiac Failure and Sudden Death," by John A. McWilliam of the University of Aberdeen, which appeared in the *British Medical Journal* in two instalments, 5 January and 16 February 1889. He was the first to suggest what was eventually achieved by Paul Zoll of Harvard University and the Beth Israel Hospital in 1952. In a series of seven articles, David C. Schecter (*New York State Medical Journal*, 1971-1972) composed the most erudite history about electrical stimulation of the heart that I have been able to find. He has assembled numerous pertinent illustrations and the seven bibliographies add up to 721 references. The instrument for applying electrical stimuli to the heart in cases of Morgagni-Adams-Stokes syndrome which Dr. A. S. Hyman introduced in 1932 received considerable publicity in newspapers when it was announced. Then nothing was seen or heard of it in medical journals or in the lay press. Of this, Dr. Schecter remarks:

> The reader will probably be startled to learn, as I was, that the Hyman artificial pacemaker was used clinically for the management of Adams-Stokes disease in the 1940s. The surprise is understandable since no report of the cases was published.

He quotes from the proceedings of a conference held on 16 February 1942 by the Brooklyn Naval Hospital Clinical Society. Among those present were Drs. Albert Hyman, George Cramp, Burton Opitz, Walter Bensel, Homer Cudmore, Franz Groedel, and Alexander Richman. A case of complete heart block was treated by Drs. Richman and Hyman. They applied needle electrodes directly to the right atrium, in the unconscious patient, and recorded ventricular contractions at 76 per minute. Dr. Opitz is quoted:

> In simple cardiac resuscitation the instrument has proved its value in any number of operating rooms and on the emergency service of our local New York hospitals. Whether the instrument can be equally successful in the management of heart block with very low idioventricular rates remains to be seen.

Another unpublished item, a preliminary report, was presented at a meeting of the New York City Clinical Society on "The Use of the Artificial Pacemaker in Complete Heart Block," on 11 February 1946 by Dr. Hyman and four co-authors. Three patients were treated, two were present at the meeting and one had died. All three had had periods of unconsciousness. There were no further reports about Dr. Hyman's instrument.

Dr. Paul Zoll's contribution is dealt with in Dr. Schechter's seventh article (May 1972) which bears the subtitle "Modern Era of Artificial Cardiac Pacemakers." Its opening sentence is,

> An incalculable debt of gratitude is owed to Paul M. Zoll, M.D. for his monumental contributions, which led to the electrical treatment of Morgagni-Adams-Stokes disease becoming firmly entrenched in medical practice.

He elicited from Dr. Zoll precious reminiscences about the genesis of the idea and its evolution in the early stages.

> The idea for electric stimulation to resuscitate patients from cardiac arrest came to me during the War, when I observed Dwight Harken doing surgical removal of foreign bodies from the cardiac chambers and walls. At that time I was impressed with the responsiveness of the heart to mechanical stimulation and the close apposition of the posterior part of the left ventricle to the oesophagus. It had also been known since Galvani, I believe, that electric currents applied directly to the heart can produce effective cardiac contractions. Therefore I thought it altogether too bad that patients with ventricular standstill,

whether caused by Stokes-Adams disease or unexpected cardiac arrest, should die for want of an appropriate stimulus to the heart. . . .

My initial idea was to supply electric stimuli from some external locus to resuscitate from ventricular standstill by a method that would be clinically easy and avoid the need for thoracotomy and direct cardiac massage. . . . I thought of passing one electrode in the oesophagus until it lay behind the left ventricle and of placing another anteriorly over the precardium. Because of my poor background in electronics I did not know what type of stimulus to use nor how to provide it.

Finally, in 1950 or 1951, I heard John Callaghan, then from Toronto, speak at a surgical meeting in Boston at which he described stimulating the sino-auricular node, with an electrode passed as a catheter by way of the jugular vein (Callaghan, 1951). I recognized that this technique was not suitable for the purpose I had in mind, as it only stimulated the atria and would not be useful in atrio-ventricular block. . . . I asked him, after the meeting, what type of pulse generator he used, and he suggested a Grass Physiologic Stimulator. . . . I think that the high spot of the whole project was when one morning we applied electric stimuli across the oesophageal and precardial electrodes in a dog under nembutal anaesthesia, and observed normal sinus rhythm interrupted by an extrasystole produced by the pacemaker. It was immediately clear to me that the problem of cardiac arrest was solved, at least in theory.

During the next two years Zoll, assisted by Dr. Leon Norman Zarsky, solved the many technical problems and in 1952 he had the instrument, the external artificial pacemaker, which proved effective in two cases of ventricular standstill. This experience was reported (Zoll, 1952). Thus, the modern era in artificial cardiac pacemakers came into being.

The story of how the Zoll external pacemaker first came to Canada begins with an apparently banal event at the Second World Congress of Cardiology, in September 1954. On the last day of the Congress, I visited the scientific exhibits. As I was leaving that area, I passed an exhibitor standing beside a longish table on which there was an instrument about the size of a large loaf of bread. He was showing it to Dr. Stirling Nichols (of Miami, Florida) with whom I was well acquainted. Nichols caught sight of me and called out, “Come and see this very interesting instrument!” This was my first introduction to Paul Zoll and to his artificial pacemaker, which was already on the market. I was unaware of the article he wrote about it in 1952. Unlike most commercial exhibitors he did not offer any brochure or reprint. Soon after returning home, a colleague, the late Dr. David Riven, called me to join him in the care of a man of about 50 who had been admitted with acute myocardial infarction. We found a faint first heart sound at the apex. This suggested partial A-V block which was confirmed by the electrocardiogram with a P-R interval of .30 sec. I spoke of the Zoll pacemaker as we discussed the possibility of complete A-V dissociation occurring in this man. Two days later on a Saturday evening he began to have convulsive seizures of Morgagni-Adams-Stokes disease. I spoke with Dr. Zoll by telephone and he arranged for an official of the Electrodyne Co. of Norwood, Mass., the manufacturers, to send us a pacemaker. It arrived Sunday morning, hours after the patient had died of cardiac arrest.

During the next nine months, Dr. Isadore Rosenfeld, the Resident in Cardiology at the Jewish General Hospital and I treated five patients with Adams-Stokes disease in our institution, one at Reddy Memorial Hospital, and Dr. Rosenfeld participated in the care of one at the Queen Mary Veterans Hospital. Our experience with the first three cases was published (Rosenfeld and Segall, 1955) and the case treated at the Veterans Hospital was reported the following year (Kaye *et al.*, 1956). These, as far as I have been able to ascertain, are the first two publications stemming from Canadian institutions, on the clinical application of the external pacemaker.

The next stage in the evolution of the pacemaker was first introduced in Canada by Dr. Arnold Johnson at the Royal Victoria Hospital following the work by Furman and Robinson (1958) with transvenous intracardiac electrodes. The first case was a patient who had been under my care for recurrent episodes of Morgagni-Adams-Stokes syndrome treated with the external pacemaker in 1958 to 1960. Dr. Johnson demonstrated the new method to me. The venous catheter in place, the electrode attached to right ventricular myocardium and the small pulse generator, solved the problem of dealing with the unpredictable recurrences of cardiac standstill. My comments dealt with balancing the possibility of serious pulmonary emboli against that of cardiac standstill. In the course of time, my fears of the emboli proved nugatory and the patient survived to enjoy the advantages of the next stage, the arrival of the implantable pacemaker (Johnson, 1962). Dr. Schechter relates the story of the contributions by the pioneer researchers in a very interesting manner, with long quotations from their "breakthrough" articles. These appeared in a relatively brief time period from 1950 (Bigelow, Callaghan and Hopps) to 1959 (Greatbatch and Chardack).

Before the introduction of the Zoll pacemaker, the physician felt virtually helpless and frustrated in the management of Morgagni-Adams-Stokes seizures. The availability of an implantable pacemaker triggered a chain of inventions designed to discover and effectively treat life-threatening arrhythmias. To electrocardiographic monitoring of the patient in the hospital, there was added ambulatory monitoring. What came to be known as CPR, cardiopulmonary resuscitation, grew out of the technique described by Kouwenhoven and associates (1960), and again Zoll and his associates (1956) contributed an effective method of ventricular defibrillation. The availability of these new techniques require specially trained personnel and new hospital procedures for efficiency in applying the new methods of diagnosis and treatment. Thus the coronary care unit came into being. All this happened between 1952 and 1962. What a fertile decade! And only a few years later, a mobile coronary care unit came into being (Partridge and Geddes, 1967). This development brings the personnel and instruments to the patient instead of losing precious time in the traditional procedure of bringing the patient to the hospital.

The first attempt to construct an electrocardiograph for recording continuously during many hours was reported by Likoff, Rappaport, and Levine (1944). They presented a calculation which showed that recording an electrocardiogram at conventional speed on film or photosensitive paper for 24 hours would result in a record, 7,200 feet in length (1.68 kilometres). They devised a photographic recording system which could record the electrocardiagram during 26.7 hours without any attention from a technician and on a manageable length of film. An enlarger rendered the miniature complexes into a conventional size. They demonstrated transient arrhythmias which could be detected only by such prolonged continuous recording.

The beginning of the modern era of such prolonged monitoring dates from the work of Dr. Norman J. Holter, a native of Helena, Montana, a graduate in science of the University of California at Los Angeles (1937). By 1942, he held the post of Associate Physicist, Radio and Sound Laboratory, U.S. Navy. During the years when he invented what is now known as Holter dynamic electrocardiography, he was President and Director of Research of the Holter Research Foundation Inc. The first, most pertinent article appeared in 1961,

"A New Method for Heart Studies: Continuous Electrocardiography of Active Subjects." The basic principle was that of radio broadcasting: the cardiac electrical potential was broadcast to nearby receiving equipment.

In London, Ontario, Cerkez, Steward, and Manning (1965) built a system of this nature which recorded the electrocardiogram of persons during activity of various kinds within a radius of ten miles. They studied 63 patients in whom 93 telemetric examinations were made, 55 in 37 patients with heart disease. They recorded arrhythmias which could not be detected by any other method.

In 1964, Dr. Holter, in association with Drs. J. S. Gilson and W. R. Glasscock, devised a portable electrocardiographic tape-recording unit. They also introduced the method of scanning the tape record at 60 times actual speed on a fluorescent screen. A disturbance in the regular, picket-fence pattern announces an abnormality. This portion of the record is then recorded on conventional electrocardiographic paper in actual time and the abnormality is displayed for analysis. Subsequent developments brought the addition of an instrument that scans the electronic tape and produces a printout with such details as the total number of beats, the frequency of ectopic beats, differentiating ventricular from atrial ectopic beats, etc.

In Canada, the first report about the use of this method of monitoring cardiac rhythm was made by K. H. Shumak, a Rykert Research Cardiologist and Kenneth W. G. Brown (1968) of the Toronto General Hospital. The project was supported by the Ontario Heart Foundation. They reported their experience with 41 patients. Well-defined abnormalities were found in 25 cases. This established the great advantages of this method in discovering events which otherwise do not declare themselves by the usual technique of recording electrocardiograms. They drew attention, also, to deficiencies in the apparatus which required correction. In the course of time the apparatus was greatly perfected and its cost grew accordingly. Nevertheless, it is now in common use, mainly since the mid-seventies. It serves not only to record arrhythmias which occur unpredictably, but also to monitor the effects of physical activity, of medication and emotional disturbance on the electrocardiogram.

Efficient monitoring revealed the need for an effective external defibrillation to treat patients whose circulation arrest is due to ventricular fibrillation. Zoll and his associates (1956) reported their experience with an effective external defibrillator and thereby added an important link in the chain of events triggered by the pacemaker.

Kouwenhoven and his associates (1957) used their ventricular defibrillator and noticed that failure to interrupt the arrhythmia occurred if more than three minutes elapsed between the onset of fibrillation and the administration of the countershocks. This led them to search for a method of lengthening this critical period without resorting to thoracotomy for cardiac massage. Their review of the literature (Kouwenhoven *et al.*, 1960) gave good promise of achieving effective blood supply to the heart and brain by external massage in children because their thoracic cages are pliable. These researchers happily found that in unconscious adults the chest becomes about equally pliable. This led to the development of their technique of cardiopulmonary resuscitation which provides time for applying a defibrillator or a pacemaker or both, as circumstances demand. In the first twenty cases they treated, the arterial pressure was raised to between 60 and 100 mm Hg. They found that sufficient pressure must be applied to move the sternum 3 or 4 cms toward the vertebrae column in order to produce an adequate blood supply to the heart and brain.

As early as 1947 Fauteux made a plea for equipping every operating room with instruments to monitor cardiac rhythm and with a defibrillator to deal with emergencies which occur during anaesthesia and surgical procedures. In that year Beck, Pritchard, and Feil reported on the abolition of ventricular fibrillation of relatively long duration by electric shock. In 1956 Zoll and associates reported on their experience with an external defibrillator in four cases of ventricular fibrillation. They demonstrated that their instrument is effective and safe for application of counter shock to the closed chest. Such instruments soon became standard equipment in the cardiology laboratories and operating rooms and before long in the mobile coronary care units.

CHAPTER FOURTEEN

Societies and Foundations

The first seed for all medical societies and foundations in the world related to promoting the prevention and relief of cardiovascular disease was sown in New York City in 1911. The seed for Canadian societies and foundations was sown in Boston, Massachusetts in 1924.

Before the early 1920s there were no such organizations anywhere in the entire world. The earliest ripples of movement that led to the creation of the American Heart Association occurred in New York City in 1912. Those men who heralded the formation of the Cardiac Society of Great Britain and Ireland could be noticed in London in 1920. In Canada, the earliest signals that a Canadian Heart Association would come into being were flashed very weakly in 1926. The events which led to the formation of the first heart clinic in New York City, most likely the first in North America, began in Boston in 1905. Dr.Richard C. Cabot led the movement to create a social service department in the Massachusetts General Hospital. He enlisted Miss Ida Cannon who became the first Director of the first hospital Social Service Department in our part of the world. Other hospitals soon followed suit. Thus, it came about at Bellevue Hospital in New York City, that Miss Mary E. Wadley, the Director of Social Service, saw a need for a special medical clinic for patients with heart diseases:

> Scores of cardiacs discharged from the wards were referred to Social Service for convalescent care and for assistance in finding suitable employment. This we could do, but continued medical oversight was imperative if they were to carry on. For most of them this oversight was obtained only in the day clinics, and day clinics and jobs were incompatible. The situation was most distressing to patients, to physicians, and to the hospital. We social workers knew that the solution for a large proportion of cases could be found in a special evening clinic, but there was prejudice against evening clinics. Dr. Hubert Guile was deeply interested in these cases and he agreed to give his time to directing an

evening clinic if the hospital authorities would consent to the innovation. They did consent to it as an experiment. This was 1911, and there has practically been no Friday evening at Bellevue since then without a Cardiac Clinic session. We chose Friday for the clinic as that would give the patient a two-day rest, if needed, with the loss of only half a working day, and he could be back on the job Monday morning before a new worker could replace him. (de la Chapelle, 1966)

Bellevue gave birth to the first cardiac clinic in North America, "The Bellevue Hospital Social Service Clinic for Working Adults" and very likely, the first in the world. The need for similar clinics in other parts of the city and the country was further identified. In 1912, Dr. Lewis A.Conner, who later became the first President of the American Heart Association and the first Editor of the *American Heart Journal,* organized in Sharon, Connecticut the Trade School for Cardiac Convalescents known as the Sharon Shop. Its objective was to promote the rehabilitation of these patients.

In 1914, Miss Katherine Tyng's "Report of the Social Service Bureau of Bellevue and Allied Hospitals" included the results of three year's work in Dr. Guile's clinic. These findings left no doubt that many adult patients with heart disease could continue at gainful occupations, provided some attention was paid to matching their work to their physical capacities and talents. Supervision along these lines resulted in reducing acute illness associated with congestive heart failure. Dr. Conner studied a selected group of patients with heart disease in the Sharon Shop. He too demonstrated that many heart patients could perform gainful work without aggravating their health condition, and indeed, with actual improvement in their general health. Several men in Boston also began to examine problems related to heart disease. Dr. Fritz B. Talbot and Dr. Richard M. Smith established a Children's Heart Clinic at the Massachusetts General Hospital in 1910, probably the first paediatric heart clinic. Their objective was to study acute endocarditis in childhood. In 1912, Dr. Joseph H. Pratt started an Adult Cardiac Clinic in the same hospital. Dr. Paul D. White later took charge of both clinics (Washburn, 1939).

Publication of Miss Tyng's observations aroused the special interest of Dr. Haven Emerson, then Commissioner of Health in New York City. He estimated that there might be as many as 20,000 children with heart disease in the public schools. In retrospect, it would seem that Dr. Emerson did more than any other man of his time to arouse interest in organizing the medical and public health resources of the country, to deal with the mounting problems of cardiovascular disease. He was Commissioner of Health from 1915 to 1917 and it was in this capacity that he played his important role. Later, from 1922 to 1943, he was Professor of Public Health at Columbia University. In the last year of his life he wrote a memorandum dated 19 March 1957 concerning the founding of the New York Heart Association. The following three paragraphs contain the essential reasons for creating this new organization.

> The most important demographic phenomenon in the whole range of public health occurring within the half-century prior to 1910 had been the remarkable decline in tuberculosis as a cause of death. In the five-year period 1911-1915 for the first time within the memory of man the annual average tuberculosis mortality rate per 100,000 of population in New York City fell to second place (201.2) with the deaths from the circulatory system taking first place (204.5). It has maintained this position ever since, more than half of deaths from all causes being now commonly attributed to diseases of heart and blood vessels.
>
> It is not unreasonable to point to a half-century of progressively effective public health effort through official and voluntary agencies as the cause of the steadily rising death rate from circulatory diseases. We had saved the infant, the youth, the young manhood and womanhood to live into the seventh decade of life and die of causes which selectively attack the aged of the population and which are not in the present state of medical science preventable to any high degree. What appeared to be a sudden and ominous shift of mortality had its gradual origins over a half-century and was in fact an encouraging and calculable result of long-sustained public health efforts.
>
> This was the background which made for the creation of a new movement intended to better the management of heart patients, to advance knowledge of the causes of a great mass of chronic disease in the community, and to make effective use of such measures of prevention as could be shown to produce tangible results. (de la Chapelle, 1966)

During the winter of 1914-1915 a number of interested physicians held meetings in the home of Dr. Walter B. James to seek ways and means of identifying and helping cardiac patients. (Dr. James was probably the first physician in North America to own an electrocardiograph for use in his private office. Some time between 1903 and

1910, certainly before he visited Einthoven, Dr. Horatio B. Williams was invited by Dr. James to assist in installing the Edelmann Model of the Einthoven electrocardiograph in his office. In conversation with Dr. Williams in 1953, I got the impression that the installation happened in about 1906.)

As a result of these meetings, Dr. Conner called a meeting on 14 July 1915 at the New York Academy of Medicine to consider forming "An Association for the Prevention and Relief of Heart Disease." Thus, the New York Heart Association was incorporated on 15 December 1915, and Lewis A. Conner was its first President. The activities of this group, plus other similar but as yet unorganized groups in Boston, Philadelphia, St. Louis, Missouri, Chicago, San Antonio, etc. led to creating the American Heart Association. The certificate of its incorporation was signed on 14 March 1924 by Drs. Robert B. Preble, Joseph Sailer, Paul D. White, Hugh McCulloch, Robert H. Halsey, and Lewis A. Conner. The formal organization was completed on 10 June 1924, when the first officers and the executive committee were elected to hold office until the First Annual Meeting in February 1925. The officers were: President, Dr. Lewis A. Conner; Vice President, Dr. James B. Herrick; Secretary, Dr. Robert H. Halsey; Treasurer, Dr. Paul D. White.

At about this time, in 1920, a small group of physicians in London formed the Cardiac Club. In telling the story of the early beginnings of organization among cardiologists in England, Dr. John Cowan wrote in 1939:

> Before the First World War, Sir James Mackenzie had suggested to a few friends who were interested in heart disease that such an organization should be made. And so the Cardiac Club, which was formed after the war, really was conceived in Burnley where Sir James Mackenzie began his notable career.

Dr. Cowan then speaks of the war as follows:

> . . . war came and our profession was scattered over the world. It was not a great war for it altered little save garden fences, but it left a terrible swathe behind it. Many men had died and many more were suffering in health from wounds or sickness for whom provision was required. During the war the pension service was necessarily a makeshift; the staff was insufficient and inexperienced and their decisions needed revision and coordination. Many cases were cardiac, at least in name. And so in April, 1920, the Ministry appointed consultants to aid the regional

directors in the assessment and treatment of the cardiac patients. The marked majority of those appointed had been associated with James Mackenzie before the war. This group of consultants gradually became aware of the fact that they could have very profitable times discussing medical subjects formally among themselves. They therefore organized what they called the cardiac club, with James Mackenzie as their first and only honorary member. This happened in 1922. (Cowan, 1939)

In New York, Dr. Robert H. Halsey took an active part in those formative meetings in the home of Dr. James and he was a charter member of the New York Heart Association. In 1938 he wrote an account of the founding of the American Heart Association. In this brief sketch he mentions that the first meting at which the subject was formally considered took place in St. Louis on 24 May 1922 at the time of the Annual Meeting of the American Medical Association. Invitations to this meeting had been sent to about 100 men in the United States and Canada. These men were selected because of their special interest in cardiovascular disease. Forty-six responded and attended a luncheon at the Hotel Claridge on Wednesday 24 May with Dr. Robert H. Halsey acting as chairman. After a brief review of the work of the Association for the Prevention and Relief of Heart Disease of New York City since 1915 and that of other recently formed associations, and an explanation of the reason for calling the meeting, Dr. Halsey asked Dr. Haven Emerson to present the tentative plan which was, in brief, as follows:

1. New or additional national associations are undesirable unless they fill an obvious and urgent need. The magnitude of the health and economic problems connected with heart disease clearly justifies the present proposal. The possibilities of prevention of heart disease alone justifies our undertaking. So little progress has been made even in the large cities that the need still applies broadly to all the people of the country.
2. The New York Association has been cautious and developed gradually and has waited for evidence of need of coordination before asking for this conference. The need has seemed clear to us for the past two years.
3. The New York Association has in a measure been acting as a national service until now but moderate changes and extensions of its activities are required to permit its office to act as host in the first stages of a national organization.
4. The big National Association or Committee should start

slowly and proceed conservatively and thus no very great enlargements of equipment or budget should be first thought of. For the present and for a year we are prepared to offer to defray the office and secretarial expenses of any national society that may be decided upon.

5. In forming a representative national Board or Committee to represent the entire country, the 50% of our population and medical practice and more than 50% of our problem which is in the rural population must not be neglected.
6. The function of such a national group would be coordination of efforts, development of research, collection and distribution of information, public health and industrial education, to develop sound public opinion as to the true meaning and seriousness of the problem.

   It is of great importance to live within our means and to rely upon the gradual expansion of our project through education of the laity.

   Each local organization should retain its independence and responsibility for development of its own resources to meet its particular problems.

At this meeting it was decided to go forward with plans for creating a national organization. These plans were consummated on 10 June 1924 at the Hotel Drake in Chicago. In addition to the officers whose names have been mentioned above, the following Executive Committee was constituted: Dr. T. Stuart Hart, Chairman; Drs. Haven Emerson, Joseph Sailer, William D. Stroud, William H. Robey; Dr. L. A. Conner, President; Dr. Robert H. Halsey, Secretary; Dr. Paul D. White, Treasurer.

As we do not have the lists of the people present at these meetings, we do not know whether any Canadians were among them. The earliest ripple of movement which led to the creation of the Canadian Heart Association occurred in the late summer of 1926 in Montreal. That was the year in which Ray Brow and I returned to Montreal after six years of postgraduate work to begin our careers as cardiologists, Brow at the Royal Victoria Hospital and I at the Montreal General Hospital. I had occupied a seat on the sidelines during the formation of the American Heart Association when I was Paul Dudley White's cardiac Fellow at the Massachusetts General Hospital in 1923-24. When I found that no local society of cardiologists and no provincial or national society existed in Canada, I undertook to initiate the formation of such organizations in emulation of what I had observed in Boston. I invited three colleagues to lunch: Dr. Cecil Birchard, who pioneered electrocardiography at the Montreal General Hospital, Dr. Albert DeGuise who had been trained in cardiology in Paris, and initiated a department of electrocardiography at the Notre Dame Hospital in 1924, and Dr. Ray Brow, who after six years of postgraduate studies was already well placed in the University Clinic of the Department of Medicine at the Royal Victoria Hospital. We had an excellent lunch at the famous restaurant, "Drury's." I, however, could not infect my colleagues with my enthusiasm. Very soon afterwards, the Depression, followed by World War II, consumed years during which one did not start organizations of this kind (Segall, 1960).

By 1946, both medical practitioners with a special interest in cardiovascular disease and some cardiologists were active in our country, and the notion that there should be a Canadian Heart Association probably occurred to more than a few. The spark that initiated the required action came suddenly one evening in February of 1946. A few days earlier, Dr. Wilder Penfield had told his cardiologist colleagues that Montreal was being visited by a distinguished cardiologist from Mexico, Dr. Ignacio Chavez, who had come to visit his son, a student at the Montreal Neurological Institute. Some professional and social events were arranged for him. Thus, on that evening in February, 1946, Birchard, Segall, Brow, and Hebbel Hoff, who was then professor of physiology at McGill, entertained Chavez — a formal dinner at the McGill Faculty Club. A very pleasant conversation, coloured strongly by Birchard's opinions on many things, including the Gold Standard, flowed throughout the meal. Dr. Chavez spoke little. Then, at the coffee and brandy stage, he suddenly interrupted our light-hearted mood by making what seemed to be a quite formal, apparently prepared speech. He announced officially, that in October, 1946, the second Inter-American Congress of Cardiology was to be held in Mexico City; he urged that a Canadian Heart Association should be formed so that it could send a delegate. The business of the luncheon of 1926 was now resumed. I instigated the next step. In order to neutralize the possible obstacles related to the local competitive spirit among members of different hospitals, I induced Hebbel Hoff to invite all those interested in cardiology in every sector of the community — English, French, and Jewish — to meet in his laboratory with a view to organizing a society of cardiologists, first in Montreal and then in Canada. The meeting took place in the McGill physiology laboratory on Wednesday, September 25, 1946. The following men were present:

Dr. H. E. Hoff, Chairman

Dr. C. C. Birchard	Dr. C. R. Bourne
Dr. G. R. Brow	Dr. W. W. Eakin
Dr. S. Eidlow	Dr. Georges Garneau
Dr. W. H. Philip Hill	Dr. A. L. Johnson
Dr. Lyon J. Korenberg	Dr. R. Lefebvre
Dr. Pierre Marion	Dr. C. F. Moffatt
Dr. J. H. Palmer	Dr. H. N. Segall
Dr. H. E. Shister	

The minutes of that meeting contain the following relevant paragraphs.

> Dr. Hoff spoke briefly and convincingly in declaring that the time was propitious for creating a Canadian society for the prevention and relief of cardiovascular disease. Segall described the formation of the American Heart Association and mentioned that 82 Canadians were then among its members in 1946. He also presented for consideration a model constitution based on that of the Canadian Physiological Society. Dr. John Palmer spoke of the British Cardiac Society and read from its constitution and regulations concerning membership which was restricted to well recognized specialists. After a general discussion I moved that those present should constitute themselves as a provisional group to undertake the creation of the Canadian Heart Association to promote the prevention and relief of cardiovascular disease. The motion was seconded by Dr. Birchard and was adopted. A committee consisting of Drs. Hoff, Palmer, Lefebvre, and Segall as secretary, was charged with the task of communicating with cardiologists throughout Canada with respect to organizing a national society. The last item on the agenda of this meeting resulted in the creation of the Montreal Cardiac Society (Société de Cardiologie de Montréal). Dr. C. F. Moffatt was appointed Chairman and Drs. Lefebvre, Brow, Birchard, and Segall as secretary, members of a committee which assumed the responsibility for preparing a constitution and outlining a plan for meetings.

About three weeks later, I travelled to Mexico City (by air for the first time) and attended the Second Inter-American Congress of Cardiology as the representative of Canada; no other Canadian attended.

The Montreal Cardiac Society has held monthly meetings in the ensuing years and continues to meet regularly. The organizers had in mind to provide opportunities for communicating the results of research and the opportunities for people working in the various hospitals of the city to meet and get to know each other. These two goals have been well fulfilled by the Society. The other objective of the meeting — to promote the formation of a national society — was also realized. Subsequent events which led to organizing the Canadian Heart Association began 16, November 1946. Dr. Palmer brought together eleven cardiologists at a meeting in Ottawa when the Royal College of Physicians and Surgeons of Canada was in session. This group formally decided: a) that the establishment of a national heart association is feasible and desirable, and b) it was considered quite possible to achieve this objective in June 1947 at the time of the annual Canadian Medical Association meeting in Winnipeg. As the Secretary of the Committee, I went to Winnipeg armed with a draft of the constitution for the Canadian Heart Association which I had composed. The ground had been prepared by letters I had sent to all the men in Canada who I thought had a special interest in cardiology. Dr. John McEachern of Winnipeg acted as Chairman at the Steering Committee meetings and at the general meeting. A committee consisting of Dr. George Strong, Dr. Francis Mathewson, Dr. David Baltzan, and Segall met for several hours on 24 June, 1947 to study the draft constitution. The general meeting took place on the afternoon of that day between 2 and 4. The following men were present:

Professor John McMichael	London, England
Malcolm Brown	Kingston, Ontario
S. M. Asselstine	Windsor, Ontario
J. M. Kilgour	Winnipeg, Manitoba
J. Margulius	New Westminster, B.C.
T. A. Ledbetter	Winnipeg, Manitoba
Richard Lessard	Quebec City
H. D. Kitchen	Winnipeg, Manitoba
I. Miller	Winnipeg, Manitoba
B. H. Lyons	Winnipeg, Manitoba
F. G. Allison	Winnipeg, Manitoba
Wm. Boyd	Toronto, Ontario
L. DeWitt Wilcox	London, Ontario

M. G. Israels	Regina, Saskatchewan
J. C. Hossack	Winnipeg, Manitoba
D. E. Roger	Regina, Saskatchewan
A. Longmore	Regina, Saskatchewan
J. B. Collip	Montreal, Quebec
J. H. Martin	Winnipeg, Manitoba
D. M. Baltzan	Saskatoon, Saskatchewan
R. E. Beamish	Winnipeg, Manitoba
G. F. Strong	Vancouver, B.C.
F. J. Sellers	Winnipeg, Manitoba
J. Antonius	
J. E. Gibson	Kingston, Ontario
J. B. Armstrong	Winnipeg, Manitoba
E. R. Gubbay	Winnipeg, Manitoba
J. F. Edward	Winnipeg, Manitoba
J. McEachern	Winnipeg, Manitoba
F. S. Brien	London, Ontario
J. A. MacDonnell	Winnipeg, Manitoba
J. Burgess	Winnipeg, Manitoba
T. Sotolov	Winnipeg, Manitoba
S. Vaisrub	Winnipeg, Manitoba
J. Hollenberg	Winnipeg, Manitoba
D. MacIntyre	Winnipeg, Manitoba
P. T. Green	Winnipeg, Manitoba
J. N. Edmison	Victoria, B.C.
S. Malkin	Winnipeg, Manitoba
J. E. Sinder	Nipawa, Saskatchewan
E. Scharf	Calgary, Alberta
W. S. Metzler	Toronto, Ontario
A. H. Neufeld	Montreal, Quebec
D. L. McNeil	Calgary, Alberta
A. Anglin	Toronto, Ontario
D. Wagner	
L. Cherniak	Winnipeg, Manitoba
R. Cherniak	Winnipeg, Manitoba
A. E. Thomson	Winnipeg, Manitoba
A. O. Edes	Prince Albert, Saskatchewan
E. O. F. Campbell	Ottawa, Ontario
H. A. Lander	Winnipeg, Manitoba
J. J. Lander	Winnipeg, Manitoba
J. D. Keith	Toronto, Ontario
H. J. Bright	Toronto, Ontario

J. Hepburn	Toronto, Ontario
H. G. Kelly	Kingston, Ontario
I. Hilliard	Toronto, Ontario
F. C. Heal	Moose Jaw, Saskatchewan
G. C. Ferguson	Thunder Bay, Ontario
J. Doupe	Winnipeg, Manitoba
W. F. Connell	Kingston, Ontario
D. M. Peterson	
J. Stephen	
M. H. Ferguson	Winnipeg, Manitoba
S. J. Bobowski	
H. N. Segall	Montreal, Quebec
A. E. Parks	Toronto, Ontario
G. E. Hall	London, Ontario

The business of the meeting began with the story of the events in Montreal that precipitated the meeting in Ottawa, and a description of actions taken in preparation for the Winnipeg meeting. The progress made in composing the constitution of the organization was given in some detail. All of which brought the proceedings to the point when Dr. G. E. Hall of London, Ontario proposed, and Dr. David Baltzan of Saskatoon seconded, "that a Canadian Heart Association be organized and that one of its functions should be to hold an annual meeting as a section of the Canadian Medical Association." This recommendation was adopted unanimously. After the constitution was read, it was generally agreed that its adoption should be postponed until the next meeting but that in the meantime it should serve as a working basis for the coming year. The following officers were elected:

President	Dr. Cecil C. Birchard
Vice President	Dr. John McEachern
Secretary-Treasurer	Dr. Harold N. Segall
Members of Council	Dr. John Scott, Edmonton
	Dr. K. A. MacKenzie, Halifax
	Dr. G. E. Hall, London
	Dr. H. Hoff, Montreal
	Dr. R. Lefebvre, Montreal
	Dr. D. Baltzan, Saskatoon
	Dr. John Keith, Toronto
	Dr. J. Hepburn, Toronto
	Dr. G. Strong, Vancouver
	Dr. F. A. Mathewson, Winnipeg

Dr. Palmer and Dr. Birchard had arranged for Professor John McMichael (now, Sir John) to be the guest speaker. He prefaced his address with encouraging remarks about the birth of the Canadian Heart Association. He tended to favour relatively small societies, especially those small enough to permit free discussion at meetings. Such societies he considered as sources of significant progress in the advancement of human knowledge and welfare. His address dealt with the pathological physiology of the circulation in cases of arterio-venous aneurysm. Professor William Boyd thanked the speaker on behalf of all those present. And so the first meeting terminated at 4:00 p.m. and the Canadian Heart Association was born.

There remained the formalities of adopting a constitution and by-laws and of obtaining a Federal Charter. An unexpected problem presented itself in connection with registering the name in both English and French. Legal advisers declared that only one language, either of the two, was required or permitted. Eventually, after considerable delay during which we sought to make both French and English official, the Charter was written in English but both languages were used for the name of the Society on our stationery and other documents: "Canadian Heart Association Inc. — Société Canadienne de Cardiologie." The Charter was issued on 13 June 1949. All those who were listed as members on 20 February 1949 were designated Charter Members.

The format of the meetings provided for transaction of business followed by the scientific program. During the first few years the meetings took place at the time of the Annual Meeting of the Canadian Medical Association which very generously provided the room and the facilities for our sessions. The program of the scientific session which took place on 22 June 1948 in Toronto at the Royal York Hotel is of historic interest. All the participants were men working in Canadian universities and hospitals.

It is here reproduced:

AGENDA FOR SCIENTIFIC SESSION: 2:00 p.m.-5:00 p.m.

1. *Dr. L. Hession and Dr. A. C. Burton, London, Ontario: "Vector Cardiograph"*
2. *Prof. D. Y. Solandt, Dr. R. Nassim and Dr. J. D. Brown, Toronto: "Electrical Localization of Myocardial Injury"*
3. *Dr. Neil Feeney, Montreal: "Ectopia Cordis"*
4. *Dr. John Keith, Toronto: "Angio-Cardiography in Congenital Heart Disease"*

5. *Prof. Hebbel Hoff, Montreal: "The Genesis of Ventricular Fibrillation: The Nature of the Vulnerable Phase of Cardiac Cycle"*
6. *Dr. Georges-Etienne Cartier, Montreal: "Three Cases of Paroxysmal Hypertension Treated Surgically"*

The Association enjoyed the special advantages of smallness. There was free discussion and decisions could be made democratically at business meetings. During the autumn of 1948, a questionnaire was prepared with five questions and was mailed to all the members on December 28, 1948, concerning the policies of the Society. The replies indicated that the members favoured the requirements for membership as already stated in the constitution. They favoured initiating a program of public education similar to that of the American Heart Association. With respect to whether the scientific session should have a duration of two, three, or four hours, the majority preferred three hours and the subjects to be dealt with should include both clinical and basic science items. The majority favoured inviting a guest speaker who would discuss a subject for about an hour. Until 1955, the meeting lasted one day. In June of 1955, Toronto was the locale for a combined meeting of the British Medical Association and the Canadian Medical Association. For this occasion the program committee arranged a combined meeting with the Canadian Rheumatism Society for the morning of June 24, followed by a panel discussion on "Is Effort a Precipitating Factor in Coronary Occlusion?" On the following day there was to be a dissertation on "Anticoagulants in Coronary Heart Disease," as well as four shorter items mainly on cardiovascular surgery, including one by W. T. Mustard on "Artificial Heart Lung Pump in Congenital Heart Surgery." The panel consisted of C.H.A. President George (Fritz) Strong as moderator, H. J. Barrie of Toronto, and J. C. Paterson of London, Ontario to deal with pathological aspects of coronary heart disease, William Evans of London, England and myself, of Montreal, Quebec, to deal with the clinical aspects. Many members of the audience engaged in the discussion. Paul Wood of London, England made an indelible impression by his sharp criticism delivered with an "acid" technique which left the panel members speechless for a noticeably longish time. Once the panel and audience recovered from this wholesome shock, discussion resumed in the usual mood. The panel discussion was followed by a business item which resulted in the appointment of Dr. William A. Oille as Chairman of a Committee of five cardiologists who would serve the public in controversial cases of coronary heart disease claimed to result from circumstances related to the individual's work.

The scientific program had been preceded by an epoch-making business meeting on 24 June. After long discussion about the great need for research funds and the means for filling this need, vigorous measures were proposed by Fritz Strong. This was the culmination of a series of events which had occurred in the years 1947 to 1955 in the United States and in Canada. Cardiologists who returned to civilian careers from service in the American armed forces transformed the American Heart Association. They created a partnership between laymen, interested in stemming the rising tide of cardiovascular disease, and the medical professionals in order to raise the funds needed to promote research effectively. The first campaign occurred in 1947. February was adopted as Heart Month (Valentine Day played a role in this choice.) The annual campaigns were eminently successful, moreover,the grass-roots support encouraged the leaders of the Heart Association to apply for funds from the Federal Government. Paul Dudley White proved to be a very effective advocate. Canadian scientists benefited from this new development. They applied for and received grants in aid of research. I recall acting as an interviewer of applicants on behalf of the American Heart Association. Among those I interviewed were Claude Fortier and Louis Horlick, both of whom received grants. Horlick was a Research Fellow of the American Heart Association, working at McGill during 1950-1952. And there were others in other Canadian centres. In 1953, Dr. Howard Sprague, then president of the American Heart Association, wrote to the Canadian Heart Association suggesting that it should take part in the fund-raising either as a chapter of the American Heart Association or independently. This intensified the debate which took place at our annual meetings between those who favoured and those who opposed undertaking fund-raising campaigns. Other means of obtaining money for research were tried.

On 20 February 1949, the executive committee of the Canadian Heart Association (Birchard, Hepburn, Keith, and Segall) met in John Keith's home. Birchard spoke of his intention to prepare a request for funds to support research, addressed to the Canadian Life Officers' Association. Keith spoke of the creation of the Ontario Heart Foundation which would function as an instrument of the Provincial Government's efforts to support research. The need for similar organizations in the remainder of Canada was clearly recognized. However, when the subject was broached at the annual meeting in 1949 and subsequently, until 1955, those who did not favour mounting yet another public campaign for funds prevailed. This resistance did not dampen the spirits of those who favoured emulating rather than joining the American Heart Association in fundraising. They were encouraged by spontaneous donations made specifically for research. The first of these, one hundred dollars, came in 1949 from Mrs. Dora Lupovitch of Montreal, in memory of the late Mrs. Abraham Victor, whose friends contributed the money. That the donation should be made to the Heart Association was suggested by the late Dr. Samuel Eidlow. Soon afterwards a donation of ten dollars was received from Mr. E. A. Roberts of Philadelphia in memory of the late Professor Hurd.

In the meantime, John Keith was making good progress in enlisting laymen and the Ontario Deputy Minister of Health to assist in organizing cardiovascular research in Ontario. At first, a committee on Cardiology was created. Out of this committee grew the Section on Cardiology of the Ontario Medical Association, and finally, the Ontario Heart Foundation came into existence in 1952, the first such unit in Canada, a partnership of laymen and medical men. At first, only funds given by the Federal to the Provincial Government were available; the Foundation regulated their distribution.

At about this time, Hugh Stansfield in Vancouver led in assembling and organizing the cardiologists there into the Vancouver Heart Association. Before long this group became aware of the need for engaging the interest of laymen which led to creating the British Columbia Heart Foundation.

In December 1951, the executive committee (Hepburn, Keith, and Segall) called on Dr. G. D. W. Cameron, the Deputy Minister of National Health and Welfare and submitted a brief on the need for financial support of cardiovascular research in Canada. No immediate practical results could be expected from this effort. At the annual meeting in June 1952, Dr. John Palmer moved and Dr. George Strong seconded a motion to the effect that a committee be formed to seek funds for cardiovascular research. The motion was given unanimous approval. Another important stimulus in this field of our endeavour was felt when the association was enriched by a legacy of $10,000 from the estate of the late Frederick Bates of Chatham, Ontario. The announcement of this legacy at the annual meeting in Winnipeg on 16 June 1953, touched off an animated discussion on the subject of how to provide more funds for cardiovascular research. The members became better informed about the problems. We had the literature produced by the American Heart Association for its annual campaign in February and in addition, Dr. Keith produced a booklet "Heart Disease in Canada . . . A Challenge," which depicted the epidemiology of cardiovascular disease in clear lay language, aided by well designed graphs. This pamphlet is of historic interest as it is the first item prepared in Canada for educating the general public on what came to be known as the number one cause of death. The pamphlet presents the latest statistics available at the time it appeared for distribution in 1954. On page 10 it declares the primary need continues to be scientific research which will result in new methods of prevention and relief of cardiovascular disease. On page 12 it indicates that the Canadian Heart Association exists to promote such research and ends with the sentence "The Canadian Heart Association provides the stimulus and guidance in the organization and creation of new Provincial Heart Associations where they are needed."

At the annual meeting in Vancouver on 14 June 1954, the subject of supporting research again aroused much discussion. Approval was given for the use of funds to mount a campaign of public education designed to enlist support of the general population. The most significant forward step taken at this meeting was the election of George Strong as president of the association. At the next annual business meeting, held in Toronto on 24 June 1955, Dr. Carl Burton spoke of the Ontario Heart Foundation's experience in obtaining funds for research. He concluded with the statement that an appeal to the general public was being planned by means of a mailing campaign. The minutes of this meeting contain the following:

> Dr. Strong remarked that the problem of fund-raising had been discussed reasonably fully at the council meeting on June 20th, 1955 and it had been the feeling of the council that a motion should be presented at the Annual Meeting to authorize the establishment of a National Heart Foundation.

Drs. David, Keith, and Stansfield had prepared such a motion and the motion was to be read by Dr. Stansfield and seconded by Dr. Mathewson. There followed discussion of how to distribute the money that the Foundation would collect. Dr. Strong then announced that together with the secretary, Dr. Keith, he had had a talk with the Minister of Health and Welfare, the Hon. Mr. Paul Martin, who had been most encouraging. They had discussed arranging for public health funds to be specifically allocated for cardiovascular research and Mr. Martin undertook to sponsor a meeting for the purpose of establishing a Canadian Heart Foundation. The Minister made it clear that he had no funds with which to finance such a meeting, but this did not prove to be an obstacle. Dr. Strong arranged for the members of council to come to the meeting and each to bring along at least one interested layman. The meeting took place in Ottawa on January 16th, 1956. Unfortunately, a written record of the proceedings is not now available. A record was made on plastic discs with a Gray audiograph. A few years later, when I was the Chairman of the Archives Committee, I requested to examine this record, but learned that the discs could not be found. From collective reminiscences of several who were present, Dr. Keith composed a description of this very important event and recorded it in the minutes of the Annual Meeting of the Canadian Heart Association, which took place on 15 June 1956. These minutes are quoted in full below.

National Conference on Heart Disease
Ottawa, January 16, 1956

At a meeting convened by the Minister of Health, the Honorable Mr. Paul Martin, and sponsored by the Canadian Heart Association in Ottawa on January 16th, 1956, these representatives took part: Dr. G. D. W. Cameron, Mr. R. E. Curran, Dr. G. F. Strong, Mrs. F. T. Rogers, Dr. Hugh Stansfield, Mr. Gordon P. Caine, Dr. R. S. Fraser, Dr. Irwin Hilliard, Mr. George Patrick, Dr. F. A. L. Mathewson, Mr. A. N. Mitchell, Dr. R. F. Farquharson, Dr. G. W. Manning, Dr. John D. Keith, Dr. A. D. Kelly, Mr. O. A. Doherty, Dr. J. A. MacFarlane, Dr. J. B. Collip, Dr. G. H. Ettinger, Dr. Harold N. Segall, Dr. John Palmer, Dr. Paul David, Dr. A. Tétreault, Dr. A. L. Johnson, Dr. Jacques Genest, Mr. A. Wesley Mason, Mr. Alfred B. Grossman, M. Lucien Hétu, Dr. L. C. Steeves, Dr. G. C. McMillan, Mr. C. P. Fell, Mr. Ewart Cather, Dr. Wallace Troup, Dr. W. V. Johnston.

As a result of the discussion at this meeting, the following resolution was passed. Moved by Dr. R. Farquharson and seconded by Dr. Harold Segall.

Whereas it is recognized that cardiovascular disease represents the leading cause of death and disability in Canada, and

Whereas a National Conference on Heart Disease assembled in Ottawa on January 16, 1956, representative of all areas of Canada and all interests in the subject, and specifically representative of the Canadian Heart Association, the Canadian Medical Association, the College of General Practice of Canada, the Ontario and British Columbia Heart Foundations, the Quebec Life Insurance Officers Association, as well as individuals representing the Faculties of Medicine of Canadian Medical Schools and certain teaching hospitals, have considered the means for further coordinated effort on the national level in research, education and community service;

THEREFORE, BE IT RESOLVED that the Conference recommends the establishment of a national organization to be known as the Canadian Heart Foundation or such other name as may be decided upon.

A second resolution was passed. Moved by Dr. A. D. Kelly and seconded by Mr. A. N. Mitchell.

That a committee of this Conference be elected for the following purposes:

(a) To draft the aims and objects of the Canadian Heart Foundation;
(b) To elaborate the constitution and by-laws;
(c) To apply for a federal charter, and
(d) To take such other steps as may be necessary to promote the organization prior to the organizational meeting on June 7, 1956 in Montreal.

Resolutions Committee suggests that the following be elected to the aforementioned committee:

Dr. R. F. Farquharson — Chairman
Dr. G. F. Strong — Vice-Chairman
Dr. John D. Keith — Secretary
Mr. Douglas Ambridge
Dr. John H. Palmer
Dr. Paul David
Mr. Alfred B. Grossman
Dr. L. C. Steeves
Dr. F. A. L. Mathewson
Dr. J. B. Collip
Mr. Gordon P. Caine

Mr. R. E. Curran was appointed Legal Advisor of the Organizational Committee.

Respectfully submitted,
John D. Keith, M.D.
Secretary.

On 7 June 1956, a meeting was held on St. Helen's Island, Montreal, at which the constitution and by-laws which had been approved by the organization committee was adopted, and the National Heart Foundation of Canada was born nine years after the birth of its parent, the Canadian Heart Association. About fifty or sixty people representing all parts of Canada were present. Dr. Ray Farquharson acted as chairman; Dr. George Strong was the unanimous choice for president. After considerable discussion related to various items of the constitution and by-laws, Dr. Farquharson, as chairman of the nominating committee, presented the following slate of officers who were elected:

President	Dr. G. F. Strong
Vice-President	Mr. D. W. Ambridge
Vice-President	Mr. Albert Deschamps
Honorary Secretary	Dr. John D. Keith
Honorary Treasurer	Mr. A. B. Grossman
Honorary Solicitor	Mr. R. E. Curran

A motion was adopted to the effect that all those who attended the meeting of January 16th, 1956, plus seven additional men were declared to be Members at Large. Dr. T. C. Routley was appointed Chairman of the Ways and Means Committee, Dr. John Palmer, Chairman of the Credentials Committee, and Segall, Chairman of the Medical Advisory Committee. Plans were discussed and approved concerning the appointment of an Executive Secretary. An advertisement was to be published in the *Canadian Medical Association Journal* calling for applicants. Dr. Routley, with the effective collaboration of Dr. Montgomery (Chief Medical Officer of Manufacturers' Life Insurance Company) and Mr. Ross Poyntz, succeeded in obtaining a Launching Fund of $30,000 a year for two years from the Canadian Life Underwriters' Association. In addition, the Canadian Heart Association loaned the Foundation $5000 from the Bates Estate Fund, interest-free. Thus, the Foundation could engage an Executive Secretary and provide him with an office and a secretary. Of the seven candidates whose applications were reviewed in detail, Dr. John B. Armstrong of Winnipeg was chosen. He had been present at the meeting on 24 June 1947 when the Association was born and had attended its subsequent meetings at which the problems of finding funds for research were discussed. He proved to be an ideal choice. He guided the foundation's activities, both medical and non-medical, working pleasantly and effectively with a great variety of personalities who held office in the foundation. As the foundation grew in size and complexity, he required and obtained the assistance of associates. At this time (1972), the tasks were divided between him as Chief Medical Advisor and Mr. E. McDonald the Executive Director.

The decision to appoint Dr. Armstrong as Executive Secretary was made at the Board meeting on 30 October 1956, which took place in the Board Room of the Canadian Medical Association in Toronto. The Ontario Heart Foundation (O.H.F.) offered to provide temporary secretarial help and the Canadian Medical Association offered temporary office space where Miss Martin of the O.H.F. would work.

The announcement of the date (27 February 1957) and agenda of the first meeting of the Executive Committee in Montreal was typed on the first edition of the Foundation's official letter-head, which also presented the names of the officers, directors, and Honorary Solicitor, but as yet no permanent address and no executive secretary. The notice was signed by John D. Keith, Honorary Secretary. To attend this meeting, "Fritz" Strong, as our president was known to all his friends, had journeyed from Vancouver and spent February 26 with John Keith in Toronto, and then travelled with him and Mr. O. A. Doherty (of the Ontario Heart Foundation) on the evening train to Montreal. Their arrival in Montreal was marked by the tragic sudden death of our President, Fritz Strong, at the CPR station when, with Mr. Doherty, he was waiting for a taxicab. The members of the executive committee who attended the meeting on the following morning were Albert Deschamps, who acted as chairman, A. B. Grossman, John Keith, and Paul David. Others present were John Palmer, H. N. Segall, O. A. Doherty, Treasurer of the Ontario Heart Foundation, L. W. Holmes of the Canadian Medical Association Public Relations Department, and John Armstrong, the Executive Director. A minute of silence was observed in tribute to Fritz Strong and we arranged to write a letter of sympathy and to send flowers to Mrs. Strong.

At this meeting the committee took stock of the assets with which the Foundation was to begin its career. Armstrong told us how the Ontario Heart Foundation, which had been incorporated in 1952, was doing its job. Its membership numbered about one hundred cardiologists and five laymen. The Board of Directors consisted of these laymen together with five cardiologists. The directors elected their chairman. The Foundation reviewed grants in aid applications for cardiovascular studies under the General Public Health Grants (Department of National Health and Welfare) for the Province of Ontario and administered an additional Provincial grant of $100,000 which began in 1956. The Foundation had not conducted a public campaign for funds.

In Quebec a group of Jewish ladies headed by Mrs. Leon Fischel and Mrs. Gladys Laxer had organized the Quebec Heart Research Society Inc. to collect funds for the support of research in cardiovascular disease. They obtained a provincial charter on 24 May 1955, and conducted a house-to-house campaign in 1955 and 1956. A Medical Advisory Committee with Segall, as chairman, and which included a representative of McGill, the University of Montreal, and of each hospital which had a cardiac clinic, guided the officers of the Quebec Heart Society in distributing about $12,000 which they collected. As all the work was done by volunteers, the overhead expenses amounted to less than $700, leaving nearly the total sum for grants-in-aid. A few weeks after the meeting which initiated the National Heart Foundation in January 1956, the ladies agreed to change the name of the organization to the Quebec Heart Foundation Inc. and subsequently to retire from its management. Eventually, a group of influential businessmen undertook to manage the Quebec foundation.

The British Columbia Heart Foundation was incorporated in May 1955. A letter campaign late in 1955 yielded $15,000, mainly from Vancouver corporations and prominent citizens. The Foundation joined the Vancouver Community Chest for 1956; a budget of $50,000 was adopted, but as the Chest did not reach its objective, the amount was reduced to $45,000. This sum proved to be the largest amount provided by public subscription for heart research in any part of Canada in that year. A full-time Executive Secretary, Mr. E. McDonald, was appointed in November 1956. During the month of February 1957 a letter campaign was conducted which reached 80,000 householders and approximately 6,500 business enterprises. Cooperation was sought and obtained from the information media. One newspaper held a public forum on heart disease with the cooperation of the British Columbia Medical Association and the Heart Foundation. A Legion branch held a St. Valentine's Day dance, the proceeds of which went to the Foundation. The campaign's objective was $50,000 from the Community Chest of Vancouver and $50,000 from outside the city. This campaign was designed largely as an effort in public education in order to facilitate the creation of ten local branches which would function in the 1958 campaign.

The creation of the National Foundation soon activated concerned men and women in the remaining provinces. The Saskatchewan Heart Foundation was incorporated in May 1958; their Board of Directors consisted of six laymen and six doctors. They acted vigorously. An Executive Director was appointed in December of the same year and in February 1957 they had a campaign for funds with an objective of $50,000.

The Alberta Heart Foundation, incorporated in December 1956, had only one medical person on its Board of Directors, the Chairman of the Medical Advisory Committee, Dr. R. S. Fraser.

On the 8th of February 1957 a meeting of medical men took place in Winnipeg; they resolved to promote the organization of the Manitoba Heart Foundation. Some months later, the foundation was incorporated.

Dr. L. C. Steeves of Halifax represented the Atlantic provinces at the meeting of the National Heart Foundation Board of Directors on 14 September 1957, thus initiating the participation of the Atlantic region which later became a Division of the National Foundation. Still later, in 1970, the Nova Scotia Heart Foundation came into existence, with the provinces of New Brunswick, Prince Edward Island, and Newfoundland as separate divisions.

In April 1958, Mr. J. Bruce Brown accepted the task of organizing the Quebec Heart Foundation – Fondation des Maladies du Coeur du Québec. He gathered about him a Board of Directors of leading citizens and he gave generously of his time, and talents. As honorary Secretary-Treasurer he performed the work on an Executive Director during the first two years.

Such were the beginnings of the Heart Foundation. In 1968, at the end of his second year as President of the national body, Mr. Arthur Fouks prepared a valedictory address to which he gave the title "To Be or Not To Be." He drew attention to the fact that although the Heart Foundations were young, only near the threshold of their teens, the time was propitious for critically examining their performance. His sound ideas entered receptive minds. A committee was appointed to carry out this task and the resulting report contains much that guided the foundations in subsequent years.

The story of the Heart Foundations in Canada requires and merits a full length treatise, a book. How volunteers dedicated themselves to community service and the brilliant results which afford them the joy of achievements for the common good, these features appear in abundance in the story of the initiation and the performance of the Heart Foundations. The author of such a book would find much of great interest to describe and discuss. Perhaps in the near future some volunteer with the sense of history required for the challenging task will undertake it and achieve its goal.

As these lines are written in the winter of 1988, reflecting on the fact that the first Heart Campaign in 1958 brought donations totalling $828,334 and for 1987 the total was $40,255,000, firmly underlines the need for a full length history of the Heart Foundations in Canada.

Canadian Cardiovascular Society

Past Presidents

Cecil C. Birchard, Montreal, Quebec	1947-48
John A. Oille, Toronto, Ontario	1949-50
John McEachern, Winnipeg, Manitoba	1950-51
John Hepburn, Toronto, Ontario	1951-52
Harold N. Segall, Montreal, Quebec	1953-54
George F. Strong, Vancouver, B.C.	1955-56
Francis A. L. Mathewson, Winnipeg, Manitoba	1957-58
Paul David, Montreal, Quebec	1959-60
W. Ford Connell, Kingston, Ontario	1961-62
Irwin M. Hilliard, Toronto, Ontario	1963-64
Robert S. Fraser, Edmonton, Alberta	1965-66
David R. Murphy, Montreal, Quebec	1967-68
Robert E. Beamish, Winnipeg, Manitoba	1969-70

Past Secretary-Treasurers

Harold N. Segall	1947-50
John D. Keith	1951-53
H. E. Rykert	1954
Francis A. L. Mathewson	1955
John D. Keith	1956-57
Robert E. Fraser	1958-61
Robert E. Beamish	1962-65
Yves Morin	1966-69
Ronald J. Baird	1970

Annual Lecturers

R. F. Shaner, Edmonton, Alberta	1961
Arthur M. Vineberg, Montreal, Quebec	1962
Gordon D. W. Murray, Toronto, Ontario	1963
Hans Selye, Montreal, Quebec	1964
Alan C. Burton, London, Ontario	1965
Harold N. Segall, Montreal, Quebec	1966
John D. Keith, Toronto, Ontario	1967
Kenneth A. Evelyn, Vancouver, B.C.	1968
Jacques Genest, Montreal, Quebec	1969
J. Fraser Mustard, Hamilton, Ontario	1970

John Keith Lecturers

John D. Keith, Toronto, Ontario	1967
Wilfred G. Bigelow, Toronto, Ontario	1968
Jean Lenègre, Paris, France	1969
Dwight E. Harken, Boston, Massachusetts	1970

Canadian Cardiovascular Society Research Award Recipients

Dr. Derek R. Boughner, London, Ontario	1970

List of Members of the Canadian Cardiovascular Society for 1971

Alberta
Hugh A. Arnold, Lethbridge
G. S. Balfour, Lethbridge
J. C. Callaghan, Edmonton
Rodney M. Chadwick, Red Deer
Cecil M. Couves, Edmonton
Neil Duncan, Edmonton
J. Dvorkin, Edmonton
R. S. Fraser, Edmonton
W. Glenn Friesen, Edmonton
J. A. L. Gilbert, Edmonton
George S. Gray, Lethbridge
C. Bruce Hatfield, Calgary
John C. Hopkyns, Edmonton
David L. G. Howard, Calgary
David W. Irving, Edmonton
Neville Jackson, Calgary
Alan S. Khan, Calgary
Simon J. Lee, Edmonton
Lawther Logan, Calgary
F. H. McInnis, Camrose
Howard McEwen, Calgary
Ian R. McLean, Calgary
H. Oh, Edmonton
R. E. Rossall, Edmonton
Stanley Rowlands, Calgary
Ludwig J. Sherman, Edmonton
Laurence P. Sterns, Edmonton
R. F. Taylor, Edmonton
R. K. C. Thomson, Edmonton

British Columbia
Peter Allen, Vancouver
Philip G. Ashmore, Vancouver
Peter J. Banks, Victoria
Dorrance Bowers, Kelowna
E. P. Carruthers, Kelowna
W. A. Dodds, Vancouver
K. A. Evelyn, Vancouver
Ronald J. Forth, Victoria
J. G. Gillis, Vancouver
Thomas F. Godwin, New Westminster
R. H. Gourley, Vancouver
Shirley G. Hazell, Vancouver
V. O. Hertzman, Vancouver
Charles L. Hunt, West Vancouver
M. G. Israels, Vancouver
D. Kavanagh-Gray, Vancouver
A. K. Mandal, Fort St. John
B. B. Moscovich, Vancouver
M. D. Moscovich, Vancouver
A. I. Munro, Vancouver
D. S. Munro, Vancouver
J. A. Osborne, Vancouver
Dwight Peretz, Vancouver
Charles S. Rennie, Vancouver
C. B. Rich, Victoria
A. G. Richards, New Westminster
L. N. Roberts, Victoria
Ross Robertson, Vancouver
C. Eve Rotem, Vancouver
Hugh Stansfield, Vancouver
K. M. Telford, Vancouver
W. G. Trapp, Vancouver
D. J. Vince, Vancouver
M. B. Walters, Vancouver
G. M. Woodwark, Victoria
M. D. Young, Vancouver

Manitoba
J. Barwinsky, Winnipeg
R. E. Beamish, Winnipeg
E. G. Brownell, Winnipeg
Stefan A. Carter, Winnipeg
Leslie J. Cera, Winnipeg
Morley Cohen, Winnipeg
Lawrence Coke, Winnipeg
R. A. Corne, Winnipeg
T. E. Cuddy, Winnipeg
Gordon R. Cumming, Winnipeg
Allan R. Downs, Winnipeg
C. C. Ferguson, Winnipeg
Peter Gaskell, Winnipeg
John C. Graham, Winnipeg
R. G. Handford, Winnipeg
R. J. Hoeschen, Winnipeg
W. Karlinsky, Winnipeg
Reubin Kaufman, Winnipeg
B. W. Kirk, Winnipeg
B. H. Lyons, Winnipeg
F. A. L. Mathewson, Winnipeg
J. D. McDowell, Winnipeg
Kannubhal Metha, Winnipeg
Leon Michaels, Winnipeg
Anthony Miller, St. Boniface
David Mymin, St. Boniface
Bal M. Sahay, St. Boniface
Victor J. H. Sharpe, Brandon
David H. Stein, Winnipeg
V. M. Storrie, Winnipeg
Paul K. Tisdale, Winnipeg
L. L. Whytehead, Winnipeg

New Brunswick
E. S. Eddie, Bathurst
Donald Macauley, Fredericton
H. H. MacKinnon, Fredericton
G. M. Moffatt, Fredericton

Newfoundland
Albert R. Cox, St. John's
Ian E. L. H. Rusted, St. John's
R. Clifton Way, Pleasantville
Robert W. Young, St. John's

Nova Scotia
Robert N. Anderson, Halifax
H. E. Christie, Amherst
A. B. Crosby, Halifax
G. D. Denton, Wolfville
R. C. Dickson, Halifax
F. G. Dolan, Halifax
D. F. Folkins, Halifax
Max M. Gorelick, Halifax
C. E. Kinley, Halifax
S. T. Laufer, Halifax
D. L. Roy, Halifax
J. A. Shaw, Halifax
Lea C. Steeves, Halifax
John W. Stewart, Halifax
C. H. Young, Dartmouth

Ontario
M. M. Abbott, Toronto
Allen G. Adelman, Toronto
Suraj P. Ahuja, London
Harold E. Aldridge, Toronto
John B. Armstrong, Ottawa
Ronald J. Baird, Toronto
Clare B. Baker, Toronto
E. A. Bartram, London
Donald Beanlands, Toronto
Franklin Berkman, Ottawa
W. G. Bigelow, Toronto
F. S. Brien, London
K. W. G. Brown, Toronto
Carl R. Burton, Toronto
S. A. Carlen, Toronto
S. E. Carroll, London
Luigi Casella, Toronto
Bruce Charles, Toronto
Edward Charrette, Kingston
Gerald Chertkow, London
Miguel A. Chiong, Kingston
Arthur W. Chisholm, Toronto
G. Cohen, Ottawa
J. C. Coles, London
W. Ford Connell, Kingston
G. G. Copestake, Ottawa
H. V. Dobson, Peterborough
Philip E. Doyle, Ottawa

Geoffrey Evans, Hamilton
John R. Evans, Hamilton
J. E. Fay, Kingston
G. C. Ferguson, Thunder Bay
Paul Field, Sudbury
G. M. Fitzgibbon, Ottawa
Peter G. Forbath, Toronto
Frank H. Flowers, Sudbury
Rodney S. Fowler, Toronto
John T. M. Fraser, Ottawa
H. Lloyd Garvey, Ottawa
Edward Gibson, Kingston
Irving H. J. Glass, Willowdale
Bernard S. Goldman, Toronto
James H. Graham, Ottawa
Joseph Greenblatt, Ottawa
William F. Greenwood, Toronto
Eric Grundy, Toronto
Ramsay W. Gunton, London
John F. Hamel, Ottawa
Frederick G. Hamilton, Toronto
J. T. Hauch, Toronto
Thora Haynes, Oakville
H.A. Heggtveit, Ottawa
R. O. Heimbecker, Toronto
E. Maurice Heller, Toronto
Irwin M. Hilliard, Toronto
G. David Hooper, Ottawa
Wanda Jegier-Rygiel, Hamilton
David W. B. Johnston, London
K. Joe Kako, Ottawa
John D. Keith, Toronto
H. Garfield Kelly, Kingston
Wilbert J. Keon, Ottawa
Alfred J. Kerwin, Toronto
James A. Key, Toronto
B. S. Langford Kidd, Toronto
Stuart W. Klein, Willowdale
Borivoj Korecky, Ottawa
Susan C. Lenkei, Toronto
John A. Lewis, London
Allan J. Longmore, Kitchener
Ross M. Lymburner, Hamilton
R. Beverley Lynn, Kingston
Robert L. MacMillan, Toronto
George W. Manning, London
George A. Mayer, Kingston
Alexander D. McKelvey, Toronto
Francesco Meligrana, Toronto
William S. Metzler, Toronto
John A. Milliken, Kingston
Samuel Mirsky, Ottawa
Donald B. Moran, Don Mills
John E. Morch, Toronto
John D. Morrow, Toronto
D. P. Murnaghan, Toronto
James F. Mustard, Hamilton
William T. Mustard, Toronto
Edward J. G. Noble, Toronto
William A. Oille, Toronto
John Page, Brockville
John O. Parker, Kingston
Evan Patrick, Ottawa
N. J. Petkovich, Clarkson
Maurice A. Pollock, Ottawa
Arthur J. Powers, Ottawa
William M. Priddle, Toronto
J. L. Provan, Toronto
P. A. Rechnitzer, London
Margot R. Roach, London
John G. Robinson, Hamilton
J. David Roger, Ottawa
Vera Rose, Toronto
Nathan Schecter, Ottawa
Gerald A. Sears, London
F. J. Sellers, Ottawa
Samuel J. Shane, Toronto
Henry M. Shanoff, Toronto
Allan Sharp, Toronto
Isaac H. Shleser, Toronto
John C. Sibley, Hamilton
Malcolm D. Silver, Toronto
H. James Smith, Thunder Bay
Albert J. L. Solway, Toronto
Balfour B. Sparks, Toronto
Y. K. Sung, Toronto
L. J. Sutherland, Owen Sound
Sallie Teasdale, Toronto
Theodore Tennunen, Sudbury
Allan S. Trimble, Toronto
G. Trobridge, Sudbury
Wallace J. Troup, Ottawa

George S. Trusler, Toronto
W. G. Waddell, Ottawa
William J. Walker, Hamilton
J. F. S. Walmsley, Toronto
David L. Watt, Toronto
E. Douglas Wigle, Toronto
L. DeWitt Wilcox, London
Ralph E. Will, Toronto
Donald R. Wilson, Toronto
John Wilson, Toronto
S. Adrian Yaffe, Hamilton
J. Edward York, Toronto
Walter Zingg, Toronto
Thomas T. Zsoter, Toronto

Prince Edward Island
John B. Downing, Summerside

Quebec
Nicholas Aerichide, Montreal
Claude Allard, Montreal
Benoit Angers, Chicoutimi
Pierre Auger, Levis
Jonathan Ballon, Montreal
Simon Barsky, Montreal
Jean Beaudoin, Quebec
Maurice Beaulieu, Quebec
Aurele Beaulnes, Montreal
Albert Bernard, Montreal
Joseph Bernath, Montreal
Emile Bertho, Chicoutimi
Henri Bilodeau, Shawinigan
Peter E. Blundell, Montreal
Marc Bois, Montreal
Jean-Louis Borduas, Montreal
M. G. Bourassa, Montreal
G. R. Brow, Montreal
Luc Bruneau, Montreal
J. H. Burgess, Montreal
Sheldon O. Burman, Sherbrooke
Lucien Campeau, Montreal
R. Cange, Longueuil
G. E. Cartier, Montreal
Y. Castonguay, Montreal
Michel Chabot, Montreal
S. Chatterjee, Montreal
G. Choquette, Montreal
G. F. N. Collins, Montreal
François Couture, Quebec
R. F. P. Cronin, Montreal
Paul David, Montreal
R. O. Davies, St-Laurent
André Davignon, Montreal
Léandre Decarie, Verdun
Charles Decary, Lachine
J. A. S. de Champlain, Montreal
J. David Dejong, Montreal
P. P. Demers, Sherbrooke
Yvon Demers, Quebec
Sylvio Desautels, Montreal
Huyghues Despointes, Sherbrooke
Jean-Paul Désprés, Quebec
Yves Desrochers, Montreal
Jean-Marie Dieudonné, Montreal
Anthony R. Dobell, Montreal
Maurice Doray, Cartierville
Guy Drouin, Quebec
Bertrand Dumais, Sherbrooke
Guy Dumont, Montreal
Ihor Dyrda, Montreal
William W. Eakin, Montreal
Ernest Fallen, Montreal
Neil Feeney, Montreal
J. C. Fouron, Montreal
Serge Gagne, Quebec
Edouard D. Gagnon, Montreal
Paul-Emile Garneau, Quebec
George Garneau, Laval des Rapides
Michel Gelinas, Montreal
Jacques Genest, Montreal
O. P. Gialloreto, Montreal
James Gibbons, Montreal
Ghislaine Gilbert, Montreal
Bertrand Giguere, Thetford Mines
C. A. Goresky, Montreal
Claude Goulet, Montreal
Yvon Goulet, Montreal
Jean D. Gratton, Montreal
J. A. Gravel, Quebec
Claude Grondin, Montreal
Pierre Grondin, Montreal
J. Michel Guay, Quebec

Eric R. Gubbay, Montreal
Thomas R. Hale, St. Lambert
Andre Houde, Jonquiere
Arnold L. Johnson, Montreal
Reginald Johnson, Montreal
Gordon M. Karn, Montreal
Gerald A. Klassen, Montreal
Claude Labrosse, Sherbrooke
G. A. Lachaine, Montreal
J. B. Lalonde, Montreal
Jean-Louis Lamy, Montreal
Albert W. Lapin, Montreal
Leonard Lapointe, Montreal
Gerard Larouche, Athabaska
Raymond Larouche, Alma
Vianny Larue, Magog
L. Léon Lebel, Montreal
Paul E. Leclair, Cartierville
Gilles Leduc, Montreal
Rodrigue Lefebvre, Montreal
Yvette Lemire, Montreal
Gilles Lepage, Montreal
Ivan Lessard, Sherbrooke
Richard Lessard, Quebec
Benjamin A. Levitan, Montreal
Jean Longtin, Montreal
Paul J. Lupien, Quebec
Donald J. Macintosh, Montreal
Lloyd D. MacLean, Montreal
Emile Marcotte, Pierrefonds
J. R. Marcoux, Tracy
Pierre Marion, Montreal
D. G. F. Marpole, Montreal
Yves Marquis, Quebec
Claude R. Martel, Trois Rivières
Andre McClish, Quebec
Maurice McGregor, Montreal
Claude Meere, Montreal
Kenneth I. Melville, Montreal
Georges Menassa, St-Laurent
Edward N. Mercer, Montreal
Claude Mercier, Montreal
Gaston Mercier, Quebec
Myrto Messier, St. Jean d'Iberville
J. de L. Migneault, Sherbrooke
Ian G. Milne, Montreal
Henry F. Mizgala, Montreal
Andre Moisan, Quebec
Jean E. Morin, Quebec
Paul Morin, Montreal
Yves Morin, Quebec
D. Alton Murphy, Montreal
David R. Murphy, Montreal
Reginald Nadeau, Montreal
Antonio Pager, St. Hermas
W. H. Palmer, Montreal
Otto A. Papp, Dollard des Ormeaux
Yvon Paradis, Levis
H. Z. Pomerantz, Montreal
Robert Potvin, Quebec
Robert E. Primeau, Montreal
Andre Proulx, Montreal
Domenico Regoll, Sherbrooke
E. A. Stewart Reid, Montreal
Serge Renaud, Montreal
Oswaldo Rico, Montreal
Guy Roberge, Montreal
Raoul Roberge, Quebec
J. Rosensweig, Montreal
Yvan Rouleau, Montreal
Paul-Emile Roy, Quebec
H. Saint-Pierre, Drummondville
Michel Samson, Quebec,
George Saulnier, Quebec
Marc Savard, Montreal
Henry J. Scott, Montreal
Harold N. Segall, Montreal
Sydney Segall, Montreal
Fernand Seguin, Montreal
Hans Selye, Montreal
John Shanks, Montreal
Hyman E. Shister, Montreal
R. L. Stanford, Montreal
Paul Stanley, Montreal
David Stubington, Montreal
Paul H. Tanser, Montreal
J.Bertrand Tardiff, Noranda
Françoise Telmosse, Montreal
Adélárd Tétrault, Trois Rivieres
Andre Tetu, Quebec
B. Tousignant, Trois Rivieres
Gerard Tremblay, Montreal

Arthur M. Vineberg, Montreal
Joseph Wener, Montreal
Donald H. Woodhouse, Montreal

Saskatchewan
J. F. C. Anderson, Saskatoon
D. M. Baltzan, Saskatoon
M. A. Baltzan, Saskatoon
W. B. Firor, Saskatoon
Robert C. Hayton, Saskatoon
F. C. Heal, Moose Jaw
Louis Horlick, Saskatoon
Jose F. Lopez, Saskatoon
John Marian, Saskatoon
J. E. Merriman, Saskatoon
A. E. Somerville, Saskatoon
H. Sugarman, Saskatoon

U.S.A.
Constantine Cerkez, Pontiac
W. Stanley Hartroft, Honolulu
Gardner McMillan, Bethesda
Syed M. Mohiuddin, Omaha
John C. Morgan, Minneapolis

Other
W. H. Philip Hill, Nairobi
Frank C. Lu, Geneva

Life Members
M. Elliott, Wolfville, N.S.
Ross Jamieson, Toronto, Ont.
Harry N. Jennings, Calgary, Alta.
Ambrose G. McGhie, Hamilton, Ont.
E. M. Nanson, New Zealand
Earle P. Scarlett, Calgary, Alta.
J. W. Scott, Edmonton, Alta.
Percy Sprague, Edmonton, Alta.
Felix Tetu, Quebec, P.Q.

Honorary Members
Professeur Jean Lenègre, Paris
L. N. Katz, Chicago, Ill.

Bibliography

Abbott, M. E. On So-called Functional Heart Murmurs. *Montreal Med. J.*, 1899, 28, 1.

Abbott, Maude E. S. Unique Case of Malformation of the Heart. From a case reported by A. F. Holmes, M.D. in 1824. *Montreal Med. J.*, 1901, 30, 522.

Abbott, Maude E. S. Andrew F. Holmes, M.D., LL.D.: A Biographical Sketch. *Univ. Mag.*, 1905, 4, 386.

Abbott, Maude E. S. Congenital Cardiac Disease. Monograph in *Modern Medicine* (Osler & McCrae), 1907, iv, 323-425. Philadelphia: Lea & Fabiger.

Abbott, Maude E., and Boothby, W. M. On the Difference Between the Carbon Dioxide Tension in the Arterial and Venous Blood as a Diagnostic Sign in Cardiac Septal Defects. *Bull. Int. Assoc. Med. Museums,* 1916, 6, 122.

Abbott, Maude E. The Osler Pathological Collection in the Medical Historical Museum of McGill University. *J. Tech. Methods,* 1935, 14, 21.

Abbot, M. E. Book Review of Cyanosis by C. Lundsgaard and D. Van Slyke. *Medicine,* 1923, 2, 1; *C.M.A.J.* 1923, 95, 601.

Abbott, Maude E. S., and Dawson, Wilfred T. The Clinical Classification of Congenital Heart Disease. *Internat. Clinics,* 1924, 4, 155.

Abbott, Maude E. (ed.). Sir William Osler Memorial Volume. *Bull. Int. Ass. Med. Museums,* 926, p. 633.

Abbott, Maude E. S. *Atlas of Congenital Cardiac Disease.* Amer. Ht. Ass'n., New York, 1936, p. 71, plate 25.

Abbott, Maude E. Obituary of Louis Gross. *J. Path. & Bact.* 1939, 49, 439.

Abbott, Maude E. S. *Classified Bibliography of Sir William Osler.* The Medical Museum, McGill University Montreal, Canada, 1939.

Abella, Irving, and Troper, Harold. *None Is Too Many. Canada and the Jews of Europe.* Toronto, Ont.: Lester and Orpen, Dennys Ltd., 1986.

Adami, Marie. *J. George Adami, A Memoir.* London, 1930.

Allen, D. S., and Graham, E. A. Intracardiac Surgery: A New Method. *J.A.M.A.*, 1922, 79, 1929-1930.

American Medical Association of Vienna. Volksbuchdruckerei (Ant. Machat & Co.), Vienna, Margaretenplatz 7, 1925, 168 pp.

Amurlee, Lord. Sir James Mackenzie. *C.M.A.J.*, 1962, 57, 551.

Anrep, G. V. A New Method of Crossed Circulation. *Proc. Roy. Soc.* 1925, B, Vol. 97.

Anrep, G. V., and Segall, Harold N. The Central and Reflex Regulation of Heart Rate. *J. Physiol.*, 1926, 61, 215.

Anrep, G. V., and Segall, Harold N. The Regulation of Coronary Circulation. *Heart,* 1926, 13, 239.

Anrep, G. V. *Lane Medical Lectures. Studies in Cardiovascular Regulation.* California: Stanford University Press; London: Oxford University Press, 1936, p. 199.

Anonymous. Book Review. *Br. Am. Med. Phys. J.*, 1848-49, 4, 128.

Armstrong, John B. The Heart Foundations of Canada. *Man. Med. Rev.*, 1960, 40, 709.

Asimov's *Biographical Encyclopedia of Science and Technology.* Second Edition, Garden City, New York: Doubleday & Co., 1982.

Atlee, H. B. Dalhousie Medical School, 1907-1957. *Dalhousie Med. J.*, 1958, 11, 21.

Bailey, C. P., Glover, R. P., and O'Neil, T. J. E. Surgery of Mitral Stenosis. *J. Thor. Surg.*, 1950, 19, 16.

Banatt, A. J. Cardiac Catheterization: A Historical Note. *Lancet,* 1949, 2, 746.

Barron, S. L. The Development of the Electrocardiograph With Some Biographical Notes on Prof. W. Einthoven. *Cambridge Monograph No. 5.* London: Cambridge Instrument Co. Ltd., pp 4 and 25.

Beaubien, Pierre. Dissertation sur le rhumatisme articulaire presentée et soutenu à la Faculté de Paris, le 16 août, 1822. Paris: Imprimerie de Didot le Jeune, 1822, p. 42.

Belisle, Louis-Philippe. Histoire de la Radiologie au Canada Français. *Un. Méd. Can.* 1959, 88, 40.

Berman, Leonard. Editorial. Harry Goldblatt, 1891-1977. *J.A.M.A.*, 1977, 238, 1846.

Bert, Paul. *La Pression Barométrique: Recherches de Physiologie Expérimentale.* Paris: Masson et Cie., 1878.

Bigelow, Wilfred. General Hypothermia for Experimental Intra-Cardiac Surgery. W. G. Bigelow, J. C. Callaghan, and W. J. Hopps. *Ann. Surg.*, 1950, 132, 53, 1.

Bigelow, W., and Lanyon E. C. G. The Modern Conception and Treatment of Frostbite. *C.M.A.J.*, 1942, 47, 529.

Bishop, L. F. Blood Pressure in Clinical Medicine. *Med. Times,* New York, 1909, xxxvii, 363.

Blalock, A., and Taussig, H. B. The Surgical Treatment of Malformations of the Heart. *J.A.M.A.*, 1945, 128, 189.

Blum, Lester, and Gross, Louis. Technic of Experimental Coronary Sinus Ligation. *J. Thor. Surg.*, 1936, 5, 552.

Blumer, George (ed.). *Bedside Diagnosis by American Authors.* Philadelphia & London: Saunders Company, 1928, 353.

Boothby, W. M., and Abbott, Maude E. On the Difference Between the Carbon Dioxide Tension in the Arterial and Venous Blood as a Diagnostic Sign in Cardiac Septal Defects. *Bull. Int. Assoc. Med. Museums* 1916; 6, 122.

Bosworth, Newton. *Hochelaga Depicta. The Early History and Present State of the City and Island of Montreal.* William Greig, 1839. Facsimile Reprints of Early Canadian Books, No. 1, Hochelaga Depicta. Toronto: Congdon and Britnell Publishers, 1901, p. 124.

Bourne, C. R. Auricular Flutter Restored to Normal Rhythm by Quinidine. *C.M.A.J.*, 1928, 19, 180.

Bowditch, Henry I. *The Young Stethoscopist or the Student's Aid to Auscultation,* 1846. New York and London: Hafner Publishing Co., p. 278. (Reprinted 1964).

Bramwell, Byrom. *Diseases of the Heart and Aorta.* Edinburgh: J. P. Young, 1884, 783 pp.

Bramwell, Sir Byrom (obituary). *Br. Med. J.*, May 29, 1931, p. 823.

Brecher, Ruth and Edward. *The X-rays: A History of Radiology in the United States and Canada.* Baltimore: Williams and Wilkins Co., 1969, p. 62.

Breckenridge, R. D. C. *Medical Selection of Life Risks.* London: The Undershaft Press, 1977, p. 10.

Brow, G. R., Long, C. N. H., and Beattie, J. Irregularities of the Heart Under Chloroform: Their Dependence on Sympathetic Nervous System. *J.A.M.A.*, 1930, 95, 715.

Brow, G. R. The Heart in Typhoid Fever. *C.M.A.J.*, 1929, 20, 606.

Brown, Percy. *American Martyrs to Science Through Roentgen Rays.* Charles C. Thomas ed. Springfield, 1936, p.17.

Brunton, L. Preliminary Note on the Possibility of Treating Mitral Stenosis by Surgical Methods. *Lancet,* 1902, 1, 547.

Burch, George E., and De Pasquale, Nicholas P. *A History of Electrocardiography.* Chicago: Year Book Medical Publishers Inc., 1964, p. 77.

Burdon-Sanderson, J., and Page, F. J. M. Experimental Results Relating to the Rhythmical and Excitatory Motions of the Ventricle of the Heart of the Frog, and of Electrical Phenomena Which Accompany Them. London: *Proc. Roy. Soc.*, 1878, 27, 410.

Cabot, R. C. A Multiple Electrical Stethoscope for Teaching Purposes. *J.A.M.A.*, 1923, 81, 298.

Callaghan, J. C., and Bigelow, W. G. An Electrical Artificial Pacemaker for Standstill of the Heart. *Ann. Surg.*, 1951, 34, 8.

Callaghan, John C., Keys, Thomas E., and Key, Jack D. *Classics of Cardiology,* Vol. III. Malabar, Florida: Robert E. Krieger Publishing Co., 1983.

Campbell, Maurice. The Early Operations for Mitral Stenosis. *Br. Ht. J.*, XXVII, 1985, 5, pp. 670-673.

Cerkez, C. T., Steward, G. C., and Manning, I. W. Telemetric Electrocardiography. *C.M.A.J.*, 1965, 93, 1187-1199.

Chauvois, Louis. *William Harvey, His Life and Times; His Discoveries, His Methods.* Foreword by Sir Zachary Cope. London: Hutchinson Medical Publications, 1957, p. 271.

Chavez, Ignacio. *Diego Rivera, Sus Frescos en el Instituto Nacional de Cardologia.* Mexico, D. F., 11946.

Comroe, J. H. Jr., and Dripps, R. D. Ben Franklin and Open Heart Surgery. *Circ. Res.*, Nov. 1974, 35, 661-69.

Comroe, Julius H. *Retrospectroscope. Insights Into Medical Discovery.* California: Von Gehr Press, 1977, p.7.

Cotton, Thomas F. L'Electrocardiographie Clinique d'Après le Recent Volume de Thomas Lewis. *Arch. du mal. du Coeur,* 1914, 7, 131.

Cotton, Thomas F. Cardiac Hypertrophy. *C.M.A.J.*, 1914, 4, 709.

Cournand, André. "Cardiac Catheterization: Development of the Technique, Its Contribution to Experimental Medicine, and Its Initial Applications to Man." Jiminez Diaz Memorial Lecture, Madrid, 1970.

Cowan, John. Some Notes on the Cardiac Club. *Br. Ht. J.*, 1939, 1, 97.

Cushing, Harvey. *The Life of William Osler.* Oxford: At the Clarendon Press, 1925, Vol. I, p. 93.

Cushney, Arthur R. *The Action and Uses in Medicine of Digitalis and Its Allies.* London: Longmans, Green and Co., New York, Toronto, Bombay, Calcutta and Madras, 1925, p. 303.

Cutler, E. C., and Levine, S. A. Cardiotomy and Valvulotomy for Mitral Stenosis, Experimental Observations and Clinical Notes Concerning an Operated Case with Recovery. *Boston Med. & Surg. J.*, 1923, 188, 1023-27.

David, Paul. Chez P. D. White et Ch. Laubry. *Un. Méd. Can.* 1947, 76, 870.

David, Paul and Gagnon, E. G. Traitment Chirurgical de la Stenose Mitrale: Commissureotomie. *Un. Méd. Can.* 1950, 79, 1142.

David, Mrs. Paul David (Anne-Marie). *L'Aube de la Joie.* Montreal: Le Circle du Livre de France, 1959.

Day, H. W. An Intensive Coronary Care Area. *Dis. Chest,* 1963, 44, 423.

Day, H. W. Effectiveness of an Intensive Coronary Care Area. *Am. J. Cardiol.*, 1965, 1551.

DeBakey, M. E., and Simeone, F. A. Battle Injuries of the Arteries in World War II. An Analysis of 2,471 Cases. *Ann. Surg.*, 1946, 123, 534-579.

de la Chapelle, Clarence, ed., *The New York Heart Association. Origins and Development, 1915-1965.* New York Heart Association, New York, 1966.

Dietlen, Hans. *Herz und Gefasse im Rontgenbild.* Johann Ambrosius Barth, Leipsig, 1923, p. 455.

Donizetti, Pino. *Shadow and Substance. The Story of Medical Radiography.* London, Toronto, Paris: Pergamon Press, 1967, p. 92.

Duff, Lyman G. The Pathogenesis of Arteriosclerosis. *C.M.A.J.*, 1951, 64, 387.

Dukas, Helen, and Hoffmann, Banesh. *Albert Einstein, The Human Side.* Princeton: Princeton University Press, 1979, p. 38.

Eidlow, Samuel, and Mackenzie, E. R. Anomalous Origin of Left Coronary Artery From the Pulmonary Artery: Report of a Case Diagnosed Clinically and Confirmed at Autopsy. *Am. Ht. J.*, 1946, 32, 243.

Einthoven, W., and Geluk, M. A. G. Die Registrierung die Herztone. *Pfluger's Arch. ges. Physiol.* 1894, 57, 617

Einthoven, W. Un Nouveau Galvanometre. *Arch. N. Sec. ex. nat.* 1901, 6, 625.

Einthoven, W. Die Galvanometrich Registrierung des Menchlichen Electrokardiogramms, Zugleich eine Beurteilung des Anwendung das Kapillar Elektrometersin der Physiologie. *Pfluger's Arch. ges. Physiol.*, 1903, 99, 472.

Einthoven, W. Le Télécardiogramme. *Arch. Internat. Physiol.*, 1906, 4, 132.

Einthoven, W. Weiteres uber das Elektrokardiogram. *Pfluger's Arch. ges. Physiol.*, 1908, 122, 517.

Emerson, A. T. Some Observations on Blood Pressure, Before the Ontario Med. Ass'n., Peterborough, Ont. 1915. *Can. Pract. and Rev.*, 1915, 40, 383.

Engel, Leonard. *The Operation. A Minute-by-minute Account of a Heart Operation and the Story of Medicine and Surgery that Led up to It.* London: Museum Press Ltd., 1959, p. 135.

Eppinger, H., and Rothberger, J. Uber die Folgen der Durchschneidung der Tawarischen Schenkel der Reizleitung Systems. *Ztschr. Klin. Med.*, 1910, 70, 1.

Etziony, M. *The Montreal Clinical Society, Montreal.* Privately printed, 1963.

Fauteux, Mercier. Volvulus du coecum chez un enfant de quatre ans. *Un. Méd. Can.*, 1935, 64, 148.

Fauteux, Mercier. L'Exploration rectosigmoidienne dans les occlusions basses d'origine néoplastique. *Un. Méd. Can.*, 1935, 64, 1411.

Fauteux, Mercier. Experimental Study of Surgical Treatment of Coronary Disease. *Surg. Gyn. & Obst.* 1940, 71, 151.

Fauteux, Mercier. Positions actuelles du traitment chirurgical de l'angine de poitrine. *Un. Méd. Can.*, 1940, 69, 829.

Fauteux, Mercier. Les conditions de la recherche scientifique en médicine. *Un. Méd. Can.*, 1940, 69, 1204.

Fauteux, Mercier, and Palmer, J. H. Treatment of Angina Pectoris of Atheromatous Origin by Ligation of the Great Cardiac Vein. *C.M.A.J.*, 1941, 45, 295.

Fauteux, Mercier. Etudes expérimentales sur le traitment chirurgical des coronaires. *Un. Méd. Can.*, 1943, 72, 1261.

Fauteux, Mercier. La neurectomie péricoronarienne associée à la ligature de la grande veine coronaire dans le traitment de certaines formes de la maladie coronairienne. Observation clinique. *Un. Méd. Can.*, 1945, 74, 424.

Fauteux, Mercier, and Orvar, Swenson. La neurectomie péricoronairienne peut-elle abolir les douleurs de la maladie coronairienne? Etude expérimentale. *Un. Méd. Can.*, 1945, 74, 1958.

Fauteux, Mercier. Pericoronary Neurectomy in Abolishing Anginal Pain in Coronary Disease. *Arch. Surg.*, 1946, 53, 169.

Fauteux, Mercier. Treatment of Coronary Disease with Angina Pectoris by Pericoronary Neurectomy Combined with Ligation of the Great Cardiac Vein. *Am. Ht. J.*, 1946, 31, 260.

Fauteux, Mercier. Traitment préventif de la fibrillation ventriculaire au cours de la maladie des coronaires. *Un. Méd. Can.*, 1946, 75, 368.

Fauteux, Mercier. Surgical Treatment of Angina Pectoris. *Ann. Surg.*, 1946, 124, 1047.

Fauteux, Mercier. Cardiac Resuscitation. *J. Thor. Surg.*, 1947, 16, 623.

Fauteux, Mercier. Chirurgie intracardiaque arrêt temporaire de la circulation par occlusion des veines caves ou de l'artère pulmonaire comme temps préliminaire. Etude expérimentale. *Un. Méd. Can.*, 1947, 76, 1036.

Fauteux, Mercier, and Ripstein, Charles. Dupuytren's Contracture Associated with Coronary Artery Disease. *C.M.A.J.*, 1948, 58, 502.

Fauteux, Mercier. "Annual Lecture in Surgery of the Royal College of Physicians and Surgeons of Canada." Report of the Annual Meeting and Proceedings of the Royal College of Physicians and Surgeons of Canada, November 26 and 27, 1948. *The Future of Cardiac Surgery,* 1948.

Finley, F. G. Spinal Deformity as a Cause of Cardiac Hypertrophy and Dilatation. *C.M.A.J.*, 1921, 36, 719.

Flexner, Abraham. *Medical Education in Europe.* New York, 1912, p. 170.

Forssmann, W. Die Sondierung des Rechten Herzens. *Klin. Wchnschr.*, 1929, 8, 2085, 2287.

Forssmann, W. Uber Kontrastdarstellung de Hohlen des Lebenden Rechten Herzens und der Lungenschlagader. *Munch. Med. Wchnschr.*, 1931, 1, 489.

Forssmann, Werner. "Die Rolle der Herzkatheterung und Angiocardiographie in der Entvicklung der Moderner Medizin." Nobel Vortrag, 11 Dezember 1956.

Forssmann, Werner. *Experiments on Myself. Memoirs of a Surgeon in Germany.* New York: St. Martins Press, 1974, p. 352.

Francis, W. W. Book review of English translation of the Canon of Avicenna by O. C. Gruner. *C.M.A.J.*, 1931, 24, 856.

Franklin, K. J. *History of International Congresses of Physiological Sciences, 1889-1968*. Sponsored by the International Union of Physiological Sciences and published by the American Physiological Society, 1968, p. 296.

Frost, Stanley Brice. *McGill University, Vol. I, 1801-1845,* McGill-Queen's University Press, Montreal, 1980, p. 172.

Fulton, John F. *Harvey Cushing*. Springfield, Illinois: Charles C. Thomas, 1946, p. 216.

Furman, S., and Robinson, G. The Use of an Intracardiac Pacemaker in the Correction of Total Heart Block. *Surg. Forum,* 1958, 9, 245.

Garrison, Fielding, H. *An Introduction to the History of Medicine.* Fourth Edition. Philadelphia and London: W. B. Saunders Company, 1929, p. 455.

Geddes, L. A., and Hoff, H. E. The Capillary Electrometer. *Arch. Intern. d'hist. des sciences,* 1961, 56-57, 275.

Gibbon, J. H. Jr. Application of a Mechanical Heart and Lung Apparatus to Cardiac Surgery. *Minn. Med.,* 1954, 37, 171-180.

Gibson, George Alexander. *Life of Sir William Tennant Gairdner With a Selection of Papers on General Medical Subjects.* Glasgow:James Maclehose and Sons, 1912, p. 817.

Gilson, J. S., Holter, N. J., and Glasscock, W. R. Continuous Ambulant Electrocardiograms and Their Analysis: Clinical Observations Using Electrocardio Recorder and AVSEP Analyzer. *Am. J. Cardiol.,* 1964, 14, 204.

Goldblatt, Harry. In Memoriam Louis Gross, 1895-1937. *Am. Ht. J.,* 1939, 17, 749.

Goldblatt, Harry. Reflections, *Urol. Clin. N. Amer.,* 1957, 2, 219.

Goldbloom, Alton, and Segall, Harold N. Auricular Fibrillation in Infancy. Report of its Occurrence in a Three-month-old Infant, Perhaps Starting at Birth. *Am. J. Dis. Child.,* 1938, 56, 587.

Goldbloom, Alton. *Small Patients. The Autobiography of a Children's Doctor.* Longmans, Green & Company, 1959, p. 316.

Griff, E. R. N. *The Trail of the Invisible Light.* Springfield, Ill.: Charles C. Thomas, 1965, pp. 265, 283.

Gross, Louis. *The Blood Supply to the Heart in its Anatomical and Clinical Aspects.* New York: Paul B. Hoeber, 1921, p. 171.

Gross, Louis, Master, Arthur M., and Silverman, G. Electrocardiographic Changes Following Coronary Sinus Occlusion in Dog's Heart. *Proc. Soc. Exper. Biol. & Med.,* 1936, 34, 70.

Gross, L., and Friedberg, Charles K. Lesions of the Cardiac Valves in Rheumatic Fever. *Am. J. Path.,* 1936, 12, 855.

Gross, L., Blum, L., and Silverman, G. Experimental Attempts to Increase the Blood Supply to the Heart by Means of Coronary Sinus Occlusion. *J. Exp. Med.,* 1937, 65, 91.

Gross, Louis, Mendelowitz, M., and Schauer, G. Hemodynamic Studies in Experimental Coronary Occlusion: Open Chest Experiments. *Am. Ht. J.,* 1937, 13, 647.

Gross, Louis, and Calef, Bension. Electrocardiographic Changes in the Dog Following Sudden Occlusion of the Left Anterior Descending Coronary Branch Under Various Experimental Conditions. *Am. Ht. J.*, 1937, 6, 677.

Gross, R. E., and Hubbard, J. P. Surgical Ligation of a Patent Ductus Arteriosus. Report of First Successful Case. *J.A.M.A.*, 1939, 112, 729.

Gruner, O. C. *A Treatise on the Canon of Avicenna, Incorporating a Translation of the First Book.* London: Luzac and Co., 1929.

Gruntzig, A. R., Senning, A., and Siegenthaler, W. E. Non-operative Dilatation of Coronary Artery Stenosis. Percutaneous Coronary Angioplasty. *N. Eng. J. Med.*, 1979, 30, 61.

Guthrie, Charles Claude. *Blood Vessel Surgery and its Applications.* London: Edward Arnold; New York: Longmans, Green, 1912, p. 360.

Hales, Stephen. *Statical Essays: Vegetable Statics, Vol. I.* Third Edition. London: W. Innys & R. Manby, 1738, p. 376.

Harrison, Samuel, and Fisher, Bernard. *Charles Claude Guthrie: Blood Vessel Surgery.* A Collected Review of Fifty Years of Vascular Surgery. A Biographical Note on Dr. Guthrie and Dr. Guthrie's Complete Bibliography. University of Pittsburgh Press, 1959, 360 pp. and Collective Review of Vascular Surgery to 1959, 65 pp.

Hektoen, L. Isoagglutination of Human Corpuscles. *J.A.M.A.*, 1907, 48, 1739-1740.

Herrick, J. B. Clinical Features of Sudden Obstruction of the Coronary Arteries. *J.A.M.A.*, 59, 2015, 1912.

Herrick, James B. *A Short History of Cardiology.* Springfield, Illinois and Baltimore, Maryland: Charles C. Thomas, 1942.

Herrick, J. B. *Memories of Eighty Years.* Chicago: Chicago University Press, 1949.

Hill, Leonard, and Barnard, Harold. A Simple and Accurate Form of Sphygmomanometer or Arterial Pressure Gauge Contrived for Clinical Use. *Br. Med. J.*, 1897, 2, 904.

Hirschfelder, Arthur D. *Diseases of the Heart and Aorta.* Philadelphia and London: J. P. Lippincott Company, 1910.

Hodgkin, T. On Retroversion of the Valves of the Aorta. *London Gazette*, 1828-29, 3, 433.

Hoff, H. E., Geddes, L. A., and Guillemin, R. *Arch. Intern. d'histoire des sciences,* 1963, 16, p. 377.

Hollman, Arthur. Thomas Lewis, the Early Years. *Br. Ht. J.*, 1981, 46, 235.

Holmes, A. F. Case of Malformation of the Heart. *Tr. Med. Chir. Soc. Edinburgh,* 1824, 1, 252-259. Republished by Maude E. Abbott, Montreal, *Med. J.*, 1901, 30, 522-533.

Holmes, A. F. Valedictory Address Delivered to the Students in the Faculty of Medicine at McGill College. *Br.-Am. Med. Phys. J.*, 1850, 6, 53.

Holmes, A. F. Cases of Heart Disease. *The Medical Record,* 1855, 2, 421.

Holmes, Oliver Wendell. "How Far Are the External Means of Exploring the Condition of the Internal Organs to be Considered Useful in Medical Practice?" Boylston Prize Dissertations. Boston: Perkins and Marvin, 1836, p. 194.

Holmes, Oliver Wendell. *The Stethoscope Song: The Poetical Works of Oliver Wendell Holmes in Three Volumes.* Boston and New York: Houghton Mifflin and Company; Cambridge: The Riverside Press, Vol. 1, 1896, p. 148.

Holter, Norman J. New Method for Heart Studies: Continuous Electrocardiography of Active Subjects. *Science,* 1961, 134, 1214.

Holter, Norman J. *American Men of Science.* Eleventh edition. New York and London: R. R. Bowker Co., 1966, p. 2373.

Howard, R. P. Observations Upon Diagnosis of Cardiac Disease. *Br.-Am. Med. Phys. J.,* 1850, 6, 63.

Howard, R. Palmer. *The Chief: William Osler.* U.S.A.: Science History Publications, 1983, p. 194.

Howell, A. A. A New Method of Determining Venous Pressure. *Arch. Int. Med.,* 1912, ix, 148.

Howell, William Boyman. *F. J. Shepherd — Surgeon, His Life and Times.* Toronto and Vancouver: J. M. Dent and Sons Ltd., 1934, p. 135.

Hun, Henry. *A Guide to American Medical Students in Europe.* New York: William Wood & Company, 1883, p. 151.

Hustin, A. Principe d'une nouvelle methode de transfusion muqueuse. *J. Med. Bruxelles,* 1914, 12, 436-439.

Jacobson, J. H., and Suarez, E. L. Microsurgery in Anastamosis of Small Vessels. *Surg. Forum,* 1960, 11, 243-245.

James, W. B., and Williams, Horatio B. The Electrocardiogram in Clinical Medicine. *Am. J. M. Sc.,* 1910, 140, 408.

Janeway, Theodor C. *The Clincial Study of Blood Pressure.* New York and London: D. Appleton and Company, 1904.

Johnson, Arnold L., Wollin, Delbert G., and Ross, Janice B. Heart Catheterization in the Investigation of Congenital Heart Disease. *C.M.A.J.,* 1947, 56, 249.

Jones, W. A. Eulogy of Gordon Earle Richards. *J. Can. Ass'n. Radiologists,* 1955, 6, 1.

Kaye, M., Schickler, O., Rosenfeld, I., and Lapin, A. W. Successful Treatment of Ventricular Arrest During Complete Heart Block by External Electrical Stimulation. *Am. Ht. J.,* 1956, 51, 450.

Keith, John. The Policy of the Canadian Heart Foundation. *C.M.A.J.,* 1957, 77, 503.

Keith, John, Rowe, Richard D., and Vlad, Peter. *Heart Disease in Infancy and Childhood.* New York: The Macmillan Company, 1958, p. 877.

Kevran, Roger. *Laennec, His Life and Times.* New York: Pergamon Press; Oxford, London, Paris, 1960, p. 176.

Koenigsberger, Leo. *Hermann von Helmholtz.* Translated by Frances A. Welby With a Preface by Lord Kelvin. Oxford: At the Clarendon Press, 1906.

Korotkoff, N. S. *Experiments for Determining the Efficiency of Arterial Collaterals, 1910.* Preface, biographical notes, and editing of translation from Russian by Harold N. Segall. Privately printed, Montreal, Canada, 1980.

Kouwenhoven, W. B., Milnor, W. R., Knickerbocker, G. G., and Chestnut, W. R. Closed Chest Defibrillation of Heart. *Surgery,* 1957, 42, 550-561.

Kraus, F., and Nicolai, G. F. Uber das Electrocardiogramm unter Normalen and Pathologischen Vershaltnissen. Berlin: *Klin. Wchnschr.,* 1907, 44, 81.

Laennec, R. T. H. *De l'auscultation médiate ou traité du diagnostic des maladies des poumons et du coeur fondé principalement sur ce nouveau moyen d'exploration.* 2 tomes. Paris: J. A. Brasson & J. S. Chaudé, 1819.

Laennec, R. T. H. *A Treatise on Diseases of the Chest in Which They are Described According to Their Anatomical Characteristics and Diagnosis Established on a Principle by Means of Acoustic Instruments.* With Plates. Translated from the French with a Preface and Notes by John Forbes. First American Edition. Philadelphia: James Webster, William Brown, Printer, 1823.

Landsteiner, K. Zur Kentniss der antifermentativen lytischen und agglutinierender wirkungen des blutserums und der lymphe. *Centralbl. Bakteriol. Parasit. Infekt.,* 1900, 27, 357-362.

Leibowitz, Joshua O. *The History of Coronary Heart Disease.* Los Angeles: University of California Press, 1970.

Lessard, Richard. Les débuts de la cardiologie à Québec. *La Société Canadienne de l'Histoire de médecine. The Canadian Society for History of Medicine. Nouvelles de l'Automne,* 1932, *Autumn Newsletter,* p. 1.

Levine, Samuel A. *Clinical Heart Disease.* Second edition. Philadelphia and London: W. B. Saunders Company, 1942, p. 147.

Levine, S. A., and Lown, B. "Arm-Chair" Treatment of Acute Coronary Thrombosis. *J.A.M.A.,* 1952; 148, 1365.

Lewis, D. Sclater. *Royal Victoria Hospital, 1887-1947.* Montreal: McGill University Press, 1969, p. 144.

Lewis, T., and Cotton, T. The P-R Interval in Human Electrocardiograms and its Relation to Exercise. *J. Physiol.,* 1913, 46, 60.

Lewis, T., Meakins, J. C., and White, P. D. The Susceptible Region in A-V Conduction. *Heart,* 1914, 5, 289.

Lewis, Thomas. The Excitary Process in the Dog's Heart, Part I. The Auricles. *Phil. Tr. Roy. Soc.,* London, 1914, Series B205: 375.

Lewis, Thomas. *The Mechanism and Graphic Registration of the Heartbeat.* London: Shaw and Sons Ltd., Third edition, 1925.

Lewis, W. H. Jr. Evolution of Clincial Sphygmomanometry. *Bull. N. Y. Acad. Med.,* 1941, 17, 871.

Libman, Emanuel. Osler and Endocarditis and Mycotic Aneurysm. *Bull. Internat. Assoc. Med. Mus.* Special Osler Memorial Number, 1926, 9, 10.

Libman, Emanuel, and Friedberg, Charles K. *Subacute Bacterial Endocrditis.* Edited by Henry A. Christian. New York: Oxford University Press, 1941, p. 113.

Likoff, William B., Rappaport, Maurice B., and Levine, Samuel A. Continuous Recording Electrocardiography. *Am. Ht. J.*, 1944, 28, 98.

Lipinski, J. K. Some Observations on Early Diagnostic Radiology in Canada. *C.M.A.J.*, 1983, 129, 766.

Lippmann, Gabriel. Encyclopedia Judaica, Vol. 11, 1972, p. 286.

Loewe, Leo, Rosenblatt, P., Greene, H. J., and Russell, M. Combined Penicillin and Heparin Therapy of Subacute Bacterial Endocarditis. *J.A.M.A.*, 1944, 124, 144.

Loudon, Julian. Clinical Electrocardiography. *Can. Pract. and Rev.* 1914, July.

Lown, B., Fakiro, A. M., Hood, W. B. Jr., and Thorn, G. W. The Coronary Care Unit. *J.A.M.A.*, 1967, 199, 188.

Ludwig, Carl. Beitrage zur Kentniss des Einflusses der Respirations bewegungen auf den Blutlauf in Aortensysteme. *Muller's Arch. Anat.*, 1847, p. 240.

MacDermot, H. E. *Maude Abbott: A Memoir.* The Macmillan Co. of Canada Ltd., at St. Martin's House, 1941, p. 99.

MacDermot, H. E. *A History of the Canadian Medical Association, 1867-1921.* Toronto: Murray Printing Co., 1935, p. 155.

MacDermot, H. E. *A History of the Montreal General Hospital.* Published by the Montreal General Hospital, 1950.

MacDermot, H. E. Obituary of Cecil C. Birchard. *C.M.A.J.*, 1951, 85, 393.

MacDermot, H. E. *One Hundred Years of Medicine in Canada, 1867-1967,* pp. 97-88. Toronto/Montreal: McClelland and Stewart Limited, 1967.

Mackenzie, James. *The Study of the Pulse, Arterial, Venous and Hepatic and of the Movements of the Heart.* New York and London: The Macmillan Company, 1902.

Mackenzie, James. *Diseases of the Heart.* London: Henry Froude, Hodder and Stoughton, 1913.

MacKenzie, Kenneth A. A Century of Medicine in Nova Scotia. *N. S. Med. Bull.*, November 1953.

MacKenzie, Kenneth A. The Beginnings of Dalhousie Medical School. *Dalhousie Medical Journal,* 1958, 11, 7.

Marey, E. J. Des variations electriques des muscles et du coeur en particulier etudiées au moyen de d'electromètre de Lippmann. *Compt. rend. Acad. Sc.*, 1876, 82, 975.

Marey, E. J. *La méthode graphique dans les sciences expérimentales et principalement en physiologie et médecine.* Paris: G. Masson, editeur, 1878, p. 661.

Martin, H. Newell, and Sedgwick, W. T. Observations on the Mean Pressure and the Characters of the Pulse-Wave in the Coronary Arteries of the Heart. *J. Physiol.* 1881, Vol. 3.

McKusick, Victor A. *Cardiovascular Sound in Health and Disease.* Baltimore: The Williams and Wilkins Company, 1958.
McWilliam, John A. Cardiac Failure and Sudden Death. *Br. Med. J.*, 1889, Jan. 5 and Feb. 16.
Meade, Richard H. *A History of Thoracic Surgery.* Springfield, Ill.: Charles C. Thomas, 1961.
Means, James H., and Segall, Harold N. The Immediate Effect of Subtotal Thyroidectomy in Toxic Goiter. *Arch. Surg.*, 1924, 8, 176.
Means, James H., Starr, Paul, and Segall, Harold N. The Effect of Iodine in Exophthalmic Goiter. *Arch. Int. Med.*, 1924, 34, 355.
Mendelowitz, M., Schauer, G., and Gross, L. Hemodynamic Studies in Experimental Coronary Occlusion: Closed Chest Experiments. *Am. Ht. J.*, 1937, 13, 664.
Miller, B. J. The Development of Heart Lung Machines. *Surg. Gyn. & Obstet.*, 1982, Mar. 154(3), 403.
Mines, G. R. On Dynamic Equilibrium in the Heart. *J. Physiol.*, 1913, 46, 349.
Mines, G. R. On Circulating Excitations in Heart Muscles and Their Possible Relation to Tachycardia and Fibrillation. *Trans. Roy. Soc. Canada (Biol.)*, 1914, 8, 43.
Editorial, The Late Professor Mines. *C.M.A.J.*, 1914, 4, 1095.
Moffatt, C. R. The Electrocardiogram in Prognosis. *The Medical Clinics of North America*, 1924, 7, 1677.
Moffatt, C. F. The Prevention of Heart Disease. *C.M.A.J.*, August 1923.
Montreal Star, Tuesday, 27 September, 1955.
Morrow, W. S. Ueber die fortplanzungsgeschwindigkeit des Venenpulses. *Arch. Gesamte Physiol.*, 1900, 69, 442.
Morrow, W. S. The Physiological Laboratory of McGill University, Montreal, With a Note by W. Mills. *Br. Med. J.*, 1903, 1, 844
Morrow, W. S. A Functional Conception of Pathology as a Basis for the Diagnosis and Treatment of Heart Disease. *C.M.A.J.*, 1919, 9, 497.
Morrow, William Stairs (Obituary). *C.M.A.J.*, 1920, 10, 394.
Moynihan, Lord M. of Leeds. *Truants, Based on the Linacre Lecture.* London: Cambridge University Press, 1936 and the Keynes Press, British Medical Association, 1983, p. 73.
Murphy, J. B. Circular Anastamosis of Blood Vessels. *Med. Record,* New York, 1897, 51, 73-88.
Murray, Gordon, Wilkinson, R. R., and Mackenzie, Ross. Reconstruction of the Valves of the Heart. *C.M.A.J.*, 1938, 38, 317-319.
Murray, Gordon. *Medicine in the Making.* Toronto: The Ryerson Press, 1960, 235 pp.
Murray, Gordon. *Quest in Medicine.* Toronto: The Ryerson Press, 1963, 185 pp.
Nathan, Otto, and Norden, Heinz. *Einstein on Peace.* New York: Simon and Schuster, 1960, p. 4.

Nicolai, G. F., and Simons, A. Zur Klinik des Electrokardiogramms. *Med. Klin.*, 1909, 5, 160.
Nicolai, G. F. *The Biology of War.* Translated from the original German by Constance A. Grande and Julian Grande. New York: The Century Co., 1919, p. 553.
O'Brien, E., Crookshank, A., and Wolstenholme, G. *A Portrait of Irish Medicine.* Ward River Press, 1984, p. 306.
Osler, William. The Goulstonian Lectures on Malignant Endocarditis. *Br. Med. J.*, 1885, i, 467-470; 522-526; 577-579.
Osler, William. The Influence of Position for Hearing Heart Murmurs. *Med. & Surg. J. of Montreal,* 1877-78, 6, p. 335.
Osler, William. Robert Palmer Howard (Obituary). *Med. News,* Phila., 1889, 54, 419.
Osler, William. Congenital Affections of the Heart. In *Cycl. Dis. Child. M. and S.* (Keating). Philadelphia, 1889, ii, 747.
Osler, William. *The Principles and Practice of Medicine.* New York: D. Appleton and Company, 1892, 1079 pp.
Osler, William. Lectures on Angina Pectoris. *N. Y. Med. J.*, 1896, 64, 177, 249, 281, 345.
Osler, William. *Lectures on Angina Pectoris and Allied States.* New York: D. Appleton and Co., 1897, 160 pp.
Osler, William. *The Student Life*. In *Aequanimitas,* 2nd Edition, Third Impression. London: H. K. Lewis, 1914, p. 413.
Osler, William. Professor Wesley Mills (1847-1915). *C.M.A.J.*, 1915, 5, 338.
Ottenberg, R., and Kaliski, D. J. Accidents in Transfusion: Their Prevention by Preliminary Blood Examination, Based on an experience of One Hundred and Twenty-eight Transfusions. *J.A.M.A.*, 1913, 61, 2138.
Ozanam, Ch. *La circulation et le pouls,* 1886. See also: *Les appareils de mesure du pouls et de la pression artérielle.* Paris: Editions Louis Parente, 1979, p. 70.
Pardee, H. E. B. An Electrocardiographic Sign of Coronary Artery Obstruction. *Arch. Int. Med.*, 1920, 26, 244.
Pardee, H. E. B. *Clinical Aspects of the Electrocardiogram.* New York: Paul B. Hoeber Inc., 1928.
Park, Libbie. *Norman Bethune, His Times and Legacy.* Canadian Public Health Association, 1982, p. 138.
Paul, Oglesby. *Take Heart. The Life and Prescription for Living of Dr. Paul Dudley White.* Boston: Howard University Press, 1986, p. 315.
Penfield, W. Edward Archibald, 1872-1945. *Can. J. Surg.* 1958, 1, 167.
Poiseuille, J. L. M. Recherches sur la force du Coeur Aortique. *J. de physiol. exp. et path.* par F. Magendie, 1828, 8, 272.
Powers, J. H. Experimental Production of Mitral Stenosis. *Arch. Surg.* 1929, 18, 1945-1959.

Powers, J. H. Experimental Cardiac Valvular Disease in Dogs, and Subacute and Chronic Cardiac Valvular Disease in Man; Comparative Pathologic Study. *Arch. Surg.*, July, 1930, 21, 1-11.
Powers, J. H., Pilcher, C., and Bowie, M. A. Some Observations on Circulation in Experimental Mitral Stenosis. *Am. J. Physiol.*, 1931, 97, 405-411.
Powers, J. H. Surgical Treatment of Mitral Stenosis: An Experimental Study. *Arch. Surg.*, 1932, 25, 505-570.
Rappaport, M. B., and Sprague, H. B. Physiologic and Physical Laws that Govern Auscultation and Their Clinical Application. The Acoustic Stethoscope and the Electrical Amplifying Stethoscope and Stethograph. *Am. Ht. J.*, 1941, 21, 257.
Rautaharju, Pentti M. A Hundred Years of Progress in Electrocardiography: Early Contributions from Waller to Wilson. *Can. J. Cardiol.*, 1987, 3, 362-374.
Redding, J. S. An Historical Vignette: Intensive Care. *Respir. Ther.*, 1979, Jan-Feb. 9(1), 74-6, 78.
Reed, J. Who Invented the Modern Hospital and Who Should Tell the Story? *Rev. Am. Hist.*, 1981 (1), 29.
Richards, Gordon Earle (Obituary). *C.M.A.J.*, 1949, 60, 318.
Richards, Dickinson, W. "The Contributions of Right Heart Catheterization to Physiology and Medicine with Some Observations on the Physiopathology of Pulmonary Heart Disease." Nobel Lecture, 11 Dec. 1956.
Riesman, David. *High Blood Pressure and Longevity.* Chicago, Philadelphia, Toronto: The John C. Winston Company, 1937, p. 133.
Riva-Rocci, S. Un nuovo sfigmomanometro. *Gaz. Med. Torino,* 1986, 981, 1001.
Rodin, A. E. Osler's Museum Specimens of Heart Disease. *Chest,* 1971, 60, 587.
Roentgen, W. K. Uber eine neue Art von Strahlen. *Vehandl. de Physik-Med. Gesellschaft,* Wurzburg, 1895, N.F. XXIX, 132.
Roesler, Hugo. *Clinical Roentgenology of the Cardiovascular System.* Springfield, Ill.: Charles C. Thomas, 1937, p. 343.
Roland, Charles G. Priority of Clinical X-ray Reports: A Classic Dethroned. *Can. J. Surg.*, 1962, 5, 247.
Rosenfeld, G. *Die Dianostik inn. Krankeiten mittels Rontgenstrahlen.* Wiesbaden: J. F. Bergmann, 1897.
Rosenfeld, I., and Segall, H. N. An External Cardiac Pacemaker in the Treatment of Stokes-Adams Syndrome. *Am. Ht. J.*, 1955, 50, 749.
Rytand, David A. The Circus Movement (entrapped Circus Wave) Hypothesis and Atrial Flutter. *Ann. Int. Med.*, 1966, 65, 125.
Sarton, G. The Discovery of X-rays. *Isis,* 1936, 26, 349.
Saxl, P., and Heilig, R. Uber die diuretische Wrikungron Novasural and anderen Quecksilberpreparaten. *Wien. Klin. Wohnschr.*, 1920, 33, 943.

Schauer, G., Gross, L., and Blum, L. Hemodynamic Studies in Experimental Coronary Occlusion: Stellate Ganglionectomy Experiments. *Am. Ht. J.*, 1937, 14, 669.
Schecter, David C. vi. Precursor Apparatus and Events to the Electrical Treatment of Complete Heart Block. *N.Y. State Med. J.*, 1972, April 15, p. 953.
Schecter, David C. vii. Modern Era of Artificial Cardiac Pacemakers. *N.Y. State Med. J.*, 1972, 15 May, p. 1166.
Scrimger, F. A. C. Removal of Needle From Heart with Electrocardiographic Records Before, During and After Operation. *J. Thor. Surg.*, 1933, 2, 629-634.
Segall, Harold N. An Experimental Anatomical Investigation of the Blood and Bile Channels of the Liver. *Surg. Gyn. and Obst.*, 1923, 152.
Segall, Harold N., and White, Paul D. Progress in the Study of Cardiovascular Disease During 1923. *Boston Med. & Surg. J.*, 1924, 190, 503.
Segall, Harold, N., and White, Paul D. Clinical Observations on the Value of Calcium Chloride as a Diuretic and Upon its Influence on the Circulatory Mechanism. *Am. J. Med. Sci.*, 1925, 170, 647.
Segall, Harold N., and Anrep, G. V. The Isometric Contraction of the Frog's Ventricle. *Heart,* 1926, 13, 61.
Segall, Harold N. Recent Advances in Knowledge of Coronary Circulation. *C.M.A.J.*, 1927, 17, 711.
Segall, Harold N. Auscultation of the Heart. *C.M.A.J.*, 1932, 27, 632.
Segall, Harold N. Obituary of Louis Gross. *C.M.A.J.*, 1937, 37, 609.
Segall, Harold N. Lyman G. Barton, Sr. *C.M.A.J.*, 1945, 52, 202.
Segall, Harold N. Rupture of Ventricular Myocardium. Report of Four Cases With Comments on Pathogenesis and on Clinical Significance of Cardiac Rupture in Prognosis of Coronary Heart Disease. *Am. Ht. J.*, 1945, 30, 39.
Segall, Harold N. The Principal Patterns of Cardiac Pain Related to Arteriosclerotic Coronary Artery Disease. *C.M.A.J.*, 1950, 62, 341.
Segall, Harold N. Laennec and His Contribution to the Evolution of Clinical Methods. *McGill Med. J.*, 23, 1954, pp. 145-154.
Segall, Harold N. History of the Canadian Heart Association. *Man. Med. Rev.*, 1960, 40, 94.
Segall, Harold N. Evolution of Graphic Symbols for Cardiovascular Sounds and Murmurs. *Br. Ht. J.*, 1962, 24, 1.
Segall, Harold N. Spoon-Feeding the Recumbent Statue in Atavia. *The Can. Nurse J.*, 1965, 61, No. 6.
Segall, Harold N. On Learning About Cardiovascular Sound. *Man. Med. Rev.*, 1967, 47, 503.
Segall, Harold, N. Introduction of the Stethoscope and Clinical Auscultation in Canada. *J. Hist. Med. & Allied Sci.*, 1967, 22, 414.
Segall, Harold N. Personal communication from Dr. Edouard Gagnon in 1970.

Segall, Harold N. L'introduction au Canada de l'électrocardiographie. *Un. Méd. Can.*, 1975, 104, 1685.
Segall, Harold N. N. C. Korotkoff, 1974-1920, Pioneer Vascular Surgeon. *Am. Ht. J.*, 1976, 91, 816.
Segall, Harold N. William Stairs Morrow, Canada's First Physiologist-cardiologist. *C.M.A.J.*, 1976, 114, 543.
Segall, Harold N. Auto-auscultation in a Patient With a Floppy Mitral Valve. *Am. Ht. J.*, 1976, 91, 816.
Segall, Harold N. Goldbloom, Goldblatt, Greenspon and Gross: The Four G's of McGill Medicine Class 1916. *Canadian Jewish Historical Society Journal*, 1982, 6, 17.
Segall, Harold N. William Osler and Thomas Browne, A Friendship of Fifty-Two Years. Sir Thomas Pervades Sir William's Library. *Koroth*, 1985, 8, 150.
Segall, Harold N. William Osler and the Genesis of Cardiology in Canada. *Can. J. Cardiol.*, 1986, 2, 320.
Segall, Harold N. Introduction of Electrocardiography in Canada. *Can. J. Cardiol.*, 1987, 3, 358-361.
Segall, Harold N. Some Aspects of the Genesis of Cardiology in Canada — The Montreal Factor, Part 1. *Annals RCPSC*, 1987, 20, 421-425.
Segall, Harold N. Some Aspects of the Genesis of Cardiology in Canada — The Montreal Factor, Part 2. *Annals RCPSC*, 1987, 20, 497-502.
Shakespeare, William. *Romeo and Juliet*, Act 2, Scene 3.
Shah, Mazhar H. *The General Principles of Avicenna's Canon of Medicine.* Printed in Pakistan at the Inter Services Press Ltd., 1966.
Shapiro, A. P. In Memoriam I. Arthur Mirsky, M. D., 1907-1974. *Psychosom. Med.*, 1975, 37(1), 1.
Shepherd, Francis J. *Origin and History of the Montreal General Hospital.* Privately printed 1924, p. 39.
Shoemaker, P., and Jones, M. V. From Infirmaries to Intensive Care Hospitals in Wisconsin. *In* Numbers, R. L., Lear, H. J. W. (eds.). *Wisconsin Medicine: Historical Perspectives* Madison: University of Wisconsin Press, 1981, p. 105.
Shumack, K. H., and Brown, K. W. G. Continuous Portable Electrocardiography. *C.M.A.J.*, 1968, 68, 139-144.
Smith, H. J., and Anthonisen, N. R. Results of Cardiac Resuscitation in 254 Patients. *Lancet* 2, 1965, 1027.
Snellen, H. A. *Selected Papers on Electrocardiography of Willem Einthoven, With a Bibliography, Biographical Notes and Comments.* Leiden University Press, 1977, p. 16.
Spinoza, Baruch. *Philosophy of Benedict de Spinoza.* Translated from the Latin by R. H. M. Elwes, with an Introduction by Frank Sewell, M.A. New York: Tudor Publishing Co., 1933, p. 70.
Stanton, W. B. A Practical Clinical Method for Determining Blood Pressure in Man, with a Discussion of the Methods Hitherto Employed. *Univ. Penn. Med. Bull.*, 1903, 15, 466.

Steeves, Lea C. Clyde W. Holland, F.A.C.P. *Bull. Am. Coll. Phys.*, Nov. 1971, p. 595.
Tandler, Julius. *Anatomie des Herzens.* Verlag von Gustav Fischer, 1913, p. 292.
Vaquez, H., and Bordet, E. *Le coeur et l'aorte. Etudes de radiologie clinique.* Librairie J.-B. Baillière et Fils, Paris, 1913, 1st ed.
Vaquez, H. *Maladies du coeur.* Librairie J.-B. Baillière et Fils, 1921, p. 23.
Veith, Ilza. *The Yellow Emperor's Classic of Internal Medicine.* Translated with an Introductory Study by Ilza Veith. Berkeley, Los Angeles, London: University of California Press, 1972, p. 159.
Vierordt, K. Die bildliche Darstellung des Menschlichen Arterien Pulses. *Arch. Physiol. Heilk.*, 1854, 13, 284.
Vineberg, Arthur M. Development of Anastamosis Between Coronary Arteries and Transplanted Internal Mammary Artery. *C.M.A.J.*, 1946, 55, 117.
Vineberg, Arthur M. *Myocardial Revascularization by Arterial-Ventricular Implants.* John Wright, PSG Inc., 1982.
Vogl, Alfred. The Discovery of the Organic Mercurial Diuretics. *Am. Ht. J.*, 1950, 39, 881.
Waller, A. D. A Demonstration on Man of Electromotive Changes Accompanying the Heart's Beat. *J. Physiol.*, 1887, 8, 229.
Waller, A. D. Introductory Address on the Electromotive Properties of the Human Heart. *Br. Med. J.*, 1888, 2, 751; and at First International Physiological Congress, Basle, Switzerland, 11 September, 1889.
Waller, A. D. *Eight Lectures on the Signs of Life From Their Electrical Aspect.* New York: E. P. Dutton & Co., 1903, pp. 175, 162.
Waller, A. D. *The Electrical Action of the Human Heart.* University of London Press Ltd., 1922, p. 103.
Warfield, L. M. The Auscultatory Blood Pressure Phenomenon. *Wisconsin Med. J.*, 1914, 14, xii, 71.
Washburn, Frederic A. *Massachusetts General Hospital, 1900-1935.* Boston: Houghton, Mifflin Company, 1939, p. 375.
Weiss, David. *Physician Extraordinary. A Novel of the Life and Times of William Harvey.* Delacorte Press/Eleanor Friede, 1975, p. 455.
Wenckebach, K. F. und Winterberg, Heinrich. *Die Unregelmassige Herztatigkeit.* Verlag von Wilhelm Engelmann. Leipzig, 1927, Textband, p. 635, Tafelband, p. 183.
White, Paul D., and Myers, Merrill M. The Classification of Cardiac Diagnosis. *J.A.M.A.*, 1921, 77, 1414.
White, Paul Dudley. *Heart Disease.* New York: The Macmillan Company, 1931, p. 143.
White, Paul Dudley. *Heart Disease.* New York: The Macmillan Company, 1944, p. 503.
White, Paul Dudley. *My Life and Medicine.* Boston: Gambit Inc., 1971, p. 55.

Williams, C. J. B. *Memoirs of a Life and Work.* London: Smith, Elder and Co., 1884.

Williams, Francis H. A Method for More Fully Determining the Outline of the Heart by Means of the Fluoroscope Together With Other Uses of the Instrument in Medicine. *Boston Med. & Surg. J.*, 1896, 135, 335.

Williams, Francis H. *The Roentgen Rays in Medicine and Surgery as an Aid in Diagnosis and a Therapeutic Agent Designed for Use of Practitioners and Students.* New York, London: The Macmillan Company Ltd., 1901, p. 658.

Willius, Frederick A., and Keys, Thomas E. *Cardiac Classics.* St. Louis: The C. V. Mosby Company, 1941, p. 699.

Yu, P. N., Imboden, C. A., Fox, S. M., III, and Killip, T. III. A Specialized Intensive Care Unit for Acute Myocardial Infarction. *Modern Concepts Cardio. Vasc. Dis.*, 1965, 34, 23.

Zoll, P. M. Resuscitation of the Heart in Ventricular Standstill by External Electrical Stimulation. *N. Eng. J. Med.*, 1952, 247, 768.

Zuelzer, Wolf. *The Nicolai Case.* Wayne State University Press, 1982, p. 463.

Glossary

Degrees and Fellowships

A.C.F.A.S.	Association Canadienne-Française pour l'Avancement des Sciences
A.O.A.	Alpha Omega Alpha Society
A.R.C.S.T.	Associate, Royal College of Science and Technology
A.R.C.S.	Associate, Royal College of Science
A.S.C.I.	American Society for Clinical Investigation
B.Ch./B.Chir./Ch.B.	Baccalaureus Chirurgiae (Bachelor of Surgery)
B.M.	Bachelor of Medicine
B.S.	Bachelor of Surgery
B.Sc.	Bachelor of Science
C.A.B.S.	Certificant, American Board of Surgery
C.A.S.S.	Coronary Artery Surgery Study
C.F.M.S.	Canadian Forces Medical Services
C.H.A.	Canadian Heart Association
C.M.	Chirurgiae Magister (Master of Surgery)
C.R.C.P.	Certificant, Royal College of Physicians
C.S.C.I.	Canadian Society of Clinical Investigation
C.P.S.Q.	College of Physicians and Surgeons of Quebec
C.S.P.Q.	Certified Specialist in the Province of Quebec
D.Phil./Ph.D.	Doctor of Philosophy
D.Sc.	Doctor of Science
F.A.A.P.	Fellow, American Academy of Pediatrics
F.A.C.A.	Fellow, American College of Anesthesia
F.A.C.C.	Fellow, American College of Cardiology
F.A.C.C.P.	Fellow, American College of Chest Physicians
F.A.C.P.	Fellow, American College of Physicians
F.A.G.S.	Fellow, American Gynecological Society
F.A.H.A.	Fellow, American Heart Association
F.A.I.N.	Fellow, American Institute of Nutrition
F.C.A.P.	Fellow, American College of Pathologists
F.C.C.P.	Fellow, College of Chest Physicians
F.I.C.A.	Fellow, International College of Anaesthetists
F.M.O.Q.	Federation des médecins omnipracticiens du Québec
F.M.S.Q.	Federation des médecins specialistes du Québec
F.R.A.C.P.	Fellow, Royal Australian College of Physicians
F.R.C.P.	Fellow, Royal College of Physicians
F.R.C.P.(C)	Fellow, Royal College of Physicians (Canada)
F.R.C.P.S.	Fellow, Royal College of Physicians and Surgeons
F.R.C.S.	Fellow, Royal College of Surgeons
F.R.C.S.(C)	Fellow, Royal College of Surgeons (Canada)

F.R.S.A.	Fellow, Royal Society of Arts
LL.B.	Legum Baccalaureus (Bachelor of Laws)
LL.D.	Legum Doctor (Doctor of Laws)
L.M.C.C.	Licentiate, Medical Council of Canada
M.A.	Magister Artium (Master of Arts)
M.B.	Medicinae Baccalaureus (Bachelor of Medicine)
M.C.G.P.	Member, College of General Practitioners
M.D.	Medicinae Doctor (Doctor of Medicine)
M.R.C.P.	Member, Royal College of Physicians
M.R.C.S.	Member, Royal College of Surgeons
R.C.A.M.C.	Royal Canadian Army Medical Corps
R.C.P.(C)	Royal College of Physicians (Canada)
R.C.P.& S(C)	Royal College of Physicians and Surgeons (Canada)
R.C.V.S.	Royal College of Veterinary Surgeons
R.S.C.	Royal Society of Canada
R.S.N.A.	Radiological Society of North America

Periodical Publications

Alberta Med. Bull.	Alberta Medical Bulletin
Am. Ht. J.	American Heart Journal
Am. J. Cardiol.	American Journal of Cardiology
Am. J. Clin. Path.	American Journal of Clinical Pathology
Am. J. Dis. Child.	American Journal of Diseases of Children
Am. J. Med. Sci.	American Journal of the Medical Sciences
Am. J. Med. Tech.	American Journal of Medical Technology
Am. J. Ophth.	American Journal of Ophthalmology
Am. J. Path.	American Journal of Pathology
A.M.H.	Annals of Medical History
Ann. Anat. Path.	Annales d'Anatomie Pathologique
Ann. I. Med.	Annals of Internal Medicine
Ann. R.S.P.S.C.	Annals of the Royal College of Physicians and Surgeons of Canada
Ann. Surg.	Annals of Surgery
Ann. Thor. Surg.	Annals of Thoracic Surgery
Arch. Anat. Histol. Embry.	Archives d'Anatomie, d'Histologie et d'Embryologie
Arch. Internat. Histoire Sci.	Archives Internationales d'Histoire des Sciences
Arch. Int. Phys.	Archives Internationales de Physiologie
Arch. Gesamte Physiol.	Archiv für die gesamte Physiologie des Menschen und die Tiere (Pfluegers)
Arch. Mal. Coeur	Archives des Maladies du Coeur et des Vaisseaux
Arch. Surg.	Archives of Surgery
B.A.C.P.	Bulletin of the American College of Physicians
B.H.M.	Bulletin of the History of Medicine
Boston Med. & Surg. J.	Boston Medical and Surgical Journal
Br. Ht. J.	British Heart Journal
Br. Amer. J. Med. Phy.	British American Journal of Medical and Physical Science
Bull. Am. Coll. Phy.	Bulletin of the American College of Physicians
Bull. Am. Coll. Surg.	Bulletin of the American College of Surgeons

Bull. Intern. Assoc. Med. Mus.	Bulletin of the International Association of Medical Museums
Bull. N.Y. Acad. Med.	Bulletin of the New York Academy of Medicine
Can. J. Biochem.& Phys.	Canadian Journal of Biochemistry and Physiology
Can. J.P.H.	Canadian Journal of Public Health
Can. J. Surg.	Canadian Journal of Surgery
Can. Pract. & Rev.	Canadian Practitioner and Review
C.M.A.J.	Canadian Medical Association Journal
Chest/Dis. Chest (before 1970)	Diseases of the Chest
Circ. Res.	Circulation Research
Compt Rend. Acad. Sci.	Comptes Rendus de l'Academie des Sciences
Gaz. Med. Torino	Gazzetta Medica Italiano, Torino
J.A.C.C.	Journal of the American College of Cardiology
J.A.M.A.	Journal of the American Medical Association
J.C.A.R.	Journal of the Canadian Association of Radiologists
J. Cardio. Surg.	Journal of Cardiovascular Surgery
J. Clin. Invest.	Journal of Clinical Investigations
J. Exp. Med.	Journal of Experimental Medicine
J.H.M.& A.S.	Journal of the History of Medicine and Allied Sciences
J. Med. Bruxelles	Journal de Médecine (Bruxelles)
J.P.S.	Journal of Pediatric Surgery
J. Path. & Bact.	Journal of Pathology and Bacteriology
J.Ped.	Journal of Pediatrics
J. Physiol.	Journal of Physiology
J. Physiol. Exp. & Path.	Journal de Physiologie Experimentale et Pathologique
J. Surg. Res.	Journal of Surgical Research
J. Tech. Meth.	Journal of Technical Methods
J. Thor. Surg. (to 1959)/ J. Thor. Cardiovasc. Surg.	Journal of Thoracic and Cardiovascular Surgery
Laval Méd.	Laval Médicale
Man. Med. Rev.	Manitoba Medical Review
Man. Med. Stud. J.	Manitoba Medical Studies Journal
McGill Med. J.	McGill Medical Journal
Med.& Biol. Eng.	Medical and Biological Engineering
Med. Hist.	Medical History
Med. J. Aust.	Medical Journal of Australia
Med. Rec.	Medical Record
Med. Times (N.Y.).	Medical Times (New York)
Med. World News	Medical World News
Mem. Acad. Chir.	Memoires, Academie de Chirurgie
Mod. Conc. Cardiovasc. Dis.	Modern Concepts of Cardiovascular Disease
Mod. Med. of Canada	Modern Medicine of Canada
Munch. Med. Wchnschr.	Müchener medizinsche Wochenschrift
N. Eng. J. Med.	New England Journal of Medicine
N.M.A. Newsletter	Newfoundland Medical Association Newsletter
N.S. Med. Bull.	Nova Scotia Medical Bulletin
N.Y. Med. J.	New York Medical Journal

N.Z.M.J.	New Zealand Medical Journal
Phil. Tr. Royl Soc.	Philosophical Transactions of the Royal Society
Proc. Royl. Soc.	Proceedings of the Royal Society
Proc. Soc. Exp. Biol. & Med.	Proceedings of the Society for Experiments in Biology and Medicine
Psychosom. Med.	Psychosomatic Medicine
Quart. Bull. Can. Assoc. Med. Clin.	Quarterly Bulletin of the Canadian Association of Medical Clinicians
Resp. Ther.	Respiratory Therapy
Rev. Am. Hist.	Reviews in American History
Rev. Lyon Méd.	Revue Lyonnaise de Médicine
Saguenay Méd.	Saguenay Médicale
Stud. Hist. Med.	Studies in the History of Medicine
Surg. Forum	Surgical Forum of the American College of Surgeons
Surg. Gyn. & Obst.	Surgery, Gynecology and Obstetrics
Tr. Med. Chir. Soc. Edin.	Transactions of the Medical and Chirurgical Society of Edinbrugh
Tr. Royl. Soc.Can. (Biol.)	Transactions of the Royal Society of Canada (Biology)
Un. Méd. Can.	Union Médicale du Canada
Univ. Man. Med. J.	University of Manitoba Medical Journal
Univ. Mag.	University Magazine
Univ. Penn. Med. Bull.	University of Pennsylvania Medical Bulletin
U. of T. Med. J.	University of Toronto Medical Journal
Urol. Clin. N. Amer.	Urologic Clinics of North America
Verh. Dtsch. Phys. Ges.	Verhandlungen der Deutschen Physikalischen Gesellschaft
Verh. Dtsch. Ges. Exp. Med.	Verhandlungen der Deutschen Gesellschafte für Experimentelle Medizin
Wien. Klin. Wohnschr.	Wiener Klinische Wochenschrift
Ztschr. Klin. Med.	Zeitschrift für klinische Medizin

Chronology

1628 William Harvey publishes *de Motu Cordis*
1661 M. Malpighi publishes *de Pulmonibus*
1665 Frederik Ruysch studies blood vessels by anatomical injection
1690 John Floyer counts the pulse by a watch
1715 Raymond Vieussens publishes *treatise on heart diseases*
1724 Gabriel Daniel Fahrenheit reports on his mercury thermometer
1726 Stephen Hales measures arterial blood pressure in a horse
1742 Anders Celsius invents 100 degree thermometer
1749 J.-B. de Senac's treatise on heart disease published
1761 G. Margagni's *de Sedibus* is published
1761 L. Auenbrugger's *Inventum Novum* is published
1768 W. Heberden describes Angina Pectoris
1785 W. Withering's treatise on foxglove (digitalis) published
1792 L. Galvani's essay on animal electricity published.
1799 Mathew Baillie describes endocarditis
1800 Library of Congress (Washington) founded
1810 W. C. Wells describes rheumatism of the heart
1816 R. T. H. Laennec invents the stethoscope for mediate auscultation
1819 R. T. H. Laennec book on mediate auscultation published
1821 Montreal General Hospital opened on Dorchester St.
1821 R. T. H. Laennec. English translation of mediate auscultation by John Forbes in first English edition.
1823 R. T. H. Laennec. Forbes translation of Laennec's book on mediate auscultation in first American edition
1823 Montreal Medical Institution founded
1824 Andrew Fernando Holmes publishes case report of congenital cor triloculare biatriatum
1827 R. Adams describes heart block
1828-29 Thomas Hodgkin describes aortic regurgitation
1828 University College (London) opened
1828 J. L. M. Poiseuille uses mercury manometer to measure blood pressure in experimental animal
1829 Montreal Medical Institution becomes first functioning faculty of McGill University
1835 P. C. A. Louis introduces medical statistics
1836 J.-B. Bouillaud correlates endocarditis with rheumatic fever
1844 Claude Bernard performs cardiac catheterization in experimental animal

1846 W.J.G. Morton introduces ether anaesthesia at the Massachusetts General Hospital
1847 Carl Ludwig invents the kymograph
1849 Royal Canadian Institute (Toronto) founded
1849 William Osler born on July 14
1850 Karl Vierordt introduces the sphygmograph
1850 R. P. Howard publishes article on *Observations on the diagnosis of cardiac disease*
1851 W. Helmholtz invents ophthalmoscope
1854 Claude Bernard discovers vasodilator nerves
1857 Pasteur makes discoveries in bacteriology beginning with work on fermentation
1859 Florence Nightingale publishes *Notes on Nursing*
1865 John Shaw Billings initiates Army Medical Library (National Library of Medicine)
1867 Joseph Lister introduces antiseptic surgery
1867 Dominion of Canada established (July 1)
1869 C. R. Wunderlich publishes treatise on clinical thermometry
1870 William Osler comes to McGill as a student to graduate in 1872
1872 G. Lippmann invents capillary electrometer
1876 R. Virchow publishes *A description and explanation of the method of performing post-mortem examinations*
1876 W. Osler appointed first pathologist at Montreal General Hospital
1878 E. J. Marey publishes *La Méthode Graphique*
1878 J. Burdon-Sanderson records an electrocardiogram of frog's heart using Lippmann electrometer
1880 H. N. Martin invents the heart-lung preparation
1884 William Osler delivers the Goulstonian Lectures on malignant endocarditis
1886 Ch. Ozanam introduces ink-writing sphygmograph lever
1887 A. D. Waller records human electrocardiogram using Lippmann electrometer
1889 Johns Hopkins Medical School opened
1892 William Stairs Morrow appointed Lecturer in Physiology at McGill
1894 Maude Elizabeth Seymour Abbott graduates M.D.
1895 W. K. Roentgen discovers X-rays in December
1896 Dr. J. Cox assembles X-ray apparatus to find site of bullet in man's leg which Dr. R. C. Kirkpatrick is to remove at the Montreal General Hospital in February
1896-1906 Dr. G. Girdwood serves as X-ray expert at Montreal General and Royal Victoria Hospitals
1896 Monseigneur J. C. K. Laflamme in Quebec City produces X-ray pictures of an infant's hand and foot
1896 Monseigneur Choquette in St-Hyacinthe applies X-rays in search of renal calculi

1896 S. Riva-Rocci invents clinical sphygmomanometer
1896 J. B. Murphy performs circular anastamosis of blood vessels
1901 K. Landsteiner discovers blood groups
1901 W. Einthoven invents string galvanometer
1902 Thomas Lauder Brunton recommends studies in search of a surgical procedure treatment of mitral stenosis
1902 J. Mackenzie publishes the *Study of the Pulse*
1902 A. Carrel introduces new methods of vascular anastamosis and organ transplantation
1904 E. F. Sauerbruch introduces pneumatic cabinet for thoracic surgery
1905 N. C. Korotkoff discovers auscultatory method for measuring arterial pressure
1907 International Association of Medical Museums founded; Maude Abbott the secretary treasurer and editor of the Bulletin
1907 F. Kraus and G. F. Nicolai publish article on clinical electrocardiography
1908 A. D. Waller introduces Thomas Lewis to electrocardiography
1910 At the Massachusetts General Hospital, Dr. Fritz B. Talbot and Dr. Richard M. Smith establish the first children's heart clinic and in 1912 Dr. Joseph H. Pratt opens an Adult Heart Clinic. Later both clinics managed by Dr. Paul Dudley White
1910-13 E. Libman describes subacute bacterial endocarditis
1911 At Bellevue Hospital, New York, Miss Mary E. Wadler (social service) and Dr. Hubert Guile found the first cardiac clinic for adults
1911 R. Ottenberg introduces blood matching for transfusion
1912-13 Thomas Cotton first Canadian to train for cardiology to practise at Montreal General Hospital
1913 J. C. Meakins trains for cardiology to practise at Royal Victoria Hospital, Montreal
1913 John Oille specializes in cardiology at Toronto General Hospital
1914 R. A. Jamieson trained for cardiology to practise at Toronto General Hospital
1914 Cambridge Instrument Co. electrocardiographs delivered to seven institutions and one private practitioner in Canada
1914 J. Loudon publishes first Canadian article on electrocardiography
1914-18 T. Cotton, J. C. Meakins and C. C Birchard associated with T. Lewis in the study of effort syndrome in soldiers
1914 Electrocardiography Department headed by Dr. Arthur Burridge in Winnipeg
1914 Death of G. R. Mines
1915 New York Heart Association founded
1919 At Montreal General Hospital C. C. Birchard chief of electrocardiography
1920 At Royal Victoria Hospital, Montreal, C. F. Moffatt, chief of electrocardiography initiates cardio-renal clinic

1920 C. W. Hurlburt introduces electrocardiography in Edmonton
1920 K. Mackenzie of Halifax practises clinical cardiology in the Maritime provinces
1920 M. A. Pollack, a general practitioner practises electrocardiography
1921 L. Gross publishes *Blood Supply to the Heart*
1921 White and Myers publish *Classification of Cardiac diagnosis*
1921-24 A. deGuise trains for cardiology in Paris and joins staff of Notre Dame Hospital, Montreal
1922-23 G. F. Strong trains for cardiology with Samuel A. Levine in Boston and joins staff of Vancouver General Hospital
1923 E. Cutler and S. A. Levine report on surgical treatment of mitral stenosis
1923 J. Hepburn joins staff of Toronto General Hospital
1924 American Heart Association formed
1924 W. Einthoven honored with Nobel Prize for contribution to electrocardiography
1925 H. Soutar performs surgical operation for mitral stenosis
1926 G. R. Brow trains for cardiology (1920-1926) and joins staff of Royal Victoria Hospital, Montreal
1926 H. N. Segall trains for cardiology (1920-1926) and joins the staff of the Montreal General Hospital; starts cardiac clinic
1927 D. Baltzan returns to Saskatoon after a year of post-graduate study in Europe to practise as internist with special interest in cardiology
1929 W. Forssmann performs cardiac catheterization on himself
1930 E. P. Scarlett, an internist, introduces electrocardiography in Calgary
1932 Gordon Murray pioneers transplantation of kidney
1932 R. D. Roach introduces electrocardiography in New Brunswick
1933 F. A. C. Scrimger reports operation on heart for removal of a darning needle
1933 Richard Lessard introduces cardiology and electrocardiography in Quebec City
1933 S. Eidlow general practitioner of Montreal attends Paul Dudley White course in cardiology and acquires Sanborn electrocardiograph
1933 R. M. Lymburner introduces cardiology in Hamilton, Ontario
1934 H. Goldblatt creates experimental hypertension model
1935 L. D. Wilcox suggests surgical ligation of patent ductus arteriosus
1936 Gordon Murray, L. B. Jacques, T. S. Perret and C. H. Best introduce heparin in treatment of venous thrombosis following injury
1936 L. Gross begins search for surgical treatment of angina pectoris
1937 A. Tétrault introduces electrocardiography in Trois Rivières
1938 Harold N. Segall initiates postgraduate course in cardiology
1940 A. Cournand and H. A. Ranges report on cardiac catheterization in humans

1940-48 Mercier Fauteux in quest for surgical treatment of angina pectoris
1943 Fraser B. Gurd performs ligature of patent ductus arteriosus and subacute bacterial endocarditus, a first in Canada
1944 L. Loewe and associates demonstrate how to administer penicillin to people with subacute bacterial endocarditis successfully
1942 W. Bigelow and E. C. G. Lanyon report on the treatment of frostbite; the beginning of Bigelow's researches on hypothermia.
1945 A. Blalock and H. Taussig report on surgical treatment of tetralogy of Fallot
1945 Charles Bailey introduces commissureotomy for mitral stenosis
1946 Arnold L. Johnson first in Canada to perform cardiac catheterization and to report results
1946 John Keith initiates cardiology department at Sick Children's Hospital and practises cardiac catheterization and angiocardiography
1946 Montreal Cardiac Society founded
1947 Canadian Heart Association founded; name changed to Canadian Cardiovascular Society in 1962
1947 William F. Greenwood introduces cardiac catheterization at Toronto General and Wellesley Hospitals
1948 American College of Cardiology founded
1948 Gordon Murray introduces surgical treatment of atrial septal defect
1949 Robert E. Beamish and John A. Hildes introduce cardiac catheterization in Winnipeg.
1950 E. Gagnon and P. P. David report mitral valve commisureotomy
1950 Arthur Vineberg performs internal mammary artery implant operation for angina pectoris
1950 First World Congress of Cardiology in Paris
1951 Hugh Stansfield founding president of Vancouver Heart Association
1951 J. B. Downing, an internist, introduces electrocardiography in Prince Edward Island
1951 Jacques Genest becomes Director of Clinical Research at Hôtel-Dieu de Montréal
1951 Joffre-André Gravel introduces cardiovascular surgery in Quebec City
1951 W. Bigelow and J. C. Callaghan invent a cardiac pacemaker
1952 Paul Zoll initiates pacemaker era in clinical cardiology
1954 W. A. Mustard invents a surgical approach to treatment of transposition of the great vessels
1952 Garfield Kelly and Donald Hatcher introduce cardiac catheterization at Queen's University
1952 Douglas Leonard Roy introduces cardiac catheterization in Halifax
1952 A. Yaffe performs first cardiac catheterization in Hamilton
1953 Osman Gialloreto introduces angiocardiography at Notre-Dame Hospital in Montreal

1953 Maurice D. Young pioneers paediatric cardiology in Vancouver
1953 Georges E. Cartier performs endarterectomy at Hôtel-Dieu de Montréal
1953 Morley Cohen, a member of Lillehei's team when he performed first open heart surgery using human donor for extra-corporeal circulation by heart-lung preparation
1953 Meeting in Montreal of International Union of Physiological Sciences
1954 Montreal Heart Institute opened with P. P. David, its founder, as director
1954 Frank H. McGinnis associated with N. Holter in creating radioelectrocardiography for continuous dynamic monitoring of heart
1954 J. B. Roberts introduces electrocardiography in Newfoundland
1954 Eric M. Nanson introduces cardiovascular surgery in Saskatoon
1954 Will Carleton Whiteside introduces cardiovascular surgery in Edmonton
1954 Ontario Heart Foundation founded
1955 Louis Horlick and John Merriman establish haemodynamic laboratory in Saskatoon
1955 Cardiac catheterization performed at Ottawa General Hospital by Dr. Frank Berkman
1955 Hugh Stansfield initiates formation of British Columbia Heart Foundation
1956 J. C. Morgan introduces cardiac catheterization in Calgary
1956 F. G. Dolan becomes first cardiovascular surgeon in Halifax
1956 A. R. C. Dobell introduces open heart surgery in three Montreal hospitals
1957 Yves Morin established haemodynamic laboratory in Quebec City
1957 G. F. Strong founding president of Canadian Heart Foundation
1957 John B. Armstrong becomes Executive Secretary of Canadian Heart Foundation
1959 D. Kavanagh-Gray introduces cardiac catheterization in Vancouver, B.C.
1960 A. L. Johnson and G. A. Klassen introduce electrode catheter for pacemaker
1960 G. A. Woodwark establishes haemodynamic laboratory in Victoria, B.C.
1960 André Louis Davignon pioneers paediatric cardiology in francophone Montreal
1962 P. Field introduces cardiovascular surgery in Sudbury
1964 Interamerican Congress of Cardiology takes place in Montreal
1967 Ontario Heart Foundation establishes the John Keith Lecture, to be delivered at the annual meeting of the Canadian Cardiovascular Society
1967 (Dec.) C. Barnard performs human heart transplant operation

Chronology of Societies and Foundations

1915 The New York Heart Association is incorporated
1920 The Cardiac Club formed in London, England
1924 The American Heart Association is formed
1926 Attempt made to form a Heart Association in Montreal
1944 Inter-American Society of Cardiology formed in Mexico City
1946 Montreal Cardiac Society formed
1947 Canadian Heart Association founded
1950 First World Congress of Cardiology (Paris)
1952 Ontario Heart Foundation incorporated
1955 British Columbia Heart Foundation incorporated
1955 Quebec Heart Society Inc. formed, the forerunner of Quebec Heart Foundation which was incorporated in 1958
1956 Alberta Heart Foundation incorporated
1956 Conference organized by Paul Martin, Minister of Health and Welfare for promoting formation of a National Heart Foundation took place in Ottawa on January 16th
1956 June: Letters patent of the National Heart Foundation of Canada (renamed the Canadian Heart Foundation in 1962) granted
1957 Manitoba Heart Foundation incorporated
1957 Maritime Provinces form a division of the National Heart Foundation
1958 First National Heart Fund campaign
1958 Saskatchewan Heart Foundation incorporated
1962 Canadian Heart Association changes its name to Canadian Cardiovascular Society
1964 7th Interamerican Congress of Cardiology meets in Montreal

Index of Persons

Index of Subjects